LIVING WITH
TINNITUS

A Practical Guide to Understanding,
Treating, and Coping with Tinnitus

Laura Cole

𝒵
ZoZo Publishing

Living With Tinnitus

Copyright 2017 © by Laura Cole

The author is grateful to Terry of Tinnitus Talk for allowing inclusion of his innovative "Back to Silence" treatment method and to Paul Hughes of Tinnitus Talk for his insights on hypnotherapy to treat tinnitus. I want to thank Techopedia.com for granting permission to use their description of "gray noise." I especially want to express my gratitude to the Tinnitus Talk forum, www.tinnitustalk.com, for everything I learned from its members, as well as their support in my journey with tinnitus.

Cover Design: Celeste Cole;
Cover Image: AnsonLu
Library of Congress Control Number: 2017914941
ISBN-13: 978-0-9994507-0-3

ZoZo Publishing
Joseph, Oregon
www.zozopublishing.com

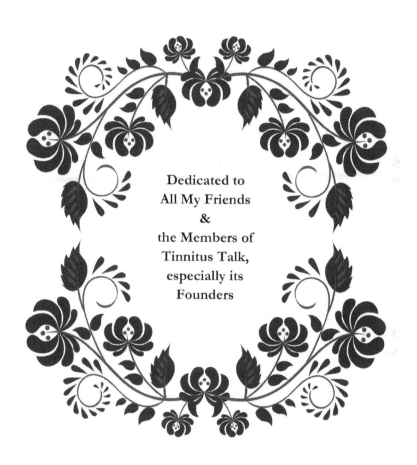

Dedicated to
All My Friends
&
the Members of
Tinnitus Talk,
especially its
Founders

CONTENTS

Table of Contents

Table of Contents

INTRODUCTION

Tinnitus, especially when it's severe, can be extremely disruptive to quality of life, affecting everything from how we interact with others, to our sleeping patterns, our work productivity, and more. Some people need only a little bit of help to get by. Others need a lot of help, up to and including professional medical assistance.

When I first acquired tinnitus in April of 2014, it was unbearably loud, intrusive, and distressing. I spent every spare moment researching online, hoping to find anything that would help. The available information about tinnitus is exhaustive and complex. I have sifted through that information and pared it down to the things that someone new to this condition really needs to know.

Living With Tinnitus does not cover each and every aspect of tinnitus. That would require thousands of pages of material, and much of it would simply not apply to most people. However, I hope you will find enough information within this book to help you understand what tinnitus is, the physical and emotional issues that may arise when you first acquire it, as well as coping methods and treatment options to lessen its impact on your life and give you long-lasting relief.

The book is divided into 11 sections:

Section I, "The Basics," will help you understand the basics of tinnitus, what it is, how it manifests, and the different types of tinnitus.

Section II, "What Causes Tinnitus," explains the most common reasons for acquiring tinnitus.

Section III, "Demographics of Tinnitus," covers who is most likely to get tinnitus, and why.

Section IV, "The First Months are the Worst Months," discusses tinnitus in the early stages, along with some guidance on how to avoid the most common mistakes made in reacting to tinnitus.

Section V, "Tinnitus Affects Your Life," talks about the effects tinnitus can have on everyday life.

Section VI, "Your Brain and Auditory System," delves into the complicated relationship between your brain, your auditory system, and how tinnitus is increasingly being viewed as a problem with the brain.

Section VII, "Coping Techniques," discusses the most popular methods that people use to cope with tinnitus, including what to expect if you use alcohol or marijuana.

Section VIII, "Treatments," reviews treatments ranging from the conventional and conservative to the leading edge of experimental techniques. I include the basis for why each treatment is believed to work, as well as do-it-yourself options for several of the treatments.

Section IX, "Food and Drink," reveals why certain foods and drinks may cause your tinnitus to worsen, and what you can do to change your food habits to improve your chances of reducing tinnitus severity or intrusiveness.

Section X, "Closing Thoughts," just a bit of advice to wrap things up and offer encouragement.

Section XI, "Appendix," features a list of Resources where you can learn more about tinnitus, including suggestions for some products that make living with tinnitus easier. Next is a Glossary of common words and terms associated with tinnitus, and Reference Links from each chapter. Following that is the Author Page, Bibliography, and Index.

There is some overlapping information in different chapters where you will occasionally see points repeated; for example, the relationship of alpha brain waves with tinnitus, and the similarities between tinnitus and epilepsy. This was done so that each chapter includes the necessary useful information, even if you skip reading prior chapters.

Tinnitus is commonly referred to as "t" in online tinnitus forums. The companion website for *Living With Tinnitus* is www.livingwitht.com. It contains highlights of information from this book and the links listed within the Appendix. I will also be posting articles of interest about tinnitus, as well as other auditory and related neurological disorders.

"Everyone has a doctor in him or her; we just have to help it in its work. The natural healing force within each one of us is the greatest force in getting well."

- Hippocrates -

SECTION I

THE BASICS

1
WELCOME TO TINNITUS

Welcome to the baffling and often frustrating world of tinnitus. If you are suffering from this condition, I want to give you a view of tinnitus that balances reality and hope. Reality means having a better understanding of tinnitus and how it may affect your life. Hope means that tinnitus isn't the end of your world as you know it, regardless of how loud or intrusive it may seem to be at this moment.

If you are reading this because you have recently acquired tinnitus, it may give you some comfort to know that you're in the company of somewhere around 360 million people worldwide who either have tinnitus now or have experienced it at some time in the past. Tinnitus respects no age, no race, no culture, no gender. It is an equal opportunity disorder. If someone you love or care about has tinnitus, I want to thank you for taking it seriously enough to try to help them with it. One way to do this is by offering your unconditional support. Another is by learning everything you can about tinnitus and how it affects those who have it.

There is a one group of people in particular that definitely needs to know about tinnitus. This group includes everyone who has either not experienced tinnitus, or who does not have it as a chronic condition. Within this group are young people between the ages of 12 and 27. They are at risk because of our sound-saturated environment that seems intent on pumping up the noise, such as earbuds with extreme volume levels and booming bass on specially-manufactured car stereo systems. As an individual's age rises, the risk of tinnitus grows exponentially. This is partially due to more frequent participation in loud venues such as nightclubs, as well as more time spent listening to music and/or playing online games while wearing earbuds and headphones, without understanding the risk of how excess volume can damage the auditory system. Of course, the natural aging process is another factor.

It's surprising how many people don't know what tinnitus is or how to protect themselves against it. No wonder it sneaks up on them. If someone has never been warned about what causes tinnitus, how can they take steps to prevent it if they aren't even aware of the danger? If you have tinnitus now and didn't know about it before, don't beat yourself up about it. Tinnitus is often a very mild condition and generally people who have it are reluctant to talk about it. This is usually because they either believe that nothing can be done about it, or because it's associated with hearing loss and they consider that an admission of "getting old." As a result, most people know very little about this condition, and even then their knowledge is restricted to their own experience with it. There are people who have never even heard of it at all. Some even confuse the word "tinnitus" with the word "tendinitis." No matter how you first learned of it, if you are currently trying to cope with tinnitus, it's important to understand what it is and what can cause it. You need to know as much as you can about it, because anything that can cause tinnitus can also make it worse if you already have it. The last thing you want is for mild or intermittent tinnitus to become severe or permanent.

Is tinnitus a serious condition? Well, yes and no. It depends on what caused it and how it affects you. Tinnitus is not a disease. It is a symptom that something has gone wrong. Even though tinnitus is classified as a symptom, it should still raise a red flag that there may be a serious underlying medical condition that could be causing or contributing to it. And even though the phantom sounds of tinnitus are generally considered by the medical community as not harmful, your reaction to it can make a very big difference in how it affects you physically, mentally, and emotionally. It's extremely important that you understand the significance of your reaction and the role it plays in the severity and intrusiveness of tinnitus. The reason for this is covered more in-depth in Chapter 15, "Don't Panic and Other Advice."

Looking for information online is a very common approach when tinnitus first appears. However, if you don't take time to learn the basic facts of tinnitus, you may end up being alarmed and/or confused by some of the horror stories and outright inaccurate information about tinnitus that is found online. Fortunately, there is also a lot of truthful and reassuring information available. I've walked through the minefield and will do my best to guide you away from the fears and the scams that will do you no good, and point you to a path where you can begin a well-informed journey with tinnitus.

2
WHAT IS TINNITUS?

The Latin word "tinnire," meaning to ring or a ringing sound, is the origin for the word "tinnitus." The word "tinnitus" is usually pronounced in two distinctive ways: "tin-EYE-tus" is the typical United States version, and "TIN-i-tus" is the typical British pronunciation. The best way to define common tinnitus is to say that it's an internal phantom sound that you hear in your ears or your head, or both. It's a phantom sound because it isn't real. It cannot be heard by others who share your environment, but you can hear it as clearly as you hear any other sound, and sometimes even more clearly. The phantom sound of tinnitus is as strange and persistent as phantom limb pain, which is the perception of pain in an amputated limb. For example, if a person has their leg amputated below the knee but continues to feel pain in the missing part of the leg, that is phantom pain. The pain is experienced and feels just as real as if the entire leg still existed.

The phantom sounds of tinnitus are likewise experienced as if those sounds actually exist. For example, a common description of one type of tinnitus sound is cicadas. There might not be a single cicada within miles, but it sounds like a swarm of them in your head. Another common description is hissing, like a radiator leaking steam, or a snake hiss. Those sounds may not be in your environment, but you hear them just the same as if they were. A brief but uncomfortable episode of ringing in the ears is common after intense noise exposure. This ringing sensation is a familiar form of tinnitus for many with intermittent tinnitus. Some people with chronic tinnitus hear a non-stop ringing, one of the many sounds that tinnitus creates.

I will refer to tinnitus as sounds, not as noise. It's very important in adapting to tinnitus to resist any negative associations with it. The word "noise" is loaded with emotional negativity, whereas the word "sound" is fairly neutral. Anything you can do to reduce negative associations with tinnitus will help you to adjust to it being a part of your world, a part of who you now are. You want to maintain a healthy emotional attitude. Emotional health plays a large part in coming to terms with having tinnitus. Research has shown that the limbic system of our brain, which handles emotion and our response to it, is a major player in the creation of tinnitus and perception of its volume. Most of us have difficulty controlling our basic emotional responses, since that's wired into the brain. However, we can make an effort to control our reaction to the emotions that arise within us. More on that later in Chapter 23, "The Amygdala and Limbic System."

There are two basic types of tinnitus, subjective and objective. Subjective tinnitus can only be heard by the person experiencing it. Neuroimaging studies show changes in neuronal activity that correlate with the presence of tinnitus. From a practical standpoint, that is the limit of their usefulness. Neuroimaging studies cannot measure tinnitus volume or intrusiveness, even though someone reading the scans may infer the level of severity depending on how much hyperactivity is being recorded. Because tinnitus is a subjective experience, just as pain is a subjective experience, there's simply no reliable and conclusive way to measure how loud any individual perceives it to be or how difficult it is for them to ignore it.

Subjective tinnitus is extremely common, but a sudden eruption of severe tinnitus in someone with no prior history of tinnitus episodes is cause for concern. It would be wise to see a medical professional to rule out an underlying physical condition. Remember that tinnitus is not a disease, it's a symptom. With severe tinnitus that follows acoustic trauma, such as exposure to a gunshot or an explosion, it's possible to lessen the damage if you seek treatment immediately or within a very narrow window of time. If sudden onset tinnitus is accompanied by a significant loss of hearing, it is imperative to seek medical treatment without delay. This type of hearing loss is known as sudden sensorineural hearing loss (SSNHL), and must be treated as a medical emergency. Standard course of treatment is a tapering course of oral corticosteroids. The sooner the treatment begins, the better.

Even if there is no appreciable hearing loss, if you are experiencing sudden moderate to severe tinnitus following acoustic trauma, an immediate course of steroids (usually prednisone) is one treatment option that may be helpful at reducing the level of severity. There is no clear evidence that this will work in the absence of SSNHL, but you can still consider it unless there are medical reasons for not doing so. In either case, the window of opportunity for steroid treatment is believed to be within the first 24 to 48 hours, although I have read accounts where it was helpful within the first four weeks.

Objective tinnitus can be heard not only by the person experiencing it, but by anyone who is close enough to hear the sounds coming from the ear. Objective tinnitus occurs when the blood vessels or muscles in the ear create an actual sound. It can be caused by atherosclerosis (where plaque has built up inside your arteries), a malformed blood vessel, a tumor, or even high blood pressure. Your body can generate clicking noises if the muscles in your middle ear twitch or spasm. Multiple sclerosis can also lead to spasms which create objective tinnitus. It's very important that if you develop tinnitus which can be heard by someone listening to your ear, that you see a healthcare professional qualified to treat it. Even then, the cause may remain undetermined.

Two other types of tinnitus are pulsatile tinnitus and reactive tinnitus. A person can have pulsatile or reactive tinnitus in addition to the sounds of subjective tinnitus. Pulsatile tinnitus is the sensation of hearing your pulse in your ear; thus the term "pulsatile." Among its causes are high blood pressure, atherosclerosis, a tumor pressing on the blood vessels in your head or neck, and other blood vessel disorders. See your healthcare practitioner if you develop pulsatile tinnitus. It's important to determine the origin and begin treatment for the underlying cause. Your ultimate treatment may be something as simple as routine monitoring, but pulsatile tinnitus should not be ignored when it first begins. Whooshers.com is an online forum dedicated to information and support for those with this unique form of tinnitus.

Reactive tinnitus is self-descriptive. This is tinnitus that typically lies dormant or at a tolerable level until something triggers its activation or an increase in tinnitus volume. Any loud and sudden noise can cause reactive tinnitus to spike, that is, jump to a much higher level. Reactive tinnitus can also be triggered by an adrenaline surge, such as in a moment of high anxiety or a panic attack. It's not unusual for people with chronic tinnitus to also have reactive tinnitus. Their tinnitus can be at a steady baseline level for hours or days at a time, and then become extremely loud when they are exposed to acoustic insults like a slamming car door, a toddler wailing, a dog frantically barking, a car honking close by, or a motorcycle revving. There are countless environmental noises that most people take for granted and seldom notice but are extreme stressors for people with reactive tinnitus.

If you either have or seem to be developing reactive tinnitus, you should carry earplugs with you in case you find yourself in a situation where you are going to be exposed to loud noise levels and are unable to leave. If the noise exposure is brief, step away, take deep breaths and try to relax, because the adrenaline surge from anxiety is just as likely to contribute to a spike as the actual noise itself. The exception of course is exposure to an intensely high decibel level, such as a fire alarm, firecracker, explosion, or gunshot close by. In that case, seek medical attention immediately. If you are worried about noise exposure as a regular occurrence in your everyday life, you might consider taking N-acetyl-L-cysteine (NAC) on a daily basis. NAC is an over-the-counter supplement that has been proven to protect ears at risk of damage from loud noises. This is covered in more detail in Chapter 58, "Popular Supplements for Tinnitus."

There is an unusual form of tinnitus that is referred to as cycling tinnitus. People with cycling tinnitus tend to experience a predictable pattern of their tinnitus shifting in intensity over the course of two or more days. For example, the tinnitus may be extremely loud one day and barely perceptible the next. Then the day after that, it's loud again, followed by another day where it can barely be heard. It's a pattern of one day on and one day off. Another pattern is where the tinnitus volume gradually increases over the course of several days, until it reaches a point where it's intensely loud. Following the loudest day, the tinnitus drops to a mild level, and the cycle begins again. Cycling tinnitus might follow a pattern of two loud days, two moderate days, and then a mild day, and then the pattern repeats. It's also not unusual for tinnitus to completely fade away by the end of a day, and then return with a vengeance the next morning. Incidentally, some people with cycling tinnitus report that their tinnitus not only changes volume, but it also creates different types of sounds throughout the cycle; for example, hissing one day, buzzing another day, a dental drill the next, et cetera.

Some people with cycling tinnitus have no discernible pattern at all.

They never know whether a day of intrusive tinnitus is going to be followed by a day of mild tinnitus or whether they'll have another day of loud tinnitus. Sometimes the tinnitus will seem to disappear for hours or even an entire day or two. This type of tinnitus is sometimes mistakenly referred to as intermittent tinnitus, but it is more aptly described as random cycling tinnitus because it's still a fairly constant presence in one's life. Intermittent tinnitus tends to arise once in a while and then disappears for a relatively long period of time. When it does occur, it can be quite bothersome or disruptive to daily activities. There's no way to know for certain if someone's intermittent tinnitus will eventually become chronic. It's important to stay on the safe side and protect your ears from further damage if you have intermittent tinnitus.

Cycling tinnitus is a mystery and certainly makes one question whether it can be attributed to hearing loss or whether some other type of neural damage or chemical imbalance is causing the tinnitus to vary its intensity from day to day. Sometimes people with cycling tinnitus will keep a daily journal of their tinnitus episodes, hoping to find a link between what they do or what they eat and the level of tinnitus severity. Very few have been able to trace the tinnitus intensity to any activity, specific noise exposure in their everyday environment, or changes in their diet, except for excess caffeine or sugar intake that can sometimes aggravate tinnitus.

Although cycling tinnitus is a known condition within the tinnitus community, there are otolaryngologists (ENTs) and even audiologists who have never heard of it and sometimes cast doubt that this phenomenon exists. This is unfortunate, because perhaps by studying those with cycling tinnitus, such as with neuroimaging studies or blood tests, there may be a correlation found that could be applied to the greater tinnitus population. The possibility of discovering a root cause of tinnitus by studying cycling tinnitus is speculation on my part; however, as noted before, it seems odd that hearing loss alone would cause tinnitus that randomly changes in intensity and character, or appears in both predictable and erratic patterns.

Another frustrating aspect of tinnitus is experienced by those with fluctuating tinnitus. It may start out loud in the morning and decrease in intensity as the day progresses, or vice-versa. The tinnitus sounds

3
TINNITUS SOUNDS AND VOLUME

I can't remember when I first heard about tinnitus, but probably sometime in my twenties. The main impression I got was that tinnitus was like a slight hum or buzz that was heard in the ears and it never stopped. At the time it seemed like tinnitus would be an extreme irritation, something that I would find very difficult to deal with on a permanent basis. Even though I mistakenly believed at the time that tinnitus was simply a mild background sound, the idea of living with a constant buzz or hum was too awful to contemplate. It never occurred to me just how intrusive and devastating tinnitus can be. No one ever talked to me about tinnitus, and I never came across any articles describing the annoying and sometimes dreadful sounds that tinnitus can generate.

For those of you who are unconcerned about acquiring tinnitus because you believe it's just a mild tone you hear in quiet environments, please be aware that only the lucky ones have that type of tinnitus. Sometimes the lucky ones take their level of tinnitus for granted, unaware that it can worsen if they take unnecessary risks. In this chapter I'll do my best to describe the unbelievable array of sounds that tinnitus can make, whether it's in your ears, your head, or both. This is not meant as a scare tactic, but just to set out the caution signs for those with mild tinnitus, and to let those with moderate or severe tinnitus know that they are not alone.

As noted in the prior chapter, not only can tinnitus be perceived as different sounds, it can manifest at different volumes from one day to the next. A sound which is rather easily ignored at low volume can be very difficult to dismiss when it's amplified many times over, just as a fly buzzing outside the room becomes much more irritating when it's buzzing around your head. Tinnitus may be one distinct sound, or it might be several sounds blended or layered on top of one another. Some days all the sounds might be heard at equal volume; on other days, one sound is heard clearly but the other sounds are faint or maybe not audible at all. The sounds can be steady, they can have a static-like nature, or they may oscillate in an endless ebb and flow.

Besides the ringing sensation that most people associate with tinnitus, here are other sounds of tinnitus:

- Tonal, like a high-pitched eeeeeeeee;
- Humming, low-pitched or high-pitched mmmmmmm;
- Whistling, like a tea kettle, high-pitched audible dog whistle, or one-note tin whistle;
- Buzzing, the sound of bees, mosquitos, cicadas, or other noisy insects;
- Hissing, like steam escaping from a radiator, a snake pit, and similar sounds;
- Squealing, like a high-pitched insect, or air leaking from the pinched neck of a balloon;
- Roaring, as if one held a conch shell to one's ear to "hear the ocean," but louder;
- Jet engine, similar to roaring but much more intense;
- Screeching, the sound of a train braking on rusty tracks;
- Droning, a low-pitched rumbling, the sound of the engine of a large diesel truck next to you, but the sound is in your head;
- Beeping, staccato tones, Morse code sounds, dial tones;
- Static, ranging from an old television CRT tube to a short in an electrical wire;
- Sizzling, a sound like something frying in oil, very similar to violet noise effect;
- Telephone ring, either constant or in pulsed tones;
- Siren, like an ambulance;
- Marching feet;
- The sound of coal being shoveled;
- Dentist's drill.

Tinnitus sounds that defy description are common. Many people have trouble adequately explaining what they're hearing because there's nothing they've ever heard before that sounds quite like it. Sometimes the descriptions will make you cringe, like the gentleman who vividly characterized his tinnitus as "monkeys banging cymbals together." The British Tinnitus Association created a video with electronic simulations of different sounds of tinnitus. You can find it on YouTube by searching for "British Tinnitus Association - Sounds of Tinnitus."

For most people, the intensity and intrusiveness of tinnitus will lessen as time goes on. The actual sounds themselves may change as the brain adjusts to the presence of tinnitus signals. I heard so many different sounds in the first few months of tinnitus that I could not believe what my brain was doing. The fact that my tinnitus was incredibly loud made it all the more difficult on those days when it sounded like pipes banging together, or curtains of tiny bells swaying back and forth in my head, or an endless telephone ring or dentist's drill. After two years, my brain decided to stick with three different sounds: a constant high-pitched hum/whine, a raspy tea kettle whistle, and a static hiss that can turn into a screech on the high-volume days. The therapies I've followed have given me more days of mild tinnitus, but otherwise I hear some combination of those sounds in my head almost every day. Many people with tinnitus experience this level of tinnitus, and worse.

There are loudness matching tests performed by audiologists which can fairly accurately determine how loud your tinnitus is. In this test, you will be seated in a soundproof booth to block out all ambient noise, and you will wear a close-fitting set of headphones. The audiologist first determines the decibel level of your hearing threshold by playing a tone until you indicate that you hear the tone. That's the HL, the hearing level. Next, she determines the decibel level of your tinnitus by increasing the volume of that tone until you indicate that it matches the loudness of your tinnitus. That's the dB SL, the decibel sensory level. The difference between those two levels is your tinnitus loudness matching level. I'll give a couple of examples to clarify how it's measured.

Johnny has severe hearing loss. He begins to hear the hearing threshold tone at 50 decibels. That's his hearing level, HL. The audiologist continues increasing the volume of the tone. Johnny indicates the tone is as loud as his tinnitus when it reaches 60 decibels. He has a decibel sensory level of 60. The dB SL of 60 minus the HL of 50 equals a tinnitus loudness matching level of 10 decibels.

Mary has excellent hearing. She hears the threshold tone at 5 decibels. Thus, her hearing level (HL) is 5. Now the audiologist plays a tone and instructs Mary to indicate when the volume of that tone is as loud as her tinnitus. The audiologist slowly increases the volume of the tone. Mary indicates that it is as loud as her tinnitus when the volume reaches 30 decibels, so her dB SL is 30. Mary therefore has a tinnitus loudness match of 25, which is the difference between her hearing level of 5 and her decibel sensory level of 30. Because her hearing threshold is excellent, even though she hears the tinnitus at 30 decibels and Johnny hears his at 60 decibels, it is likely that Mary will perceive her tinnitus as louder than Johnny will perceive his. A tinnitus loudness matching level of 25 is rather extreme. 70% of people have a tinnitus loudness matching level of 6 decibels or less.

If you've ever been with someone who needs the television volume turned up to the point it's uncomfortably loud for you, that's probably because of the difference in your hearing threshold. Maybe tinnitus seems to lower in volume as time goes by not because it's actually decreasing, but because the hearing threshold itself is higher as more hearing loss occurs due to the natural aging process. In other words, the difference between the hearing threshold and the decibel sensory level is narrowing, so the tinnitus doesn't seem as loud.

The Online Audiogram Hearing Test, which you can access at www.audiocheck.net, will give you a very good idea of your hearing threshold at different frequencies. You can even use it to try to match the loudness of your tinnitus by comparing the difference between your hearing threshold and the perceived volume of your tinnitus. After you've determined your hearing threshold, play the tones again at increasing decibel levels until one of them is the same volume as your tinnitus. Then subtract the hearing threshold level from the tinnitus level. Please note that matching tinnitus loudness is not the intent of the creator of the Online Audiogram Hearing Test, but it may give you some comfort to know that your tinnitus is not as loud as you perhaps fear it to be. For example, if you discover that your dB SL is 30 decibels, compare it to the noise level chart of decibel ratings at www.noisehelp.com. You will see that 30 decibels is the same volume as a whisper. In other words, the actual volume of your tinnitus is not that loud, even though it may be intrusive and annoying because it's always there or the sound itself is harsh or otherwise unpleasant. For a true tinnitus loudness matching, though, the test needs to be performed by an audiologist in a proper testing environment.

An individual's perception of tinnitus loudness and their perception of its severity do not necessarily go hand in hand. Someone with a tinnitus loudness matching level of 12 might be only slightly bothered by their tinnitus, whereas someone with a level of 2 may suffer extreme distress and find it very difficult to cope. The source of tinnitus distress is usually due to complicated factors based on one's psychological makeup and stress response. I cover this phenomenon in Chapter 6, "Tinnitus is Everywhere." Perceived distress also has a lot to do with how a person's brain is wired and the processing of emotions, as explained in Chapter 23, "The Amygdala and Limbic System."

The next chapter covers the odd but common experience of initially hearing tinnitus in one or both ears, and then gradually the tinnitus shifts to being perceived as located inside the head.

4

TINNITUS IN THE EARS,
TINNITUS IN THE HEAD

Typically when tinnitus strikes, the phantom sound seems to be in the ears. When the sound first appears as a subtle high-pitched whine or a droning type of hum, it's not unusual for people to walk around their home with their hand cupped to their ear, listening intently for the source. Sometimes they'll press their ear against the wall, trying to figure out where the sound is coming from. This is because tinnitus definitely can mimic the hum of electrical wiring or perhaps a malfunction in a computer system. After a while it dawns on them that the sound is internal, not external. Depending on the volume and nature of the sound, their reaction can range from shrugging it off to an all-out anxiety attack. It may be easier for someone to casually dismiss the sounds if they've had bouts of tinnitus in the past. They understand what's going on and aren't too concerned because they think it's just another episode. That is, unless the sound is much louder and/or more intrusive than before, and that's when they become worried.

When tinnitus generates sounds that are discordant or completely different from past experience, when a person hears clashing cymbals, the stomping sound of marching feet, a jet engine's roar, or a train's brakes screeching on railroad tracks, that's when panic can easily set in. Those types of sounds often seem to be located in the head. They can be extremely loud, leading to confusion and fear. That is not the typical experience, though. The more common sounds of tinnitus, such as a hum, whine, static, or buzz, tend to be experienced as being in one or both ears.

Tinnitus can be perceived in one ear or both, it can be perceived as being in one or more locations in your head, or it can seem to be in both your head and your ears. Some days it can sound like it's in your ears, and then other days it's in your head. It can even move around in your head, changing its perceived location from the side to the front, from the front to the back, through the center from temple to temple, or filling the entire head.

There are a couple common beliefs as to when tinnitus is considered chronic or permanent. One belief is that after six months, if the tinnitus continues to be heard constantly or if it has begun to establish a regular cyclical pattern, then it's chronic. The other belief is that when you perceive your tinnitus has moved from your ears to inside your head, it has now reached the chronic stage. It's very common to experience the phantom sound first in your ears and then, as time goes by, the sound becomes centralized in your head. This can make the tinnitus feel more intrusive, and therefore more difficult to mask. Masking means you listen to a constant sound of your choice, usually white noise or some sort of nature soundscape, to distract yourself from the tinnitus. This helps to ease the discomfort or annoyance of hearing your tinnitus. Masking as a coping technique is discussed in Chapter 31, "Masking."

5
CHRONIC TINNITUS AND SPIKES

Most people have had the experience of hearing a high pitched tone that suddenly appears out of nowhere, lasts for a few seconds, then fades away. That is a form of tinnitus, but it's really nothing to be concerned about. However, when that high pitched tone appears and doesn't fade away as the days, weeks, and months go by, then it's possible you've now got chronic tinnitus. In other words, it's a constant presence, and tends to have the same characteristics from one day to the next, although that may gradually change.

A common term in the tinnitus world is "baseline." Baseline is the typical volume level and type of sound that someone with tinnitus has. In other words, it's what a person can generally expect of their tinnitus from day to day. Many people with tinnitus will occasionally experience a sudden dramatic increase above the baseline. This is what's known as a spike. It may be caused by an extreme acoustic event, such as a slamming door or screaming toddler, or it may occur out of the blue for no apparent reason at all. Spikes can be difficult to deal with because they are unpredictable both in volume and intensity. They may last for hours, or they may persist for days or even weeks. It isn't always the case, but sometimes a spike heralds the worsening of tinnitus. This is more likely if a spike is caused by sustained noise exposure or severe acoustic trauma. A random spike may also foreshadow an improvement in tinnitus once the spike passes, as if somehow the brain has discharged an excess of hyperactive neural energy and then resets the tinnitus at a lower baseline. It's also possible for the pattern of mild, moderate and severe days to change following a spike. In most cases, however, the tinnitus simply returns to where it was before, both in volume and sound characteristics.

There's a tendency to panic when a spike hits, because the first fear is that your tinnitus has suddenly gotten worse and it's going to remain at that spike level. It's very important to stay as calm as possible. You want your brain to know that its tinnitus alarm system is malfunctioning beyond its normal level (the baseline), and that you are fine and not in

y is a form of fear, which puts the limbic system on
thing you want is your limbic system overreacting to a
tinnitus volume or intensity. Do your best to ease the
anxiety, ...   n that will help put the brakes on the spike as soon as
possible.

That being said, if you have tinnitus and are exposed to a traumatic
acoustic event, and especially if it's accompanied by a spike, seek medical
help immediately. A tapered regimen of prednisone can go a long way in
stopping the cascade of damage. Some examples of acoustic trauma are a
gunshot close to your ears without hearing protection, someone yelling
directly into your ear, a firecracker exploding at close range, or a car trunk
(bonnet) slammed down too hard. Remember that if you have tinnitus,
you are at greater risk of harm than someone who does not have tinnitus.
It's no different than someone with a damaged vertebra in their back who
is likely to be injured far worse in a car accident than someone with a
strong, healthy back. In short, if the acoustic trauma is painful or
irritating, that's a warning sign. It's far better to obtain medical help and
discover you don't need it, than to casually brush it off and wish later
that you had sought treatment.

When is tinnitus considered to be chronic? In the prior chapter I
noted that tinnitus is sometimes considered to be chronic when it moves
from the ears to the head. Timewise, tinnitus is generally thought to be
chronic if it has persisted for at least six months. This assumes that the
tinnitus is not caused by a treatable underlying condition, such as
temporomandibular joint disorder, in which case treatment of the
condition may resolve the tinnitus as well. However, even in the absence
of an underlying condition, remember that everyone is an individual with
a unique physiology. There have been cases where tinnitus has been
reported to simply go away after two years or more, even after a decade. I
don't want to spread false hope, because the chance of it spontaneously
disappearing is rare, but we can never know what hidden healing
mechanisms are going on inside our body that may eventually result in a
life free from tinnitus. In the meantime, if you've had tinnitus for at least
three months, and certainly if it has persisted for six months or more,
approach it as though you will have tinnitus for at least the next few
years. Many people with tinnitus will tell you that's the wrong way to look

at it. They'll tell you to face the fact that after a certain period of time, you'll have tinnitus for the rest of your life and you need to accept the finality of it. There are three reasons why I disagree with that approach.

The first reason is that it's too emotionally overwhelming to think of dealing with a negative or debilitating condition for the rest of one's life. Psychologically, humans like to deal in small chunks of time; that is, units such as this hour, this day, this week, this month, this year. We usually feel more comfortable when we can confront problems one step at a time. The idea of tinnitus for the rest of your life can feel like a tidal wave coming at you. However, if you make a determined effort to think of it as one month at a time, you reduce the tidal wave to a disturbing wake in the water. If you've ever been in a small motorboat and gotten in the wake of a larger boat, you know that the wake can be strong enough to toss you about a bit, but you hang on and ride it out. With tinnitus, you need to hang on by staying focused on the here and now. You can deal with the long-term future when it arrives, because things are likely to have changed by then.

The second reason to set aside the idea that you'll have tinnitus for the rest of your life is because no one can honestly tell you that you will be affected by it to the same degree as time goes on. It's definitely possible that you will gradually habituate to it to the point where you rarely think about it. With that degree of habituation, the tinnitus loses its importance in your conscious thoughts. Your brain sends the sound so far into the background that it's like you don't have it at all. For example, the prevalence of tinnitus in the elderly has always been a problem, but you generally don't hear them complaining about it. They've lived long enough to understand that we're all susceptible to one sort of disorder or another, particularly as we age, and the best thing to do is to not make that disorder the center of one's attention. Obviously a disease like diabetes demands conscious attention because it requires medication, monitoring of one's diet, and visits to a physician. But with tinnitus, the less attention you pay to it, the better your chances are that you will no longer notice it unless you deliberately shift your focus to it. In other words, you still have tinnitus lying in wait, but it needs to be activated by your attention.

Third, there is an increasing possibility that neuroscientists will

6
TINNITUS IS EVERYWHERE

No one really knows the number of people worldwide who have chronic tinnitus, but the Hearing Health Foundation places the number at approximately 360 million. In the United States, it is estimated that somewhere around 50 million people have experienced tinnitus at one time or another. Of those 50 million, approximately 16 million people have sought medical help. For every person who has sought medical attention, there are likely two or more people who have not sought treatment. It's not uncommon for someone to simply hope for the best because they figure nothing can be done about it. People with intermittent or mild tinnitus are less likely to be troubled enough to seek treatment. In one Australian study of 2,015 adults aged 55 to 99 who described their tinnitus as mildly to extremely annoying, 37% sought professional help. Of that 37%, only 6% actually received treatment. A.J. Heller, in the article "Classification and Epidemiology of Tinnitus," states that prolonged (chronic) tinnitus requiring medical evaluation is present in 10 to 15% of the adult population.

Because of the Internet, people now have a tendency to search for information and solutions online before contacting a healthcare practitioner. For those who do eventually seek professional help, the results can be discouraging. Many physicians have so little familiarity with tinnitus that they simply don't know what to do for a patient. The prevalent attitude is that tinnitus is an ailment for which very little, if anything, can be done to relieve it. Patients are often advised that they need to learn to live with it. Sometimes a patient is referred to an otolaryngologist, commonly referred to as an ENT, an ear, nose and throat doctor. Unfortunately, even specialists in the medical profession do not have a wide range of options for treating tinnitus itself; rather, they tend to treat a patient's response to tinnitus. Either way, it can be an expensive and long-term process. If funds are limited, a person who develops tinnitus may take a wait and see attitude, hoping that either the condition improves over time or that they will get used to it and find a way to live with it. This is easier said than done.

Of the 50 million in the United States who experience tinnitus, 2 percent suffer from severe and intrusive tinnitus, designated as catastrophic tinnitus. This 2 percent population, roughly 1 million people, is significantly affected, sometimes to the point where they absolutely cannot function on a day-to-day basis. They lose their jobs because they are unable to concentrate. They lose their desire to socialize because normal conversation or activities cannot mask the volume of sound in their head. They find it very difficult to enjoy anything in life because the torment never stops. A few of them commit suicide, feeling helpless and discouraged because they have given up on any hope for relief. It is particularly devastating to this 2 percent group if they are simply told to go home and live with it.

I don't believe that anyone with tinnitus should ever be told to go home and live with it. If you or someone you care about is in that 2 percent group, it's important to have professional counseling and perhaps medication to ease the sense of panic or anxiety that often accompanies severe tinnitus. This is most critical when severe tinnitus first strikes. Your initial reaction, for better or worse, can set the stage for how your brain continues to generate tinnitus. Anxiety is a major component in the perception of tinnitus volume, the degree to which it causes distress, and the role it plays in the brain itself. This topic is covered in Section VI, "Your Brain and Auditory System."

Fortunately, most people who acquire tinnitus have a mild version. They often adapt to it quickly and are able to either ignore it completely as if it doesn't exist, or are completely unbothered by it when they do hear it. This doesn't mean you have a character deficiency if you cannot cope with your tinnitus. It doesn't mean that you somehow aren't tough enough to put up with it and go on with your life. There are people with mild tinnitus who are in mental agony because the sound that never stops makes them miserable to the core of their being. They deserve our compassion, not our judgment. The experience of having tinnitus can involve complex psychological components, including but not limited to anxiety, depression, fear, anger, resentment, frustration, and grief. Tinnitus can be an emotional hardship that affects a person as much as a physical disorder. This is why it is often notoriously difficult to deal with in the beginning, no matter the degree of severity or level of intrusiveness.

Like any disease or disorder, we can sympathize with the person enduring it, but we really can't understand what they're going through unless we have that same disease or disorder. Tinnitus goes one step beyond that. It is an intensely personal affliction. The types of sounds and combinations of sound that tinnitus generates, the different volumes and frequencies, as well as the confounding nature of fluctuating and cycling tinnitus, all these factors conspire to make tinnitus a very different beast from most other human ailments. Two people may hear the same type of sound but at different volumes and frequencies. One person may have a cycle of two days of loud tinnitus followed by a day of very mild or nonexistent tinnitus, then the next two days it's loud again. Someone else may have an erratic cycling tinnitus, never knowing if they're going to wake up to a dog whistle blaring in their head or a soft hum. Some people hear tinnitus in their ears, others hear central head noise, and many hear both. If you have tinnitus and it doesn't bother you, please be compassionate with those who have tinnitus and call it torture.

How exactly does tinnitus develop, though? Section II covers the typical causes of tinnitus, which can be as varied as originating from an ear infection, all the way to being exposed to the enormous sound wave impact of a detonated explosive.

SECTION II

WHAT CAUSES TINNITUS

7
TINNITUS HAS MANY ORIGINS

Tinnitus can creep up on you, little by little, if you are exposed to noise levels that exceed your safe limits. People who have had episodes of ringing in their ears following a night of clubbing or a loud concert may wake up one day to discover that the ringing will not go away in the same short time span as it did in the past. They didn't take the ringing seriously before, because it only lasted for a few hours or maybe a day, and also because it's a common after-effect of clubbing. Then they become alarmed when the ringing persists for days, weeks, or months. What's happened is that their auditory system has finally had enough cumulative trauma to cause irreversible damage.

With cumulative trauma, there doesn't have to be one specific event, something a person can point to and say, "This noise exposure caused my tinnitus." Over the years, listening to unsafe levels of music or environmental noise finally tipped the delicate balance. It's commonly understood that there is a risk of hearing loss with noise exposure, but that's usually where the concern ends. Most people believe everything is okay as long as they seem to hear as well as they always have. What they don't realize is that exposure to unsafe decibel levels can lead to acquiring tinnitus. Even if they have heard of it, they don't yet understand how frustrating and difficult it can be to live with intrusive tinnitus.

Imagine waking up one morning to discover an annoying sound in your ears or head that refuses to go away. That's what happened to David Letterman, the popular former talk show host. In one show where his guest is the actor William Shatner, Letterman says, "I don't know what caused mine, but one morning it starts waking you up. You awaken to the sound of your head." He adds, "I don't know where it came from, but mine is getting progressively worse over the years. But mine is a combination of two sounds. This shhhhhhhhh, that's one, and then on top of that — and this goes on 24 hours a day — and the other one is eeeeeeeee ... I'm testing the Emergency Broadcast System in my head, every minute of my life."

Tinnitus can be caused by your own unintentional negligence, such as being unaware of the need to protect your ears at loud nightclubs or concerts, or failing to use adequate ear protection at a gun range. It can be caused by the negligence of others. William Shatner and Leonard Nimoy developed tinnitus following an explosion on the set of Star Trek while filming the episode "Arena." One example of negligence by others is an incompetent physician's assistant who performs an ear syringing incorrectly. Another all-too-common example is someone firing their gun without first checking to see if everyone nearby is wearing sufficient hearing protection, or someone setting off a loud firecracker or yelling directly into your ear.

Harmful negligence can be completely unintentional. Parents are taking a great risk with the auditory systems of their children when they drive around with the stereo blasting while transporting the kids or if they frequently take them to sporting events in loud arenas. The ear canals of children are narrower than adults and much more sensitive to the pressure of incoming sound waves. In fact, an infant's extremely small ear canal means they can perceive noise as 20 decibels louder than the same noise as it's perceived by an older child or an adult.

Tinnitus can be caused by the natural aging process, by disease, and by ototoxic medications (drugs that are harmful to your auditory system). You can get tinnitus from a virus, an ear infection, a concussion or whiplash, or even barotrauma from an airplane flight. "Barotrauma" is the medical term for injury to bodily tissue because of changes in barometric pressure, such as when an airplane changes altitude. It's sometimes referred to as "airplane ear." Barotrauma to the ear can also occur during scuba diving due to increased water pressure.

There is some disagreement among professionals as to whether stress can directly cause tinnitus. One study, "Stress and prevalence of hearing problems in the Swedish working population," determined that there is a clear relationship between stress and the development of tinnitus. Some of the stressors include occupational stress, poor health (including chronic illness), and long-term inadequate sleep. Another major stressor is the psychological feeling known as burnout, when one simply has nothing left to give after exerting tremendous emotional, mental, or physical energy over a sustained period of time. Some audiologists agree that stress can cause tinnitus, particularly emotional stress, such as grief.

Based on the number of members of Tinnitus Talk who list stress as a contributing factor, I think it's safe to say it most definitely plays a part. (Tinnitus Talk is an online forum for people with auditory disorders.)

It's widely accepted that unrelenting stress negatively affects the immune system. The cochlea, where the inner ear hair cells reside, is susceptible to oxidative stress. Perhaps the connection to tinnitus is the body's decreasing ability under extreme or prolonged stress to combat reactive oxygen species (ROS), which are chemically reactive molecules containing oxygen. When ROS levels are too high, oxidative stress occurs. Incidentally, ROS levels rise in the cochlea when someone is exposed to excessive noise. This increased level has been linked to hearing loss. Oxidative stress has been shown to impair the effectiveness of antioxidant defenses, including glutathione, an important nutrient and antioxidant.

When you consider all the possible causes, and especially when you factor in stress, is it any wonder that 50 million Americans have tinnitus? Let's review some of the causes and what, if anything, can be done about them.

Mild traumatic brain injury (TBI), such as a concussion or a fracture to the skull, is not a typical cause of tinnitus, but it does happen. Mild TBI in the civilian population is most often caused by falls, vehicular collisions, and physical assault. Military personnel in war zones are more at risk from mild TBI caused by weaponry and explosive devices. In fact, traumatic brain injury has been called the signature injury of Operation Iraqi Freedom, the conflict with Iraq that began in March 2003. TBI, particularly in a closed head injury, is not always obvious. Symptoms can mimic PTSD (post traumatic stress disorder). If you or someone you know has suffered a head injury followed by tinnitus, or if they exhibit behavior changes that are consistent with the symptoms of PTSD, this is a critical situation requiring the services of a healthcare professional to rule out the possibility of brain injury. Learn more about this in the article "Tinnitus Evaluation and Management Considerations for Persons with Mild Traumatic Brain Injury" on the American Speech-Language-Hearing Association website.

Tinnitus can be caused by physical disorders that affect the auditory system. The most common disease associated with tinnitus is Ménière's disease, which is a serious disorder of the inner ear. The primary symptoms are vertigo, hearing loss, and tinnitus. There are some physical abnormalities that may be associated with Ménière's disease, but no one knows why any person in particular develops it. It is not a disease that is limited to any gender or age group. Famous people past and present afflicted with Ménière's disease are: Beethoven, composer; Jonathan Swift, author of Gulliver's Travels; Marilyn Monroe, actress; Mamie Eisenhower, former First Lady; and Bryan Adams, singer/songwriter/musician and accomplished photographer. Along with tinnitus, other symptoms of Ménière's include hearing loss, aural fullness (a feeling of fullness in the ears), and intermittent vertigo, the feeling that your environment is spinning around you. Ménière's can be an extremely distressing and debilitating condition, with tinnitus adding another layer of misery. Anyone with Ménière's disease must be under a doctor's care.

I know of one woman who insists that there is some electrical interference in her apartment, so she periodically has the maintenance folks come in and listen for themselves. Obviously the folks who arrive to check for electrical interference don't hear it and thus are unable to help her because there is nothing for them to fix. This woman has a mild case of Ménière's disease and cannot accept that the sound she hears is being made by her own brain. If someone you care about has Ménière's, please keep in mind that they may also be struggling with tinnitus, even if they don't mention it. People sometimes won't admit to a physical impairment simply because they don't want pity, and prefer to appear as healthy as possible.

When tinnitus is related to dysfunction in structures of the body other than the auditory system, it is said to be somatic. ("Soma" means "body" in Greek.) Temporomandibular joint disorder is one of the most likely causes of somatic tinnitus. If you have jaw pain or swelling, or if you can change the pitch or frequency of your tinnitus by opening and closing your jaw or manipulating it sideways, you should suspect TMJ disorder. There are close connections between the chewing muscles, the ligaments of the jaw, and the nerve supply of the temporomandibular joint with the parts of the brain that process and interpret sound. Your doctor or dentist can help you to diagnose TMJ disorder and begin a course of treatment that might help alleviate or remove the tinnitus. The British Tinnitus Association website describes TMJ's connection to tinnitus in their article, "Tinnitus and disorders of the temporo-mandibular joint and neck." Somatic tinnitus is also used to describe any tinnitus which can be changed in pitch or intensity by deliberately moving the jaw, head, neck, or shoulders in a particular manner or direction. In this regard, 60 to 70 percent of people have what may be called somatic tinnitus.

Grinding your teeth (bruxism) at night or during the day can also contribute to somatic tinnitus. A properly-fitted mouth guard will not only save the surfaces of your teeth from wear and tear, it might also reduce or eliminate your tinnitus. If you live alone or your partner is a heavy sleeper who won't notice, how can you tell if you're grinding your teeth in your sleep? Check to see if you have raised ridges on the inside of your cheek that correspond with your bite. That's one of the clues. If you know you have the tendency to clench your jaw or grind your teeth throughout the day, try sugarless chewing gum instead. Chewing can be a substitute for grinding, which can help you to avoid a tendency toward bruxism. Pay closer attention to how you respond to stress. If you catch yourself frequently clenching your jaw or grinding your teeth, you need to take steps to address whatever is happening which causes that reaction.

Another cause for somatic tinnitus is dysfunction in the cervical vertebrae or other problems with your neck. If your tinnitus began with an episode of neck pain or injury, there is a strong likelihood that they are connected. If you have a stiff neck, or if your posture produces unnecessary strain on your neck, you can investigate that as a possible link to your tinnitus. There is evidence to support that the nerve endings in the neck are connected to hearing centers in the brain. If you take a pain reliever for neck pain and you discover that it lessens the severity of your tinnitus, you might find that taking better care of your neck is part of the solution to your tinnitus troubles. Start with improving your posture, particularly when you're using your computer. With the guidance of your healthcare provider, you might want to consider beginning a program of gentle neck exercises. The WebMD website article, "Neck Exercises - Topic Overview," is a good place to start. These exercises will help you to strengthen and improve your neck function.

A rare cause of tinnitus is an acoustic neuroma, also known as vestibular schwannoma. This is a benign tumor, which means it is noncancerous. Typically it is slow-growing. Sometimes an acoustic neuroma develops and then stops growing. Despite being benign, an acoustic neuroma is serious because it is located on the main nerve that leads from the inner ear to the brain. Pressure from an acoustic neuroma can create tinnitus, plus it can affect your hearing as well as your sense of balance. Diagnosis is by MRI, followed by monitoring with regular imaging studies. If the neuroma becomes too advanced, radiation or surgical intervention will be necessary to avoid permanent hearing loss and partial facial paralysis. Fortunately, it's uncommon to need such extreme measures, and regular monitoring is generally all that is required once an acoustic neuroma has been diagnosed. Of course, the tinnitus will remain as long as the neuroma is present on the nerve. Note that one symptom of acoustic neuroma is unilateral tinnitus; in other words, tinnitus in only one ear. If you have unilateral tinnitus, especially in the absence of other possible causes, consult with your physician about the possibility of an acoustic neuroma.

Excess ear wax in some people can lead to tinnitus. Usually people are aware if they have a tendency to develop too much ear wax. Either they have a history of it, or their hearing becomes increasingly muffled and their ears have a sensation of fullness. This condition is fairly easy to treat. If you suspect ear wax buildup, and if your doctor examines you and confirms it, be sure to have the ear wax removal procedure done by someone qualified to perform the procedure. Ask the person what their qualifications are and how many years of experience they have. Don't be shy about expressing any concerns. Be courteous and ask straightforward questions. If they have little to no experience, politely excuse yourself and find someone else. Don't ever take chances with your ears simply because you're afraid you might hurt someone's feelings.

Ear syringing to remove ear wax has been blamed for causing or worsening tinnitus, particularly with the older method of using a metal syringe. The more modern method of syringing involves sitting in a chair, and an electronic irrigator is used to clean your ear with warm water. A basin held by your ear captures the water and wax that runs out.

Even though the reports that syringing can be harmful may not be statistically significant, proceed with caution. You don't want to be the rare person for whom syringing causes tinnitus. Do not allow syringing if you have had ear surgery or recent ear infections, if your eardrum is perforated, or if you have problems with dizziness.

Carefully applied micro-suction is another method to remove ear wax, and a third method is a clinician using a headlamp and instruments to basically scrape out the excess ear wax. If you have no pain and no discharge from your ears, you might want to first try an over-the-counter remedy of ear wax softening drops. There is also an old-fashioned home remedy of using olive oil to soften the wax, as explained in the article "Olive Oil for Ear Wax," published on www.med-health.net. In either case, be sure to read instructions carefully and observe all precautions.

A partial list of other physical disorders that can cause or contribute to tinnitus are:

- Hypothyroidism, which is an underactive thyroid;
- Otosclerosis, an abnormal bone growth around the stapes bone in the middle ear;
- Hypertension, commonly referred to as high blood pressure;
- Labyrinthitis, which is an inflammation of the labyrinth structure within the inner ear;
- Bell's palsy, a sudden onset of unexplained one-sided facial paralysis;
- Foreign object on the eardrum, such as dust or an insect fragment;
- Ear infection; and,
- Ruptured eardrum.

If you have any of the medical conditions mentioned in this chapter, or suspect that you may have them, please seek professional advice. Your tinnitus may reduce or fade away with proper treatment, and it could help you to avoid serious future complications. For example, it's possible for tinnitus to be associated with hypothyroidism. A few blood tests to determine the accurate dosage of medication is usually all it takes to get your thyroid in proper working order. If an underactive thyroid is in fact contributing to your tinnitus, there is a good chance it will resolve when your thyroid is once again functioning as it should.

Some people acquire tinnitus and have no idea why. Their hearing is fine, they aren't experiencing undue stress, they haven't been exposed to dangerous levels of noise, they don't use earbuds or headphones, they have always listened to music or the television at reasonable levels, and all the medical tests and evaluations come back negative for anything that might have triggered the tinnitus. In this case, they are said to have idiopathic tinnitus, meaning of unknown origin.

One clinical study noted high serum levels of reactive oxygen species (ROS) in subjects with idiopathic tinnitus. ROS are implicated in several pathogenic processes, including the inner ear as mentioned earlier in this chapter. In the study, treatment consisted of an 18-week course of oral antioxidants. The result was a decrease in discomfort and reduction of perceived tinnitus intensity. Perhaps this explains why some people experience improvement when they take over-the-counter lipoflavonoids and bioflavonoids, whereas others notice no difference at all. If you have idiopathic tinnitus, it may be due to a high ROS level, which is more likely to respond to this type of supplement. I discuss bioflavonoids in Chapter 58, "Popular Supplements for Tinnitus."

8
SALICYLATES AND NSAIDS

An ototoxic substance is any medication, supplement, or additive that can cause temporary or permanent harmful effects to the auditory system. These effects can include hearing loss, balance issues, and tinnitus. The tinnitus can be as harsh and intrusive as when it's caused by severe acoustic trauma. It may surprise you to learn that some ototoxic substances are ordinary over-the-counter (OTC) pain relievers.

Salicylate is a plant-based chemical which is one of the components of aspirin. High daily doses of aspirin have been known to cause tinnitus. (In fact, for laboratory studies, research scientists sometimes give mice extremely high doses of aspirin to induce tinnitus.) The higher the dose, the greater the risk. A person who is taking eight to 12 aspirins each day is more likely to develop tinnitus than someone who occasionally takes two to four a day for a headache, or someone who regularly takes one aspirin every day for heart health. Even so, if you regularly take aspirin, no matter how low a dose, there is a chance you might develop tinnitus. Keep in mind that as we grow older, we can become more sensitive to certain substances. Some ingredients that our bodies were able to easily process in the past may now trigger an adverse reaction.

Other OTC pain relievers that contain salicylates are nonsteroidal anti-inflammatory drugs, commonly referred to as NSAIDs. Among these are Motrin (ibuprofen), Advil (ibuprofen), and Aleve (naproxen). They are also available in higher-strength prescription form, along with other prescription NSAIDS like Relafen (nabumetone). Salicylate is present in willow bark, a popular naturopathic remedy for headache and joint pain.

It is often recommended that if you have tinnitus, you should not take ibuprofen and similar NSAIDs. Because of this, many people with tinnitus avoid them for fear of worsening their tinnitus. However, some people with tinnitus can take them and it makes no difference. Occasionally people take ibuprofen and notice a reduction in tinnitus volume. If an NSAID brings you temporary relief, your tinnitus may be related to inflammation or muscle tightness you might not be consciously aware of. You can try other approaches to help ease that inflammation or muscle tightness without relying on pain relievers. Physicians recommend against taking ibuprofen or any other NSAID on a regular basis, as they can have some serious side effects when taken long-term. People over 60 and those with certain medical conditions need to exercise even more caution. Always read and follow the warning label as a guide.

If you eat a lot of foods with high salicylate content, there's a very slight chance that salicylate sensitivity could be contributing to your tinnitus. Fruits which contain a high salicylate content include blueberries, blackberries, boysenberries, oranges, pineapples, raisins, strawberries, and tangerines. Some vegetables also make the list, including peppers, tomatoes, and canned green olives. Other popular foods which are salicylate culprits are almonds, peanuts with skins left on, coconut oil, olive oil, corn syrup, honey, and jams. For an extensive list, read the article, "Salicylate Content of Foods," on the www.failsafediet.com website.

Salicylic acid is a key ingredient in many skin-care products because it causes the epidermis cells of the skin to shed more readily. If you're sensitive to salicylates, you may be sensitive to salicylic acid. Check the ingredients if you're using a product to treat acne, psoriasis, calluses, corns, warts, seborrhoeic dermatitis, or if you're using a dandruff shampoo.

The article "What Is a Salicylate Allergy?" on the WebMD website explains salicylates in more detail. It also includes a list of medications, foods, and cosmetics with salicylate as an ingredient. I wouldn't pin too much hope on salicylates being the cause of your tinnitus, but you can try avoiding them in your OTC medications and other products to see if doing so might reduce the intensity. If aspirin has been prescribed by your physician, talk with her about whether it might be contributing to your tinnitus. Do not stop taking prescribed aspirin, or any other medication, without first discussing it with your healthcare provider.

9

MYCINS, MICINS, AND CHEMOTHERAPY

When it comes to your auditory health, NSAIDs aren't the only drugs where you need to be cautious. The medications referred to as mycin and micin drugs often include tinnitus as a side effect in the package warning. Drugs whose names end in "mycin" or "micin" are derived from Streptomyces, a nonpathogenic bacteria found in soil. (Nonpathogenic means it is incapable of causing disease.) Mycins are powerful antibiotics and are extremely helpful in preventing or fighting infection, but there is a risk of ototoxicity when using them. Because of the known correlation, there is a lot of confusion surrounding just how ototoxic they are. One common belief is that all mycin drugs are ototoxic. This is not true.

First, there is a class of drugs known as aminoglycosides that are certainly ototoxic to varying degrees. Aminoglycosides are also derived from Streptomyces. The reason for confusion is that some mycin drugs are aminoglycosides, but not all aminoglycosides are mycin drugs. In fact, only about 50 percent of mycin drugs carry a risk of ototoxicity. There are also varying degrees of ototoxicity associated with each drug. Therefore, just because you've been prescribed a mycin drug, it doesn't mean that particular drug is highly ototoxic. On the other hand, you should not assume any drug is safe for your auditory system simply because it doesn't have the "mycin" or "micin" suffix. Quinine is known to be ototoxic, and as you can see, it doesn't have the suffix "mycin" or "micin."

The different degrees of risk associated with ototoxic drugs means that some are mildly ototoxic, whereas others pose a very high risk. For example, neomycin is the worst offender for cochleotoxicity, meaning toxic to the cochlea, the part of the inner ear which contains the organ of Corti where the hair cells are located. Whenever you are prescribed a medication, be sure to check the package insert for ototoxicity risk. Always let your doctor know if you have hearing loss, balance issues, or tinnitus. It's possible that she can prescribe a different drug that won't cause additional damage. Be proactive when it comes to protecting your delicate auditory system. Never assume that your healthcare practitioner will be aware of all the information necessary to protect you from unintended consequences.

As previously mentioned, it's the aminoglycosides class of drugs that are ototoxic, not the mycin drugs per se. These drugs include:

- Capreomycin, for drug-resistant tuberculosis;
- Kanamycin (brand name Kantrex), for serious infections such as caused by the E. coli bacteria;
- Neomycin sulfate, for infections that are proven to be caused by or strongly suspected to be caused by bacteria;
- Paromomycin, for intestinal infections and some liver problems;
- Streptomycin, which can affect the vestibular portion of cranial nerve VIII, resulting in tinnitus, vertigo, and ataxia;
- Erythromycin, when administered via IV in high doses;
- Gentamicin, vestibular toxicity that can occur within two weeks.

If in doubt about any drug, there are some excellent websites which will give you all the information you need for any prescription or over-the-counter medication you are taking, including its potential ototoxic effect. One of the best sites is www.drugs.com. It is written in a manner that is thorough but still easy to understand. Simply enter the name of the drug in the search bar, then click the name in the dropdown list or click the magnifying glass icon to get to its information page. Then scroll down the page and look for the heading "Side Effects," which may or may not be on the first page, depending on how much information is available for the drug. Under "Side Effects," read what's listed under "Nervous System." That's where you'll find any comments about ototoxicity. Remember that ototoxicity is more common in cases where the drug is either taken long term, in higher doses than recommended by the drug manufacturer, or intravenously.

Keep in mind that it's in your best interest to research if a medication could affect your auditory system, whether temporary or permanent, especially if you already have a pre-existing condition. Sometimes there are substitutes with a lesser risk of ototoxicity. Physicians don't always take ototoxicity into account when prescribing drugs. When you have a chronic condition, it makes sense to be as informed as possible in protecting your health. Even if the condition is mild, you don't want it to become worse. If you have concerns, ask if an effective alternative remedy is available.

The most ototoxic drugs are those used in chemotherapy. Cancer has many treatments, and science is constantly seeking a cure in the form of more and more powerful drugs. It's ironic that some people with tinnitus say that they would rather have cancer than tinnitus. They believe there are only two outcomes for cancer: either a cure, or death. The truth is, there's a chance someone can survive cancer and have tinnitus as a side effect of the treatment. Depending on the type of cancer and the drugs used to treat it, tinnitus caused by chemotherapy ranges from 20% for colon cancer treatment to as high as 60% for testicular cancer treatment. Sometimes the tinnitus recedes when the chemotherapy course is ended, and sometimes it's a permanent side effect.

A common chemotherapeutic drug which is severely ototoxic is Cisplatin. It's known as the "penicillin of cancer" because of its broad range of applications. Cisplatin is used to treat sarcomas, small cell lung cancer, germ cell tumors, lymphoma, and ovarian cancer. Carboplatin is another chemotherapeutic drug with ototoxic risk, but to a lesser degree. It's most commonly used to treat ovarian cancer.

If you or someone you love is receiving chemotherapy, please advise your oncologist immediately if any symptoms develop that are related to hearing, balance, or tinnitus. Obviously the recommendation of the oncologist must be followed when it comes to medications for a disease as serious as cancer, but perhaps there are steps that can be taken to reduce the ototoxic effects. Do not take any supplements for tinnitus without discussing them with the physician first, as certain supplements may interfere with the effectiveness of the chemotherapeutic drug. If the tinnitus is extremely distressing, it might be a good idea to arrange sessions with a cognitive behavioral therapist. This will help to cope with anxiety caused by tinnitus, as well as the anxiety associated with the cancer diagnosis and treatment.

Some over-the-counter remedies can be ototoxic. For example, tea tree oil is an extremely popular home remedy touted as being anti-microbial and anti-fungal. It is added to products like shampoo, toothpaste, and chewing gum, as well as application straight from the bottle. (Tea tree oil is one of the few essential oils that can be applied directly to the skin without first diluting it with a carrier oil.) However, a study by Zhang and Robertson concluded that tea tree oil may be toxic to the cochlea; specifically, the hair cells associated with higher frequency hearing. Although this is only one study, it would be wise to avoid applying tea tree oil within the ear canal in the hopes of curing an ear infection or some other disorder. Any time you consider using a home remedy for an ear problem, please be sure to research it for possible ototoxicity. Use reputable online sources such as www.WebMD.com. Do not rely on articles from a website that may be publishing inaccurate and harmful information. Avoid websites selling products which are advertised to cure tinnitus.

10
NOISE EXPOSURE

Without question, the number one cause of tinnitus is noise exposure. For now, let's use the definition of noise as any sound that aggravates or exceeds the comfort level of your auditory system. You may not be aware of it while it's happening, but there is a noise level that your auditory system can tolerate within a specific period of time. Beyond that limit, it can cause temporary or permanent damage. We usually don't know when we've crossed the line until it's too late. For example, two people of the same age and in good health can go to a nightclub and be exposed to the same noise level for the same amount of time. One person will leave the nightclub with ringing in his ears, but the other person will not. That's because of the difference in their noise exposure tolerance. Even though we all have basically the same structures in our auditory systems, there can be a lot of variance in tolerance level. This is why it's so important to always protect your ears from noise exposure. If you are a hyperaesthetic person, meaning one or more of your senses are more sensitive than the average person, then it's even more critical that you wear hearing protection in loud environments. Autistics also tend to have sound sensitivity issues. Temple Grandin, author of *The Autistic Brain*, explained how loud noises like a school bell were painful to her, like a dentist drill in her ears. Hyperaesthetics can relate to the pain she feels, which most people do not experience under the same conditions.

Noise exposure that results in tinnitus generally doesn't happen overnight, but tends to develop over the course of years. One example is a twin-engine aircraft pilot whose ears are exposed for long periods of time to the roar of the engines. After flying for many years, he notices that his hearing has diminished considerably and tinnitus is now present. Another example is a long distance truck driver who not only hears the diesel engine for hours on end, but has to endure road noise as well. While on the road, she might be listening to a CB radio and maybe some music on a CD player to help pass the time. To combat the road noise, the volume of the music might be kept higher than normal. Even though the decibel level is within acceptable range, the accumulated exposure over time within close quarters makes that person more susceptible to auditory damage. Some studies have suggested that the closer to the ear the sound is, and the longer the accumulated exposure in time, the more likely it is that there will eventually be some sort of negative outcome. You can think of it as similar to the wind blowing sand across a rock, year after year. It can take a very long time before you notice that the rock has eroded. By then, it's too late to undo the damage.

Anyone who plays online games with headphones or listens to music through earbuds is at risk for hearing loss and/or tinnitus. Even if the volume seems to be set at a perfectly acceptable level, it probably isn't. It's doubly unfortunate that so many people will turn the volume up on their earbuds or headphones until it's just below their pain threshold. They think if it doesn't hurt, it means that it's safe to listen to. The reality is, it isn't safe at all. The pain threshold and the damage threshold are two completely separate things. If you've been listening to music through headphones with the volume turned up to drown out the sounds of your environment and you're now struggling with tinnitus, you would be wise to limit your use of headphones and earbuds. Be very careful with the volume level. Your auditory system is now much more likely to suffer additional damage because it's already been traumatized. As mentioned in Chapter 5, "Chronic Tinnitus and Spikes," it's like comparing someone with a damaged vertebra to someone with a healthy back. In a vehicular accident, the person with a damaged vertebra is at risk for greater injury because one component in the back has already been weakened. If you currently aren't experiencing tinnitus but you've previously had tinnitus episodes, especially noise-induced tinnitus, use headphones and earbuds at safe volume levels and limit your time using them. Don't take unnecessary risks with your hearing.

If your job requires you to wear headphones, be careful with the volume. Be sure to give your ears a break of at least five minutes every hour. It's not the best solution, but it's better than nonstop exposure.

11
DECIBELS AND SAFE LEVELS

How can you tell when sounds exceed recommended exposure limits? This chapter covers what you need to know regarding safe levels of sound in your everyday life, as well as the decibel levels of certain noises that rarely occur in most people's lives but can be extremely dangerous.

A decibel is a unit of measurement for volume of sound. Research in the field of hearing safety has given us measures of decibel levels with corresponding recommended daily exposure limits. These exposure limits are based on the average person with a reasonably healthy auditory system. Whether you already have hearing loss or not, there is no way to tell whether you will have a higher or lower threshold of safety. Sustained exposure to any sound above 85 to 95 decibels can cause hearing loss. The loss occurs from both the power of the sound as well as the length of exposure. Tinnitus is closely correlated with hearing loss. Anything that can cause hearing loss can also cause tinnitus.

The following is a list of some common sounds and their decibel levels. This will give you an idea of the significant difference in safe exposure limits. Remember that these are cumulative exposure limits within 24 hours. For example, the safe level of exposure to a hand drill is two hours, meaning two hours total in a 24-hour period. In other words, it isn't safe to operate a hand drill for two hours, take a break, then expose yourself to the same 100-decibel level for another one or two hours. When you know your exposure time will put you in the danger zone, wear adequate hearing protection.

- Soft whisper, 30 decibels, no limit to exposure;
- Conversation at three feet, 60 decibels, no limit to exposure;
- Dishwasher, 55 - 70 decibels, no limit to exposure;
- Vacuum cleaner, 60 - 85 decibels, up to eight hours;
- Sounds of city traffic inside your car, 75 to 85 decibels (depending on the vehicle), up to eight hours;
- Hand drill, 100 decibels, two hours;
- Power mower at three feet, 107 decibels, 45 minutes to an hour;

- Crying baby, 110 decibels, 30 minutes;
- Gas-powered weedeater, up to 115 decibels, 15 minutes;
- Typical rock concert, 115 to 120 decibels, 15 minutes.

At 112 decibels, damage can occur within one minute of exposure, even though the limit for exposure time is 15 minutes. The pain threshold is reached at 125 decibels. There are certain noises that people willingly expose themselves to, such as sporting events, but they don't wear ear protection because they are unaware that even very short-term exposure is dangerous. In the case of grenades and explosive devices, note the extreme decibel level that military personnel may be exposed to. There is no safe exposure limit for the following:

- Stock car race, 130 decibels;
- 40,000-watt car speakers, 135 - 154 decibels;
- Jet engine at 100 feet, 140 decibels;
- Fireworks, 140 - 170 decibels;
- IED (improvised explosive device), 140 - 170 decibels;
- 12-gauge shotgun blast, 165 decibels;
- Airbag deploying, 170 decibels;
- M84 stun grenade, 170 - 180 decibels. Death of hearing tissue occurs at 180 decibels.

With fireworks, distance matters. For example, 170 decibels is excruciatingly loud, but at 50 to 60 feet away (15 to 20 meters), the risk of hearing damage in adults is greatly reduced. Children need a distance of 164 to 196 feet (50 to 60 meters) from such fireworks. As noted before, the ear canals of children are smaller than those of an adult, which increases the level of sound pressure and makes them more susceptible to damage. If you have a young child or an infant in your home, they may be at risk for hearing loss from exposure to noise levels that would be considered safe for teens and adults.

There is one type of noise exposure that most people don't even think about because it's usually in the context of a party. The popping of a balloon can register an astonishing 125 decibels. Think about how much fun kids have when they're popping a lot of balloons at a birthday party. For the sake of their hearing (and yours), give them another way to express their excitement.

The potential for injury from airbags deploying has gained increasing attention from the public. The statistics show that in most cases they save lives. Unfortunately, there is a genuine risk of trauma that an airbag can inflict when it deploys, or "explodes" as some refer to it. Hearing loss and/or tinnitus are two potentially permanent injuries that have been proven to be caused by airbags. However, the University of Michigan Transportation Research Institute conducted a study and determined that the risk of hearing damage is small at 1.7%. Some people prefer not to take a chance of hearing loss or other injuries associated with airbags, and elect to have them deactivated. Please research the laws in your state, and certainly discuss it with your vehicle insurance company before you deactivate any airbags.

You don't always have a choice when it comes to airbags deploying, but you do have a choice about which rock concerts you'll attend. There are bands that have been measured at up to 130 ear-splitting decibels. Among these are AC/DC, Led Zeppelin, and Mötorhead, and these particular bands' concert decibel levels were measured decades ago. In 1987, U2 performed in Rome, Italy, registering seismic waves that triggered earthquake alarms. It's not surprising that Bono, the lead singer of U2, has tinnitus. The British group Leftfield performed at an ear-blistering 136 decibels in 1996, causing plaster chunks and dust to fall from the ceiling of South Brixton's London Academy. There are plenty of people who think nothing of attending concerts with such brutal decibel levels, but online tinnitus forums are filled with people who deeply regret doing so.

As sound levels go up in our environment, it's more important than ever to know when the volume is getting into the danger zone. Apps that measure decibel levels are available for both iOS and Android devices. Some of the apps are free; others have a very modest price. Sound Meter by Abc Apps is a free Android app which appears to be highly rated. You can find it on https://play.google.com/store. A popular free app for iOS devices is Decibel 10th, available through https://itunes.apple.com. Be mindful that apps are not a precise measurement. Their results may vary by as much as 8 to 20 decibels from one app to another in the same environment. If you want precision, look for a handheld decibel meter. Most of these devices are in the $15 to $70 range, depending on features, and can be found both locally and through online retailers. If you decide to monitor decibel levels to guide you when to wear earplugs, remember that each increase of 3 decibels is roughly equivalent to a doubling of volume.

In an environment where it's likely that the noise will keep getting louder, and where there are bursts of extremely loud noise, a decibel meter isn't necessary to understand what you're exposing yourself to. For example, there's a YouTube video of a cheering crowd at a Seahawks versus Packers game, "Decibel Meter of Roaring Crowd Noise." The smartphone app measured the crowd at 119 decibels. Total safe exposure time at that level is 15 minutes in 24 hours, but anyone who's gone to a game like this knows that the excitement with whistles, screams, and cheers adds up to much more than 15 minutes. Use common sense and protect your hearing by inserting earplugs when the crowd first begins to roar.

SECTION III

DEMOGRAPHICS OF TINNITUS

12
WHY ME?

Hearing loss is positively linked with developing tinnitus. The number of Americans afflicted with hearing loss is staggering: 1 in 5 adults, 1 in 3 adults over the age of 65, and 3 in 5 veterans returning from war. The incidence in teens is particularly troubling. Nearly 1 in 6 teens between the ages of 12 and 19 have reported hearing loss from loud noise.

As your hearing worsens, you lose the ability to hear at higher frequencies. For example, a healthy 18-year-old should be able to hear up to 20kHz. By the age of 50, that drops to 12kHz. The website www.noiseaddicts.com has a quick and easy online test, "Hearing Test - Can You Hear This?," to check how high of a frequency you can hear. The comments posted by teens and older adults are interesting, and a good indication of the seriousness of protecting one's ears to avoid hearing loss that occurs for reasons other than the natural aging process. You can also try a frequency level hearing test on YouTube. One of the most popular ones, "Cool Hearing test," is on the Science Forum channel. Always wear enclosed headphones to eliminate ambient noise when testing your hearing. Check the volume first to ensure that it's at a safe level before putting on the headphones. Incidentally, if you have high-pitched tinnitus, it may cover up the higher frequencies played. In other words, you won't be able to detect any tone on the test which is in the same range as your tinnitus frequency. If you have cycling tinnitus, take the test when your tinnitus is mild, which will give you the most accurate reading.

Generally speaking, there are certain demographics who seem to acquire tinnitus more than others. Males are more likely to get tinnitus than females. This may be due to males traditionally working in jobs where noise exposure is more prevalent; for example, construction, long haul truck driver, railroad engineer, etc. Caucasians are more likely to get tinnitus than other races, for reasons unknown. Seniors and the elderly are more susceptible to acquiring tinnitus, particularly after the age of 60. People who engage in motorsports and hunting have higher rates, probably due to lack of adequate hearing protection. Again, these are more likely to be males, who tend to be more dismissive of the notion of protecting themselves against noise, especially when they're younger. Most people are simply unaware how easy it is to damage the auditory system and cause hearing loss.

Who is most at risk for acquiring tinnitus? That would be anyone who is routinely exposed to loud noise in their environment. Think of long distance truck drivers, spending day after day with the sound of road noise and a diesel engine. Long-term exposure at a lower decibel level can do just as much damage as a brief exposure at a higher decibel level. Construction workers are at risk, with daily exposure to nail guns, hammers, blasting operations in demolitions, back-up alarm beepers on heavy equipment, and of course the general overall loud environment caused by operating machinery and people shouting to be heard above the noise. Ironically, it's been proven that exposure to back-up beepers has become so commonplace, many people have learned to ignore them, which of course defeats the purpose of using them.

Musicians, especially those who perform in concerts, and in particular rock musicians, are very much at risk. The Tinnitus Talk board has many members who are musicians. Tinnitus doesn't spare the famous, either. A few celebrity musicians with tinnitus are Eric Clapton, Bob Dylan, Trent Reznor, Phil Collins, Barbra Streisand, Moby, Phil Young, Pete Townshend, Chris Martin, Lars Ulrich, KT Tunstall, and Ayumi Hamasaki, to name just a few.

will.i.am of the Black Eyed Peas has tinnitus, and in April 2013 he revealed that he also has ADHD (Attention Deficit Hyperactivity Disorder), a condition with some neurological similarities to tinnitus. He has posted a video online about his ADHD and his tinnitus, which includes his simulation of the high-pitched tone he hears constantly. You can watch the video by going to YouTube and searching for "will.i.am tinnitus." (The video is blocked for playing outside of YouTube.) It's inspiring to know that a musician is able to create extraordinary music despite having both ADHD and intrusive tinnitus. Musicians are passionate about composing and playing music. As much as possible, they tend to treat tinnitus as an annoyance but not a barrier to doing what they love. Beethoven was afflicted with severe tinnitus and profound deafness. In a letter to a friend, he wrote, "Of course, I am resolved to rise above every obstacle, but how will it be possible?" Beethoven did manage to rise above, composing some of the most loved and enduring music of all time.

Aside from occupational hazards and the risk of acquiring tinnitus after decades of noise exposure, one particularly troubling trend is the increased incidence of tinnitus in teens and young adults. Tinnitus can occur after years of clubbing in loud venues, or it can arise after one night from the simple mistake of perhaps standing too close to an amplifier at a concert. If you have ever had your ears ring the day after partying all night at a loud nightclub, you are already at risk of getting chronic tinnitus with each additional exposure. Some lucky people seem to be able to abuse their auditory system to no end and never experience anything beyond mild hearing loss. Other unfortunate folks find that they have permanent tinnitus after one loud exposure which exceeds their body's tolerance level.

Larry Roberts is a senior researcher in the Department of Psychology, Neuroscience and Behavior at McMaster University in Canada. He co-authored a study which indicates that nearly 30% of teenagers have experienced tinnitus. The World Health Organization sees a looming crisis on the horizon, with over 1.1 billion young people at risk for hearing loss, with much of the blame placed on earbuds being jammed into ears while playing music at unsafe levels. Hearing loss is often a precursor to tinnitus, so we can expect the rates of tinnitus to rise accordingly. It's one thing to get tinnitus when you're 50 or 60 and have learned some coping skills to help you deal with life's adversities; it's another thing entirely when you're between 16 and 25 years old and are unexpectedly hit with a major challenge like constant intrusive tinnitus.

War takes its toll and can inflict much more than psychological damage or the kinds of physical injuries we normally think of when considering the cost of war in terms of human suffering. Tinnitus is now the number 1 disability reported by soldiers returning from Iraq and Afghanistan. Thirty percent of soldiers deployed in Iraq report having tinnitus. For those exposed to IEDs (improvised explosive devices), that number jumps to 50 percent. In 2014, the Department of Veterans Affairs concluded that tinnitus now affects more veterans than PTSD. Veterans Administration audiologists who conduct tests on veterans estimate that there are approximately 710,000 veterans with hearing loss, and more than 841,000 veterans with tinnitus. Try to imagine what it's like for these men and women coming home from a war zone. Not only do they have the disturbing memories and possibly physical injuries, but now there's also a whine, buzzing, hissing, whistling or static in their ears and/or head. These veterans are struggling to cope, and their families and friends are at a loss how to help. When you realize the number of veterans affected by tinnitus, and by extension their families who do their best to share the burden, it makes you wonder why the majority of people have never heard of tinnitus. Or, if they do know what it is, they don't understand how serious it can be unless they have some kind of firsthand experience with it.

Sometimes a person's genetic makeup predisposes them to being vulnerable to developing hearing loss and/or tinnitus. A person with a high-strung personality or one who is subject to bouts of depression or anxiety attacks is potentially more susceptible. Anxiety disorders can include generalized anxiety disorder. This is when someone cannot name a specific reason for their anxiety, and yet they are burdened with an unexplainable feeling of apprehension or fear. An extreme level of anxiety can manifest in panic disorders. These are experienced as panic attacks, which can feel frighteningly similar to a heart attack. Some of the symptoms of panic attack are weakness in the extremities, shortness of breath, chest pain, sweating, a racing heart, and a feeling of impending doom. Panic attacks are terrifying, to say the least, and the first one that strikes can be emotionally devastating. Research has not conclusively determined whether panic attacks are genetic, but studies have shown that anxiety disorders do tend to run in families. If either or both parents have an anxiety disorder, the odds are greater that the children may develop one.

There's no way to tell how likely you are to develop an anxiety disorder. However, it does seem quite unfair that a person has a greater chance of acquiring tinnitus simply because they are genetically predisposed to developing an anxiety disorder. It also makes them more susceptible to experiencing elevated anxiety caused by the tinnitus. This is one reason why it's so important to learn about the basics of tinnitus and what you can do to relieve the anxiety. Understanding as much as you can about tinnitus will help you to cope with the early stages of tinnitus and hopefully keep it from becoming worse simply because it's feeding off your anxiety.

Obsessive compulsive disorder is another form of anxiety expression. It isn't unusual for someone with tinnitus, particularly severe tinnitus, to also have some form of obsessive compulsive disorder. This can be seen in people who exhibit what appears to be irrational repetitive behavior, such as having to wash their hands three or four times in a row instead of just once. Other examples are being hypervigilant about germs or other perceived threats, or an insistence on everything being in precise order and becoming angry if someone moves something out of its designated spot. Sometimes OCD manifests in the form of obsessive thoughts, being unable to let go of something which triggers a negative emotional reaction, or engaging in worrisome thought patterns which are basically endless loops from which there is no escape. If you lie in bed night after night, unable to sleep because you can't stop thinking of something which troubles you or something that you're worried will happen, that's a form of OCD.

In the 1980s, with the advent of the AIDS epidemic, public health officials began a campaign to encourage adults in non-exclusive sexual relationships to wear condoms. In addition to AIDS, other sexually transmitted diseases were reaching epidemic proportions. Among these were HPV (human papillomavirus), herpes, chlamydia, gonorrhea, trichomoniasis, and syphilis. It took a while to overcome the ingrained resistance, but now the use of condoms among sexually active adults is both accepted and expected. Common sense and the desire to protect one's health, as well as preventing unwanted pregnancy, finally became a stronger motivation than the desire for unrestricted pleasure. Sales of condoms have skyrocketed, which is a good thing. We can look back and wonder what took us so long to accept using something as simple as a condom to protect our health and well-being.

Now consider what's going on with sounds around us. Our everyday environment is becoming progressively louder each year. Theaters are much louder than in the past. In action films, the volume is noticeably increased, sometimes to what feels like deafening levels, in order to emphasize adrenalin-pumping scenes. Monster truck rallies and drag races are louder. Go into almost any store in a mall that caters to youth and the decibel level can be disturbingly high. This is a reflection of modern marketing, the notion being that loud music conveys excitement about their products. The truth is, you just about can't get away from music in any retail establishment. It's in almost every store and restaurant. Modern society subjects its inhabitants to a constant unrelenting exposure to sound and noise. Decibel levels in some environments, such as nightclubs, regularly reach levels that far exceed safe hearing thresholds. The people in charge of setting those levels are showing very little concern for the auditory health and safety of their customers. Again, it's because they believe louder volume equals more excitement, and because their customers either expect or demand it.

In this kind of noise-drenched atmosphere, when you never know what your ears are going to be exposed to, it's up to every individual to adopt a responsible attitude of protecting themselves. Earplugs should be accepted as the smart thing to use whenever there is activity involving extreme noise or loud music, just as condoms are accepted as the smart thing to use in moderate to high risk sexual activity. Some STDs are permanent, and could have been avoided with the use of condoms. Likewise, a person may find themselves struggling with hearing loss and/ or tinnitus for the rest of their life, when both could have been prevented or lessened by wearing basic hearing protection.

Wearing earplugs doesn't mean you will have good hearing forever, and it's not a guarantee you'll never get tinnitus. However, it will improve the odds that you will continue to enjoy a healthy level of hearing and possibly avoid tinnitus completely. You can get glasses or contacts to correct your vision, and you can wear hearing aids to amplify sound if you have hearing loss, but we don't have any comparable devices to reliably turn down the volume on intrusive tinnitus. No matter what your current level of tinnitus is, whether it's none, intermittent, constant, mild, moderate, or severe, it's up to you to be safe and protect your hearing.

One word of caution: only wear earplugs as needed. If you wear them constantly, you run the risk of oversensitizing your hearing and developing hyperacusis, a condition in which every sound is amplified to an uncomfortable or even painful degree. Hyperacusis is explained in more detail in Chapter 20, "The Pain of Hyperacusis."

13
BLAME THE BRAIN

It's not just the structures within your ears that are causing the trouble. There's a lot going on in the wiring of your brain that contributes to it as well. Scientists are finally coming to an agreement that no matter what causes it, tinnitus is primarily a disorder of the brain. The simple explanation is that the hair cells that line the cochlea of the ear and the sensory cells of the brain begin miscommunicating. A more detailed explanation is that when there is damage to the inner ear hair cells, sensory input is reduced in the auditory pathways of the brain. This causes alterations in synaptic connections. Those alterations are part of a process called brain plasticity, which is an adaptive development whereby the brain essentially reorganizes itself and its functions in response to the environment, events experienced, or injury.

The brain transmits information through its neurons. Information flows from one neuron to the next across a synapse. Think of neurons and synapses as the communication network of the brain. When specific neurons become hyperactive, when they don't shut off properly, this leads to changes in the neural impulses which signal the presence of sound. This can result in tinnitus, whereby the brain perceives sound despite the absence of actual external sound.

Some researchers believe that it doesn't matter what triggered the tinnitus. Their theory is that whether it be auditory trauma or infection or extreme stress or age-related hearing loss that's responsible for tinnitus, that the root cause of the phantom sound is hyperactivity of the neurons in the brain. This has led to all sorts of theories and research into why these neurons become hyperactive in some individuals but not in others. This hyperactivity and resultant tinnitus manifest at varying levels of intensity, with no specific relationship to the degree of acoustic trauma, the aging process, or any of the numerous other causes that are blamed for tinnitus taking hold.

Let's say you've had all the medical examinations that can possibly be given to rule out disease as the cause of your tinnitus. Maybe you've had an acoustic insult from loud noise exposure, or taken a medication that adversely affected your hearing, or had an ear infection, or any number of countless reasons why people get tinnitus. Despite the reassurance that you have no serious ongoing illness causing the phantom sound, you might still be wrestling with anxiety because you perceive the tinnitus to be extremely loud, intrusive, or distressing. Maybe you only hear it when you're in a quiet room, but the fact that it's always there is seriously getting on your nerves. You can't concentrate, your sleep is affected, you begin withdrawing from social activities because you're frustrated and angry at this affliction. You can't imagine living like this the rest of your life. You wonder why you're having such a hard time dealing with it. If you express how you're feeling, a friend or family member might say, "Oh, yeah, my tinnitus is really loud, but it doesn't bother me." Now you feel worse. Not only do you have this beast in your ears or head, you begin to feel like a failure for letting it get to you and affect your life.

Medical science is pointing the way to a new understanding about why tinnitus is so nerve-wracking to some people but not to others. It's not your fault that you can't shrug off the tinnitus. In fact, research increasingly shows that it likely has a lot to do with how your brain is wired, particularly the limbic system. The intrusiveness and severity of your tinnitus also depends upon the levels and interaction of neurotransmitters, the chemical messengers that deliver information to the nerve cells in your brain. That's the bad news. The good news is, with some effort, dedication, and patience, you can train your brain to essentially rewire its circuits and tame the tinnitus beast. You can build new food habits that will deprive tinnitus of some of its energy. You can engage in activities to help restore a healthy balance in your neurotransmitter levels. There are helpful treatments and sound therapies ranging from zero cost to very expensive, but all of which require an investment of time and dedicated effort. It's up to you to decide whether you're going to be proactive or reactive in dealing with your tinnitus, regardless of the level of its severity. You may not get rid of it entirely, but it's quite possible for you to gain significant relief that allows you to begin living a more normal life again.

Whether you've had tinnitus for one week, one year, or one decade, and whether your tinnitus is mild, moderate or severe, you can still benefit by taking the time and effort to reduce its influence on your life.

If you're one of the lucky ones who can dismiss the sounds of tinnitus, or if it's something that simply does not bother you, it's still a good idea to explore possible treatments. Even though for most people the perception of their tinnitus improves gradually over time, the opposite can happen. Tinnitus can remain mild for many years and suddenly change for the worse. Taking the time to understand what tinnitus is, and what you can do about it now, can make a big difference in how much it affects you in the future.

SECTION IV

THE FIRST MONTHS
ARE THE WORST MONTHS

14
HOW IT BEGINS

Some people know precisely when their permanent tinnitus began, and can point to the exact reason for why they have it. This is usually the case when there's been an isolated incident of a sudden sharp burst of high decibel sound, like a gunshot or explosion. In that instance, the tinnitus can happen immediately. That's what happened to Jacob Everett. He relates the experience in his YouTube video, "The Exact Moment I Got Tinnitus." It's definitely worth watching, but turn the volume down first. Be sure to read what he posted below the video.

Other people may acquire tinnitus when they've been too close to a constant high decibel level. As I mentioned previously, one example of this is standing next to an amplifier at a concert. When they wake up the next morning with their ears still ringing, and as time goes by the ringing hasn't stopped, they realize the mistake they made by not moving away from the amp. Unfortunately, it can be far worse than a basic ringing sound, as noted in Chapter 3, "Tinnitus Sounds and Volume."

It isn't always the case, however, that tinnitus immediately follows extreme noise exposure. Sometimes the damage doesn't show up for weeks. In addition, it's not uncommon to have a feeling of fullness in the ears or a sense of muffled hearing before the tinnitus appears. If you or someone you know has occasional tinnitus and also a feeling of fullness in the ears from time to time, that's a warning sign that the tinnitus can easily become permanent within the near future. It's just a matter of what's going to cause the tipping point to occur.

Musicians tend to be aware of the danger of excess noise exposure, but even they sometimes fail to wear adequate ear protection. When tinnitus strikes, they know why they have it, even if they can't pinpoint a specific music session that caused it. The same is true for anyone who is frequently exposed to high decibels in their occupation. One day the brain and/or the auditory system reach a point of no return, and tinnitus sets in. It may take years or it might take decades, which is why it's so important to consistently wear ear protection even if you feel like nothing is wrong. This is especially true for younger people who are more likely than any other group to take risks with their hearing.

For reasons that researchers don't quite understand yet, tinnitus appears to be intricately linked with the sleep cycle. A common trait of sudden tinnitus is that it erupts after sleeping. You can fall asleep feeling perfectly fine, but when you wake up you hear tinnitus in your ears or head. The volume can be anywhere from a slight hum to a devastating cacophony of sounds. It doesn't matter if you had a full night's sleep or only a nap; somehow the tinnitus is triggered by the brain during sleep. One would hope that with the next sleep session the sounds would go away, but that rarely happens. It's as if a switch has been flipped on in the neural circuitry, and it won't turn off.

My tinnitus began following an evening nap. In the past, I sometimes fell asleep on the couch while watching a movie or television show. Usually I'd wake up within 15 or 20 minutes. Then I would continue watching whatever was on, or call it a night and go to bed.

One night in April 2014, things went terribly wrong. I woke up from that evening nap to what sounded like a riot surrounding my house. What I heard was a blend of yelling and screams, and it was unbelievably loud. There were other roaring and clanging noises I couldn't identify because they were all jumbled together. I was dazed and disoriented because what was happening didn't make any sense. It was almost on the same level as waking up to realize your house is on fire. No one is prepared for that, just as no one is prepared for sudden catastrophic tinnitus.

Within a few moments, I realized with horror that the sound wasn't coming from outside at all. It was inside my head! I pressed my palms to the sides of my head, as if that could somehow squeeze out the sounds and make them go away. I closed my eyes and shook my head, thinking for some strange reason that would put a stop to it, the same way we shake our head when we're dizzy in an attempt to stabilize ourselves.

Most of all, I just couldn't believe how loud it was, how chaotic. I took deep breaths, trying to calm myself the only way I knew how. Mercifully, after a few minutes it died down to a soft rumble, then a buzz, then a faint hum. It was like a tornado had rampaged through my head, leaving behind only some debris and rubble. I wondered if it was just the remnant of a bad dream, where my body had awakened but my mind still held onto some part of a nightmare. I chalked it up to an odd glitch in the brain, went to bed, and fell asleep without any trouble.

The next morning when I woke up, the buzzing sound was back, but it was in my right ear instead of my head. I thought to myself, What in the world is going on? Could this be tinnitus? I went through a checklist in my mind and decided no, it can't be. I've always taken care of my hearing, exercised regularly, and eaten healthy foods. I don't drink and I don't smoke. I get a decent amount of sleep every night. I had been stressed with work, some personal matters were worrying me, but it seems like life has always been that way. A few times, maybe once or twice a year, I had heard a soft, eerie high-pitched whine in my left ear that came out of nowhere and faded away within a few seconds, but I've never had ringing or buzzing or hissing in the ears, not even for a minute. The common experience of tinnitus had simply never happened to me before. I hoped that whatever was going on, that it was temporary. Once again, I thought it was just a brain glitch and it would work itself out.

The buzzing continued in my right ear all day long, every day. Sometimes the volume dropped significantly. I'd plug my fingers in my ears to see if it's still there, hoping it wouldn't be. Yep. Still there. Sometimes the buzz would get louder, and I'd tell myself I could get used to it as long as it didn't get any worse. The truth is, I was annoyed and incredibly frustrated. The tinnitus was intrusive. It was hard for me to concentrate on work. It interfered with me going to sleep, and my anxiety level was slowly beginning to rise.

A week later, I woke up one morning to sweet silence. The buzz was gone! I couldn't even hear it by sticking my fingers in my ears. Not a trace left behind. It was like a miracle. I told myself that the tinnitus must have been a freak occurrence. I was so grateful that it had now passed, and felt tremendous compassion for anyone who had to live with tinnitus every day for the rest of their lives.

That same night, feeling relaxed from the peace and quiet, I fell asleep on the couch while reading a book. A short time later, I was awakened by the sounds of hammering noises in my head, the kind that water pipes sometimes make when their air pressure changes. This time, it didn't ease off like it did before. I went into full-blown panic mode, scared out of my wits that the "symphony from hell" was in my head to stay. I paced the floor, took deep breaths, did everything I could to calm down, but nothing helped. The tinnitus continued at its mind-shattering volume. I went to bed and tried to read, hoping to distract myself from the intruder in my head. After a few hours I fell asleep, if you can call it that. It was more like passing out from exhaustion.

The next morning, the hammering noise began the moment I woke up. That awful sound, and others just as bad, were in my ears and head every day, all day long, for the next eight months. Hammering, dentist drill, sizzling, the buzzing of bees, mosquitos or cicadas, swaying curtains of bells, cymbals resonating, an endless telephone ring, a rain of needles falling on metal, the sound of maracas being shaken. I never knew what was going to invade my head next. It felt like torture. How in the world can the human brain create such horrid sounds?

I spent every spare minute online, obsessed with studying articles about tinnitus, trying to find the magic formula to make it go away. I bought countless supplements and stopped drinking coffee. I even took time off work to reduce stress, something I really couldn't afford to do, but I was desperate. I visited Internet forums dedicated to tinnitus, bought books about it, looked up which professionals treat tinnitus and even talked to a couple of them. I read hundreds of online stories of other tinnitus sufferers who have sought help for their tinnitus. It finally dawned on me that finding a solution to tinnitus is like making your way blindfolded through an intricate maze. The saddest thing is that over and over, people are told, "Learn to live with it." It doesn't have to be that way. There is a better way forward than simply learning to live with it.

That second episode of tinnitus was the perfect opportunity for me to have turned things around, or at least prevented the tinnitus from escalating to such a severe degree. I simply didn't understand what I was dealing with. In the next chapter, I'll tell you some things I wish I had done at the very beginning, as well as things I wish I hadn't done.

15
DON'T PANIC (AND OTHER ADVICE)

Imagine a thundering of hooves as a team of horses pulling a carriage careens around a bend on a winding muddy road in the middle of the night. Their eyes are wide and their nostrils flared, they froth at the mouth as they frantically rush full speed towards a destination unknown. The driver sits atop the carriage, a determined but manic look on his face as he lashes the whip over the horses, driving them on. The mud from the pounding hooves splashes everywhere, splattering the window of the carriage compartment, where a terrified passenger is tossed about from side to side. He can't understand how he ended up in a situation like this, with no control in this alarming turn of events.

At another time, on a pleasant sunny afternoon, someone is out for a ride on her favorite horse. Without warning, a fox darts out from the brush and runs directly in front of their path. Her horse is spooked and rears up, then begins to gallop madly away from what frightened him. The rider stays calm as she gently but firmly pulls back on the reins, calling for the horse to slow down. She is deliberate in her actions and stays focused. Soon the horse is under control, and the rest of the ride goes smoothly.

The first scene describes what it's like to panic when tinnitus strikes. You are the terrified passenger, believing that you have no control and that something terrible awaits. In the second scene, you are the rider, someone who knows that the best way to handle the situation is by remaining calm and taking deliberate action. Because of my lack of knowledge about tinnitus, my initial reaction when tinnitus reappeared was to panic. This was absolutely the worst thing I could have done. If I had stayed relatively calm and not let my fear take over, my tinnitus may never have reached its level of severity. In response to my panicked reaction, my brain amplified the volume of the tinnitus, in a misguided primitive attempt to protect me. You'll learn more why this happens in Chapter 23, "The Amygdala and Limbic System." Basically, the tinnitus signal is like a switch that's stuck in the "on" position. Because it's beyond your conscious control, you can't just simply flip it back to the "off" position. However, there are things you can do to modulate it, to tone it down, even if you can't completely shut if off.

I don't want you to panic the way I did. The most important thing you can do is to keep calm. Once you understand the strange nature of tinnitus, you can begin to take away its power over you.

Think of tinnitus as a mindless beast. It stomps around in your head or curls up over your ears and yowls for your attention. The louder the tinnitus, the bigger the beast is. For some people it's smaller in the morning and gets bigger during the day, whereas others have the opposite experience. For many people the tinnitus beast is pretty much the same size all day and all night. It clings to you wherever you go. It can be downright mean and nasty, and it doesn't care about you one bit. But here's the interesting thing about that mindless beast. It feeds on your anxiety and panic. The more you panic, or the more anxious you are, the bigger and louder it gets. You panic, the beast gets bigger. Then, when it gets bigger, you panic more. It becomes a vicious cycle. You need to break that cycle any way you can, as quickly as you can. That's easier said than done, but it isn't impossible.

Try to avoid the attitude that you're going to beat the beast. That just engages the amygdala, a primitive part of your brain, and puts you into a fight or flight mode. You don't want that. The amygdala is part of your limbic system over which you have no conscious control. Instead, what you need to do is shift your attitude away from the misguided thinking that you're going to fight and defeat tinnitus. It's very important for you to defuse the powder keg of your emotional response to tinnitus. Learning to control your emotional reaction is key to diminishing the power of tinnitus. Instead of giving in to your emotions, instead of being at the mercy of your limbic system, you can access the analytical part of your brain. I'm referring to the frontal lobe, and it's your best ally when it comes to taming the tinnitus beast. In other words, don't fight tinnitus. Instead, outsmart it. More on that in Chapter 64, "Train the Brain - Basics."

Tinnitus experts advise that you should never seek out your tinnitus. If you don't hear it, then don't plug your ears and listen for it. That was another big mistake on my part. When you actively listen for your tinnitus, it reinforces the message to your brain that the tinnitus is an important sound. Whenever your tinnitus subsides, do your best to think of other things, and just go about your business as if it doesn't exist.

As time goes by, your tinnitus likely will calm down somewhat. By December of 2014, my tinnitus was still loud and intrusive, but I was beginning to have days when the tinnitus volume was a 7 out of 10 instead of a constant 9 out of 10. Sometimes it dropped even lower. If you feel like your tinnitus is beginning to improve, resist the temptation to monitor it. Many of us with tinnitus, at the first sign of improvement, will monitor our tinnitus relentlessly. "Is it getting better?" "It's not as loud today as it was yesterday." "Oh, no, it seems to be louder now." Tell yourself that no matter what, you are going to live with your tinnitus day-by-day without comparison to how it's been before, or how you hope it will be in the future.

Remember that the more attention you give your tinnitus, the more importance your limbic system will assign to it. Find something else to focus on and switch your attention to that, even if it means focusing on how your shoes feel on your feet, the number of red objects in the room, anything at all which will shift your attention. If you can focus on something that engages you emotionally, that's even better. It takes a while to learn the skill of deliberate attention, but by doing so, you will eventually push the tinnitus into the background of your consciousness. The exception of course is catastrophic tinnitus, which for most people requires professional intervention and treatment. Even so, there are people with catastrophic tinnitus who have gradually learned to completely ignore it until something brings it to their conscious awareness. Chapter 28, "Habituation," mentions one instance of this, a woman with tinnitus as loud as a siren in her head.

In the next chapter, I discuss the sensitive issue of suicide and how it is generally viewed in the tinnitus community.

16
THOUGHTS OF SUICIDE

The subject of suicide is uncomfortable to talk about, but it needs to be addressed because it is not uncommon for people who have recently acquired tinnitus to consider ending their life in order to end the tinnitus. This is more likely to be expressed by those afflicted with severe tinnitus. However, it's not unheard of for someone with mild tinnitus to consider suicide if they become distraught by the thought of having to live the rest of their life with the phantom sounds. Particularly in the first few months, tinnitus can be such a disturbing presence that it may seem like the only option left is to simply end it all and be done with it.

There are no reliable statistics to show a strong connection between tinnitus and suicide. Billy Martin has been the clinic director of the Tinnitus Program at Oregon Health & Science University in Portland, Oregon (www.ohsu.edu). With over 9,000 patients through the years, he knows of eight who have committed suicide. That's approximately .088 percent, compared to .013 percent for the general population. It sounds like a much greater percentage for tinnitus patients. However, keep in mind that most of those patients likely had the more severe levels of tinnitus. They were also struggling with insomnia, anxiety and depression. These are the same burdens shared by many in the general population who consider and/or attempt suicide.

There have certainly been a few headline-grabbing instances of tinnitus sufferers committing suicide, like the case of Robert McIndoe. He acquired tinnitus after attending a concert of Them Crooked Vultures, a rock group whose music has been described as "punishingly loud." Mr. McIndoe, who lived in London, sought help but apparently was unable to connect consistently with the right resources to help him with his affliction. This is a very sad situation that should never have been allowed to progress to the point where he endured such despair. McIndoe committed suicide only three months after the onset of his tinnitus. His psychiatrist explained his suicide as stemming from the sense of helplessness and a belief that the tinnitus would never get better. Perhaps if McIndoe had known of the coping methods and treatments for tinnitus, or if he had simply given it more time, there's a good chance his condition would have improved, at least to the point of being tolerable. Instead, he was caught in the trap of believing that his tinnitus would never get better and therefore his life wasn't worth living. The story of Mr. McIndoe's ordeal is on www.telegraph.co.uk, "Coroner slams delays over tinnitus sufferer who stabbed himself to death."

Another well-known case in the tinnitus community is the story of Gaby Olthuis, whose initial mild tinnitus developed within three years into an unrelenting severe tinnitus that she described as "train screeching or nails on a chalkboard." A YouTube video, "I have tinnitus and I want to die," tells her story as related by the journalist who interviewed her. At 5:50 on the video, you will hear what her tinnitus sounded like. Be sure to turn down the volume before listening to this section of the video. To make matters worse, Gaby also had a severe case of hyperacusis. Everyday ambient sounds that most people never notice were deafening and painful to her. She saw doctors in several countries, hoping to find something to help her condition, but nothing worked. (The video does not mention what therapies she tried.) After 13 years of tinnitus and the additional burden of hyperacusis, Gaby took the drastic step of contacting a euthanasia clinic in her country of South Holland. Her request was eventually granted. She was given a lethal potion to drink at home, with one of the clinic's doctors attending her. A medical reason for Gaby's tinnitus was never determined.

On the other end of the spectrum is the encouraging and uplifting story of Zoe Cartwright, a creative and courageous young woman. She produced and directed a video, "Tinnitus Short Film - 24.7.52.10," on YouTube, expressing her interpretation of living with both deafness and loud persistent tinnitus. Because tinnitus involves the brain, people who are deaf can also have tinnitus. One of the poetic phrases in her short film expresses the experience of tinnitus well: "Torn between the reality around me and the surreal within me." This particular line reflects the disparity between looking absolutely normal, yet having the "beast" of tinnitus living in one's head, as Zoe describes it. Although the film itself is somewhat melancholy, Zoe continues to pursue her art and self-expression. After losing her hearing at age 15 and then acquiring tinnitus, she could have sunk into the depths of despair, but instead chose a brighter path. She has stated that she loves her life and enjoys it. Zoe

Cartwright is truly an inspiration to everyone who struggles with the day-to-day reality of severe tinnitus.

In searching online tinnitus forums, you will occasionally come across posts by people who relate the disheartening news that a member of the forum has chosen to end their life. Generally speaking, though, it is not the tinnitus itself but rather the accompanying depression and sense of helplessness which leads someone to take such an extreme step. As explained in Chapter 21, "Meet Your Neurotransmitters," there are chemicals in your brain which can affect your mood and outlook. These neurotransmitters may be exerting a strong influence on the negative emotions you are experiencing. This is why it's so important to seek professional help if your tinnitus is causing you to live in a constant state of despair, where you feel there is no hope and that life is not worth living if you have chronic and/or severe tinnitus.

If you are in the early stages of tinnitus and feeling overwhelmed, wondering how you'll cope for the next day, much less the rest of your life, you're not alone. Many people have walked in your shoes and understand exactly how you're feeling. It's a natural part of being human that we tend to focus on the worst scenario possible when it feels like our sense of well-being is in jeopardy. More than ever, now is the time to assess your thoughts and how they may be contributing to your depression or anger about your condition. One thing you really need to be aware of is whether your thoughts are falling into the all-or-nothing category. If you're saying, "I'll never be able to live with this," that's one example of an all-or-nothing type of statement. Try saying to yourself, "I know the first few months are hard, maybe even the first year, but in time my brain will harden to the noise. In time, I will be able to distract myself from it and not notice it as much. One day I'll look back and wonder why I ever thought of ending my life because of tinnitus."

This isn't just rose-colored glasses talk. These more optimistic statements are based on what countless people have posted on Internet forums, people who at one time believed they would rather die than live with tinnitus, but now lead productive and satisfactory lives. For some of them, it's a matter of counting their blessings. For others, sheer perseverance gets them through the initial stages. Some people keep trying different treatments or methods to cope until something clicks and they begin to experience relief. Then there are those for whom time simply has a way of diminishing the intensity of the tinnitus.

If you are in a state of mind that no words can comfort you and life feels completely empty of meaning, please seek professional help immediately. Do what you can to relieve the stress, anxiety, or depression. As noted in Chapter 59, "Prescription Drugs," there are medications aimed at reducing anxiety which also have the benefit of decreasing tinnitus volume. Sometimes that's all it takes to bring some light into your life. Tinnitus can be an enormous challenge for anyone, no matter how strong that person may have been in overcoming other adversities in life. **It is not a character flaw if you find yourself struggling with despair, nor is it a sign of weakness to ask for help.** If you cannot afford professional help, or if you need emotional support at any time, please consider joining the Tinnitus Talk support forum at www.tinnitustalk.com. As of August 2017, Tinnitus Talk has over 20,000 members, with usually hundreds of them online at any given time. You will find them very willing to share your burden, and to be a friend when your thoughts turn dark.

Please seek professional help immediately if you are thinking of harming yourself. You can also call the following hotline numbers:

- United States: 1-800-SUICIDE (1-800-784-2433), or dial 911
- United Kingdom: 08457 90 90 90
- Australia: Lifeline, 13 11 44

SECTION V

TINNITUS AFFECTS YOUR LIFE

17
HOW TINNITUS AFFECTS YOU

Tinnitus can have a wide range of effects on one's social life and family relationships. It can profoundly affect a person's quality of work, their creativity as well as their productivity, and it can interfere with their ability to study and learn. Much of this depends upon the severity of the tinnitus; that is, how loud and/or intrusive a person perceives it to be. How one reacts emotionally to their tinnitus has a lot to do with the degree to which they are affected. People who value peace and quiet, those without a supportive network of friends and family, or those who live and/or work in a highly stressful environment may find it much harder to cope. However, even when a person is able to get through their day by keeping themselves distracted and trying to maintain a sense of calm, tinnitus is capable of disrupting normal sleep patterns. It may not only be harder to go to sleep, tinnitus can also awaken you one or more times during the night, making it difficult to feel fully rested. Fatigue can set in, leading to a lower threshold of tolerance for the intrusive sounds and making it even more of a challenge to cope with the stresses and strains of everyday life.

The most common physical reactions from living with tinnitus day after day are fatigue, inability to concentrate, headache and earache. Yes, believe it or not, tinnitus can cause physical pain. It's not uncommon for someone with moderate to severe tinnitus to complain of an earache at the end of the day, brought on by nonstop sound located in one or both ears. Occasional or frequent headaches are a side effect of loud tinnitus that is heard in the head, or there may be a sensation of being "foggy-headed." Both the ears and the head can feel as if the nerves in those regions are in an inflamed state. A buzzing feeling is another common complaint, and it can be felt either in the ears or the head. In short, tinnitus is not just a sound for many people, it can carry with it the same physical sensations as if that sound were caused by a real physical stimulus. For example, try to imagine a trapped insect buzzing against an eardrum all day long. It would be understandable that at the end of the day your inner ear might feel sore or irritated by the constant feeling of something buzzing in it.

There are other potential negative side effects as a result of feeling overwhelmed by chronic tinnitus, including but not limited to high blood pressure, bruxism (teeth grinding), overeating, and breakdown of your immune system. For an in-depth look at the potentially devastating effects of unrelenting high-level stress, go to YouTube and watch the 2009 National Geographic documentary, "Stress: Portrait of a Killer."

Fortunately, not everyone with tinnitus experiences unpleasant physical effects. However, it's hard to escape the emotional impact it can create. One's emotional state can negatively affect their mental and physical states and spill over into almost every aspect of life. The most common emotional reactions associated with tinnitus are anxiety, depression, anger, frustration, grief, irritability, and self-pity.

Let's start with anxiety. It isn't unusual for other people to be dismissive of tinnitus and say, "Why do you let it bother you? It's just a sound!" Well, it is and it isn't. As mentioned in Chapter 23, "The Amygdala and Limbic System," the amygdala plays a major role in the perception and persistence of tinnitus. When we hear a sound, our brain processes that sound and classifies it as either pleasant, neutral, or threatening. The sound of rain, for example, is pleasant or neutral if it's a gentle rainfall outside one's house, but rain that suddenly pours down in torrents when you're on a hike in the woods would definitely be interpreted by your brain as threatening. You would instinctively perceive it as a warning and immediately seek shelter to protect yourself. And even though light rainfall is usually appreciated and enjoyed, most people would find it very difficult to live in an area where it almost constantly rains. It isn't just the lack of sunlight, it's having to deal with the seemingly never-ending rain that wears them down. Tinnitus evokes the same reaction, in that one feels like there's no escape from it.

One problem with tinnitus is that often there is nothing in the soundscape of our environments that prepares us for its onset. So how does the brain react when a person hears something they shouldn't be hearing, something that they've never heard before? The brain interprets that unknown sound as potentially threatening. This in turn causes the amygdala to initiate a cascade reaction of fight or flight, a state of anxiety. Unless that anxiety is properly and immediately addressed, your brain will continue to classify the sound as threatening. When we feel threatened, our body goes into a state of high alert. All our senses operate at peak performance, especially hearing. In that state of heightened anxiety, we hear the tinnitus even more acutely, leading to greater anxiety and distress. The tinnitus, through no fault of your own, now has an emotional component of fear and/or anxiety added to it and becomes entrenched further in the brain. Anxiety is an extremely powerful emotion that very few people can control through simple willpower. Anxiety can easily intensify if you believe you can't get away from or do anything about the source of your anxiety. For example, post traumatic stress disorder following extreme emotional or physical trauma can manifest as intense anxiety in social settings.

No one knows why some people develop PTSD (post traumatic stress disorder) while others find a way to live with the memories of their trauma, but it is a medically recognized condition that most likely is tied into how the brain is wired. PTSD is a serious condition that requires treatment with compassionate therapy and usually medical intervention. Incidentally, brain imaging studies have shown that people with PTSD have smaller hippocampi, which is highly suggestive of damage to the hippocampus caused by chronic severe stress. This is the part of the brain associated with emotions, forming memories, and learning. Tinnitus is also associated with a decrease of grey matter in the hippocampus. (Like other parts of the brain, you have one hippocampus on each side.)

People who are trying to be helpful sometimes make the suggestion to think of tinnitus as no more of an annoyance than the sound of a refrigerator running in the background. That might be useful advice for someone with mild tinnitus, but for someone with a high-pitched dog whistle sound, or an angry swarm of bees, a siren, or train brakes screeching on rails, it's just not possible to imagine those sounds to be as benign as the distant hum of a refrigerator in the background. It's very important to never belittle or dismiss someone who shows signs of suffering from tinnitus, especially if it's severe. Everyone is wired differently in how they respond to different stressors. It can take a long time to gain emotional control over something that we cannot physically control. If you are experiencing anxiety due to tinnitus, remember that it's a normal reaction stemming from a primitive part of your brain. If your anxiety is seriously interfering with your physical, mental, or emotional health, seek treatment to address the anxiety. Lowering your anxiety through medication (or alternative treatment such as guided meditation), can also help to reduce your perception of tinnitus severity and intrusiveness.

In the beginning, particularly with severe tinnitus, there can be genuine disbelief that this is actually happening, accompanied by a thread of hope that the tinnitus will go away. At this stage, a person might have a fighting attitude, such as, "I'm going to beat this." It's also not unusual for there to be anger, a sense of hopelessness, or even despair at having this affliction. As time goes on and the tinnitus becomes chronic, depression is an extremely common reaction. Many people frequently break down and cry because they feel helpless or trapped; they fear that there is no chance of living a happy or normal life with the constant disturbing sound in their ears and/or head. The impact on one's sense of well-being can be greater for people who value peace and quiet, who have always tried to create surroundings of tranquility. They may feel like they have been cheated of something very precious, something that others seem to take for granted.

One serious aspect of depression is that it's related to a decrease of grey matter by as much as 10% in the hippocampus, part of the limbic system. People with a history of depression seem to be more susceptible to developing tinnitus, just as people with long-term anxiety disorder are at greater risk of developing tinnitus. Since the hippocampus plays an important role in memories and emotions, and because perception of tinnitus severity is related to emotions, it's no wonder that the hippocampus itself would actually show changes corresponding with tinnitus. Professor Poul Videbech is a specialist in psychiatry at Aarhus University Hospital in Denmark. His studies have shown that depression not only affects the regulation of neurotransmitters in the brain, but it also affects the balance between nerve degeneration and neurogenesis. In other words, there is an imbalance between dying neurons and new neurons. The hippocampus seems to be particularly sensitive to this imbalance. I address the relationship between hippocampus decrease and tinnitus in Chapter 55, "Neurogenesis." Even without depression, there is a proven correlation between having tinnitus and a reduction in grey matter of the hippocampus. If you are depressed, be mindful that your emotional health is not only affecting the way you feel, it quite likely is having an adverse effect on the health of your brain as well. Getting help is not a character flaw and it doesn't mean you're weak. Do what you can to lift your spirits, whether it be through medication, meditation, light therapy (phototherapy), or even something as simple as a regular daily walk or other forms of exercise.

Aside from the emotional impact of dealing with anxiety, depression, anger, and grief, tinnitus affects your cognitive health as well. The University of Western Sydney conducted research and concluded that tinnitus affects working memory and concentration. You can think of working memory as the system in your brain that temporarily stores information and utilizes it to perform complex cognitive tasks. For example, when you hear a phone number and then recall it later so you can write it down, that's working memory. Another example is driving, where your brain retrieves information so that you remember the rules of driving and how to handle your particular vehicle. Concentration is the ability to stay focused on a task, such as studying for an exam.

Think about what this means to students who develop tinnitus while in university. Not only are they dealing with all the attendant emotions of being in a more competitive learning institution than they experienced in high school, not only must they deal with the emotions of being separated from family and friends as they navigate the waters of independent living, now they have the additional burden that their entire future is possibly being affected by the sounds in their ears and/or head. Poor concentration and/or memory can lead to inadequate retention of curriculum material, which in turn results in poor performance on exams and can negatively affect their future to a significant degree. In other words, there is a real risk to their eventual earning potential if they are unable to cope with their tinnitus. This is serious business.

Impaired concentration with chronic tinnitus affects the working class as well, whether white collar or blue collar. Anyone whose work demands attention to detail and the ability to retain and retrieve data may find herself at risk of deficient performance. I know from personal experience that tinnitus has significantly affected my ability to concentrate. It's a challenge to retain the research material I read and then try to express it in everyday language. Web designers, software engineers, composers, nurses, physicians, teachers, and welders are just a few examples of people who need to consistently operate at peak mental efficiency in order to do their job well. They are at risk of suffering poor performance caused by the interference of tinnitus.

The University of Western Sydney study also concluded that the more complex the cognitive task, the more likely that chronic tinnitus will have a negative impact. It stands to reason that, likewise, the greater the intensity or intrusiveness of the tinnitus, the more likely it is that someone will experience significant negative effects on their working memory and ability to concentrate. Hopefully, the knowledge that this is a common experience for people with tinnitus will help you to view it as a physical challenge and not a personal flaw. If your job, your school studies, or even your social interactions are being affected by memory impairment or an inability to concentrate, employ mindfulness and pay greater attention to the here and now. Be patient with yourself, just as you would be patient with someone who needs time to heal from an injury.

Tinnitus is not like other chronic and serious health problems, such as diabetes, cancer, congestive heart disease, arthritis, fibromyalgia, Chron's disease, and all the other difficult and potentially life-threatening conditions. It's often hard for people to sympathize with an affliction like tinnitus, because it seems like such an insignificant matter compared to, say, diabetes or Parkinson's disease. Lack of proper sleep over a period of time can cause someone to lose their vibrance, it can challenge their immune system, but that isn't considered by most to be a significant health issue. Tinnitus also has no specific outward signs to indicate degree of severity, and so people may be suspicious of just how serious a person's individual tinnitus condition is. They may view someone who complains of the loudness as being a hypochondriac, or exaggerating their symptoms to get attention. Unless you've experienced it yourself, it's impossible to understand how distressful and nerve-wracking severe tinnitus can be.

When people first get tinnitus, if they're unfamiliar with it, they usually look for a medical solution. One disappointing aspect of tinnitus is that the medical world for the most part doesn't assign a lot of importance to it, certainly not with the same degree of attention that they give to hearing loss. One reason for this is because hearing loss has an array of potential treatments, but treatment options for tinnitus are very limited. Hearing aids can be quite effective at restoring hearing, whereas restoring a normal state of silence to someone with tinnitus is a much greater challenge. There are certainly researchers who are determined to find a treatment that will shut off the sounds of tinnitus, but so far nothing has proven to be effective and safe. It's not unusual for people who have had tinnitus for more than a year to express extreme anger and frustration that medical science keeps advancing with regard to treatment of other conditions, but tinnitus seems to be stuck on a treadmill. It feels like a reflection of a society that simply doesn't take tinnitus seriously. This can lead to feelings of hopelessness and despair, compounding the emotional burden of living with tinnitus.

I sincerely believe that someday medical science will find a way to put an end to the affliction of tinnitus. There is certainly more awareness and urgency now, with so many military personnel returning home with tinnitus, the number one disability amongst veterans. The staggering complexity of the condition makes an actual cure a nearly impossible goal, but we can look forward to the development of a medical solution that will reduce the volume and give people true relief. In the meantime, there are things you can do on a daily basis to protect your mental and emotional health and your physical well-being. Coping techniques, as well as potential helpful treatments, are covered in Sections VII and VIII.

18
TINNITUS SEVERITY QUICK ASSESSMENT

For a simple 1 to 10 scale of rating tinnitus, the following descriptions are a guideline to the degree of severity. It may help to reduce your anxiety if this assessment reveals that your tinnitus is not as severe when compared to others who are further up the scale. However, if you rate your tinnitus at a catastrophic level on a continuous basis, please seek medical attention from an audiologist or otolaryngologist and do not attempt to go it alone. You wouldn't try to walk with a broken leg, and even if you did attempt it, you wouldn't get very far. Likewise, catastrophic tinnitus places too great a burden on your ability to function and sleep, and will take a toll on you emotionally, mentally, and physically.

Reactions to tinnitus are not included in this list, such as whether it causes emotional or mental trauma. I have also not included sleep difficulties as a measure of severity. This guideline is simply to categorize the level at which tinnitus can be heard and its perceived volume. I created this list using measures from online Tinnitus Handicap Inventory questionnaires. I have also factored in the countless descriptions of people who have tinnitus and the level of intrusiveness they assign to its volume in different environments.

Category 0 - No Tinnitus Detected

Categories 1 - 2, Very Mild
1 - borderline presence, must plug ears to hear it
2 - soft presence, detectable only in quiet surroundings by focusing on it

Categories 3 - 4, Mild
3 - can be heard in quiet surroundings without focusing on it; fairly easy to ignore while engaged in activity
4 - can be heard during conversation between two people but not disruptive; barely noticeable while watching television or listening to radio

Categories 5 - 6, Moderate

5 - noticeable in most environments; intrusive in quiet environments, but can be masked by shower, city traffic, or noisy restaurant

6 - almost always aware of its presence; usually a shower is the only place where tinnitus cannot be detected; easier to cope with when attention is focused on conversation, music, a movie, or any activity where ambient sound is present at sufficient volume to distract from the sound of tinnitus

Categories 7 - 9, Severe

7 - always aware of its presence; loud enough to compete with any environmental sounds; interferes with concentration

8 - cannot be masked; interferes with concentration and with sleeping; work and home life are negatively affected

9 - cannot be masked; competes for attention with every sound in the environment; depression and/or anxiety set in; feels like a constant drain on energy

Category 10 - Catastrophic

10 - cannot be masked under any circumstances; loud, discordant, and/or intrusive enough that one seriously considers suicide

The next chapter covers the Tinnitus Handicap Inventory, to help you assess your tinnitus and its impact on your life.

19
TINNITUS HANDICAP INVENTORY

The Tinnitus Handicap Inventory questionnaire is a standardized industry form designed to help you score your tinnitus on a scale from mild to catastrophic. Please answer this questionnaire when you have had enough sleep to feel rested, or when you believe your reaction to your tinnitus is somewhat under control. This will enable you to obtain a more realistic and objective assessment, which will be helpful when considering treatment options. You can download a PDF file of this questionnaire at www.livingwitht.com/thi.

Assign 4 points for each "Yes," 0 points for each "No," and 2 points for each "Sometimes." Use a sheet of paper and write the numbers 1 through 25 down the side of the page. Beside each number, write "Y," "N," or "S" in response to each question. The total points will indicate your tinnitus severity level as described at the end of the Inventory.

You will notice some differences in the descriptions of severity for the Quick Assessment compared to the Handicap Inventory. That's because the Quick Assessment is based more on a layperson's interpretation, whereas the Handicap Inventory was designed to help professionals who treat tinnitus patients. The Starkey Hearing Technologies online blog has an editorial discussing the THI, with additional helpful information regarding outcome and treatment. An easy way to find it is to go online to www.duckduckgo.com and do a search for "Starkey + THI."

It may be helpful for you to take the Inventory every two to three months, to measure how well you're coping or habituating to your tinnitus. (Habituation is discussed in Chapter 28.) I would recommend that you not review the Inventory any more often than that, because you don't want to give too much attention to your tinnitus.

TINNITUS HANDICAP INVENTORY

1. Because of your tinnitus, is it difficult for you to concentrate?
   Yes ____ No ____ Sometimes ____

2. Does the loudness of your tinnitus make it difficult for you to hear people in conversation?
   Yes ___ No ___ Sometimes ___

3. Does your tinnitus make you angry?
   Yes ___ No ___ Sometimes ___

4. Does your tinnitus make you confused?
   Yes ___ No ___ Sometimes ___

5. Because of your tinnitus are you desperate?
   Yes ___ No ___ Sometimes ___

6. Do you complain a great deal about your tinnitus?
   Yes ___ No ___ Sometimes ___

7. Because of your tinnitus do you have trouble falling asleep at night?
   Yes ___ No ___ Sometimes ___

8. Do you feel like you cannot escape from your tinnitus?
   Yes ___ No ___ Sometimes ___

9. Does your tinnitus interfere with your ability to enjoy social activities; for example, going out to dinner or to the movies?
   Yes ___ No ___ Sometimes ___

10. Because of your tinnitus do you feel frustrated?
    Yes ___ No ___ Sometimes ___

11. Because of your tinnitus do you feel that you have a terrible disease?
    Yes ___ No ___ Sometimes ___

12. Does your tinnitus make it difficult to enjoy life?
    Yes ___ No ___ Sometimes ___

13. Does your tinnitus interfere with your job or household responsibilities?
    Yes ___ No ___ Sometimes ___

14. Because of your tinnitus do you find that you are often irritable?
    Yes ___ No ___ Sometimes ___

15. Because of your tinnitus is it difficult for you to read?
    Yes ___ No ___ Sometimes ___

16. Does your tinnitus make you upset?
    Yes ___ No ___ Sometimes ___

17. Do you feel that your tinnitus has placed stress on your relationships with members of your family and friends?
    Yes ___ No ___ Sometimes ___

18. Do you find it difficult to focus your attention away from your tinnitus and onto other things?
    Yes ___ No ___ Sometimes ___

19. Do you feel that you have no control over your tinnitus?
    Yes ___ No ___ Sometimes ___

20. Because of your tinnitus do you often feel tired?
    Yes ___ No ___ Sometimes ___

21. Because of your tinnitus do you feel depressed?
    Yes ___ No ___ Sometimes ___

22. Does your tinnitus make you feel anxious?
    Yes ___ No ___ Sometimes ___

23. Do you feel like you can no longer cope with your tinnitus?
    Yes ___ No ___ Sometimes ___

24. Does your tinnitus get worse when you are under stress?
Yes ___ No ___ Sometimes ___

25. Does your tinnitus make you feel insecure?
Yes ___ No ___ Sometimes ___

SEVERITY GRADE LEVEL

0 - 16 points:
Grade 1 - Slight (only heard in quiet environments)

18 - 36 points:
Grade 2 - Mild (easily masked by environmental sounds and easily forgotten with activities)

38 - 56 points:
Grade 3 - Moderate (noticed in presence of background noise, although daily activities can still be performed)

58 - 76 points:
Grade 4 - Severe (almost always heard, leads to disturbed sleep patterns and can interfere with daily activities)

78 - 100 points:
Grade 5 - Catastrophic (always heard, disturbed sleep patterns, difficulty with any activities)

Reference:
A. McCombe, D. Bagueley, R. Coles, L. McKenna, C. McKinney, and P. Windle-Taylor (2001), Guidelines for the grading of tinnitus severity: the results of a working group commissioned by the British Association of Otolaryngologists, Head and Neck Surgeons, 1999, Clinical Otolaryngology 26, 388-393.

20
THE PAIN OF HYPERACUSIS

Hyperacusis is a condition of intense painful sensitivity or intolerance to everyday sounds. People who develop severe hyperacusis discover that even a soft-spoken voice is unbearable to listen to. The light rustling sound of someone turning the pages of a magazine can be agonizing. This condition may arise on its own from various causes, such as post traumatic stress disorder, depression, or head injury. Because it is typically a disorder of the auditory system, it is more likely to occur in people with tinnitus than the general population. Approximately 25% of people who have tinnitus also have some degree of hyperacusis. Conversely, approximately 85% of people who suffer from hyperacusis also have tinnitus. It is not uncommon for people who have both tinnitus and hyperacusis to say that the hyperacusis is much harder to deal with. Many people with tinnitus develop mild hyperacusis and learn to adapt by avoiding sounds that may cause pain or intense discomfort. For example, they walk away from a microwave oven before it beeps, they make sure to be extremely gentle in handling pots and pans, cutlery and dinnerware, and they avoid places where they know from experience that noise levels will be intolerable. However, for the unfortunate few with severe hyperacusis, the sensitivity to sound is at such an extreme level that being able to live a normal life is almost impossible.

Hyperacusis is not just a temporary reaction to noise that is perceived as too loud. The pain lingers long after the sound stimulus has died away. Imagine walking down the street and suddenly someone nearby slams a car door. Most people might experience a temporary sensation of annoyance but are able to shrug it off as no big deal. Someone with moderate to severe tinnitus may possibly feel some pain, and perhaps accompanied by a rush of anxiety that the slamming car door might set off a spike. But the unlucky person with hyperacusis will certainly feel an immediate sharp stabbing-type pain, and continue to feel a burning type of pain for hours afterward.

For many years scientists were uncertain what was causing hyperacusis. One theory was that the extreme hypersensitivity to sound was possibly psychosomatic, a psychological reaction to anxiety. In the absence of any observable physical trauma or disorder, it seemed that there was no plausible reason for the hyperacusis. Like many ailments that were once dismissed as merely manifestations of neurosis or expressions of hypochondria, it turns out that psychosomatic has nothing to do with it. Most cases of hyperacusis do in fact arise from a physical basis, and its origins are in the cochlea.

Scientists were aware of the presence of mysterious fibers within the cochlea, the sophisticated snail-shaped organ located in the temporal bone of the skull. These fibers resembled pain fibers located elsewhere in the body, but more studies needed to be done to conclusively determine their role. Over the course of 15 years, Jaime García-Añoveros, Ph.D., of the Northwestern University Feinberg School of Medicine in Chicago, Illinois, worked with strains of deaf rats. He discovered that intense noise activated these fibers. Coincidentally, experiments at Johns Hopkins University showed that there are sensory cells within the cochlea that release a chemical when exposed to loud noise. This chemical activates the pain fibers. Hyperacusis develops when these pain fibers fail to shut off and instead remain permanently activated.

Treating mild to moderate hyperacusis is a delicate balancing act. You need to be careful not to shut yourself off from the everyday sounds of life, such as washing dishes or having the television on at a moderate volume. If you avoid any and all noise exposure, you run the risk of making your auditory system even more sensitive or intolerant to everyday sounds. The general consensus seems to be that the best treatment for hyperacusis involves a gradual reintroduction of typical environmental sounds, combined with wearing a sound generator for several hours a day to provide auditory stimulation. The sound generator volume should be set to a comfortable level, whereby one is aware of the generated sound but not irritated by it. If you have tinnitus and hyperacusis, set the volume just below the threshold of your tinnitus. If that's too painful, gradually work up to that level.

Sound therapy can take from six months to two years before the full benefits are reached. It may seem to you that your hyperacusis developed suddenly, but it likely was a long-term process that finally reached a tipping point, similar to the way tinnitus often occurs. It's only natural and to be expected that reducing or eliminating the hyperacusis will take a long time as well.

Using a sound generator to treat hyperacusis doesn't work for everybody, but it has been shown to be successful in some subjects with mild or moderate hyperacusis. If your hyperacusis is severe, it's important to seek professional help. There may be a physiological disorder, for example, a recent physical trauma to the head or neck. Similar to tinnitus, stress can heighten the perceived effects of hyperacusis. Your healthcare provider might recommend a short-term medication for anxiety. This will help you to cope with the mental and emotional distress that often accompanies hyperacusis. When you feel better emotionally, it increases your motivation to stick with a long-term treatment regimen.

If you have a friend or family member with hyperacusis, it's important to understand that this is not a psychological condition where they're looking for attention or being emotionally dramatic. The plain truth is that this condition hurts, and it hurts a lot. It isn't necessary to walk on eggshells when you're around someone with hyperacusis, just be mindful of their sensitivity. If you have barking dogs, train them to bark only when someone is at the door. A dog's bark can feel like needles piercing the eardrum, particularly the high-pitched yappers. Keep your speaking voice at a moderate level. The television or radio volume should be set to their comfort level if possible. A nice gesture would be to give them a tabletop fountain, as gentle water sounds seem to be the most soothing to an overreactive auditory system. Be understanding when they don't want to go to cafes or restaurants that have loud background music or poor acoustics that amplify conversations and laughter. Don't take it personally if they avoid get-togethers that they once enjoyed attending. In time, they may gradually become more tolerant of sound and will be able to socialize more often. Until then, do what you can to ensure they aren't exposed to sudden loud noises, but otherwise carry on with normal life as much as possible.

To learn more about the devastating effects of hyperacusis, please read the article, "When even soft noises feel like a knife to the eardrums," on www.statnews.com. It's the story of Tom Maholchic, a young man who has suffered for years from severe hyperacusis. His condition is beginning to improve slightly, but it's still debilitating enough that it basically controls his life. The article also provides some insight into the causes of hyperacusis and what medical researchers are doing to better understand this baffling condition.

The American Tinnitus Association recommends undergoing a Loudness Discomfort Level (LDL) test if you suspect or know that you are developing or already have hyperacusis. LDL refers to the level at which sound results in discomfort or pain, and is useful for gauging severity of tinnitus and/or hyperacusis. This test needs to be administered by a hearing health professional.

The Tinnitus Talk online forum has a subforum on Hyperacusis and Ear Pain. They share their experiences, keep up with research, and discuss the latest developments. If you have hyperacusis, I highly recommend that you visit the forum and read some of the threads. Please don't hesitate to reach out for help if you're suffering. The link is www.tinnitustalk.com/forums/support.55/.

The Hyperacusis Network, at www.hyperacusis.net, is a website dedicated to hyperacusis and other sound sensitivities and disorders. Among these are recruitment, which is sensitivity to sounds within the pitch range of one's hearing loss. It is thought to be caused by the still functioning hair cells being "recruited" to handle incoming sound, but because of the proximity to damaged hair cells, the sound is perceived as much louder. Another condition is misophonia, best described as hatred or strong aversion to certain sounds. The problem with misophonia isn't the volume of the sound, it's the very nature of the sound itself. The hatred can be so intense that someone who suffers from misophonia may become instantly enraged upon hearing that sound. A common trigger for misophonia is hearing someone chewing, or the crinkling sound of a bag of snacks. An extreme degree of misophonia is phonophobia, a fear of sound itself. The level of anxiety is just as severe as for someone who has acrophobia, a fear of heights. The difference is that sound is everywhere; thus, phonophobia can lead to extreme isolation and requires professional help from specially trained clinicians.

❖

Section VI discusses the brain and its relationship to the auditory system, as well as the critical role of neurotransmitters and how they relate to the generation and perception of tinnitus.

SECTION VI

YOUR BRAIN AND AUDITORY SYSTEM

21
MEET YOUR NEUROTRANSMITTERS

As mentioned in the prior chapter, "Blame the Brain," scientists have determined that tinnitus is a malfunction of the brain, often operating in tandem with nerve cell damage within the ear. To get a better understanding of what could be going wrong in your brain, it's helpful to cover the basics of neurons (nerve cells), how they function, and what can impair their performance. Depending on the severity of your tinnitus and your ability to cope with it, your healthcare provider may recommend a temporary course of prescription drugs. Neurotransmitters are often the target of prescription drugs used to treat tinnitus. Understanding the role of neurotransmitters will help you to be more proactive in your treatment regimen. It will help you to be aware of what is happening in your brain and your body when neurotransmitters are under the influence of certain medications.

Your body and brain are communication highways, constantly sending messages back and forth to be received, interpreted, and acted upon. The communication signals travel from neuron to neuron. The gap between the neurons is a synapse. Think of synapses as invisible bridges that communication signals must cross over to keep the message moving onward to its intended destination. Sometimes these signals can be suppressed too much along the way. They can also be increased too much. If the signals are suppressed, then they are *inhibited*. If the signals are increased, they are *excited*.

Neurotransmitters are chemicals that enable the signals to travel across the synapses in a healthy manner. Inhibitory neurotransmitters create a sense of relaxation, and calm the brain. Excitatory neurotransmitters stimulate the brain. When the level of one or more neurotransmitters is out of balance, particularly for a sustained period of time, it can result in a disturbance in functions of the brain and/or body. The relationship between the brain and the body is intricately intertwined. This is why a problem which begins in the ears can end up being a problem in the brain. Neurotransmitters play a major role in this complex relationship. There are over 200 neurotransmitters in the brain, but only a few of them are thought to have a strong influence on tinnitus. Among these are GABA (gamma-aminobutyric acid), dopamine, serotonin, and glutamate.

There are also neurotransmitters that contribute to making changes in the brain that relate to the perception of tinnitus. Acetylcholine and norepinephrine are two that are thought to be significant in helping to make those changes, but the research is in the early stage. For now, let's focus on the neurotransmitters that have received a lot more attention for their role in the development and experience of tinnitus.

GABA is the most abundant neurotransmitter in the brain. It is the major inhibitory and relaxing neurotransmitter. When GABA levels are normal, there is a reduction in stress, anxiety, and nervousness. GABA decreases beta brain waves, the brain waves associated with high alertness, fear, and tension. It increases alpha brain waves, which are most active when you're in a state of relaxation. GABA blocks the nerve impulses associated with anxiety from reaching the motor centers of the brain. It does this by attaching to specific receptors in the brain, the same receptors that are targeted and affected by benzodiazepine drugs. Benzodiazepines, nicknamed "benzos," are drugs that work on the central nervous system. They are typically prescribed for anxiety. One of the best-known benzos is Xanax, which is sometimes prescribed to ease the anxiety that accompanies the onset of tinnitus.

The importance of sufficient GABA has been demonstrated by studies measuring the neurochemistry levels in the brain. Measurements of GABA levels reveal that the presence as well as the severity of tinnitus correlates with a significant reduction of GABA in the auditory cortex. As an inhibitory neurotransmitter, GABA also appears to protect the cochlea from excitotoxicity. Another benefit is that it helps to reduce the stiffness and increase the motility of the inner hair cells. **A decrease in GABA therefore represents a reduction in the protection of hair cells**, making them more susceptible to the influence of excitatory neurotransmitters such as glutamate, a known culprit in hair cell damage.

Over-the-counter GABA supplements are a popular sleep aid. While it's true that these supplements do not cross the blood-brain barrier, they are still effective for many people to induce relaxation and ease the anxiety that often accompanies insomnia. GABA supplements are relatively inexpensive. Although they have been sold over the counter for years and appear to be safe, there is only limited information about possible interactions with other supplements or drugs. Pregnant and breastfeeding women are advised not to take GABA supplements.

Dopamine is a neurotransmitter that helps to monitor metabolism. It's often referred to as the "feel good" chemical. It controls our energy, contributes to our sense of excitement about new ideas, and ramps up our motivation when tackling a project which we are passionate about. It also supports brain and heart health. The neurons which create dopamine are located in the substantia nigra of the midbrain, and other dopamine neurons are located in the ventral tegmental area (VTA), which is also situated in the midbrain. The VTA is part of the reward circuitry of the brain, and plays a critical role in motivation, addiction, and how one experiences intense emotions associated with love. Too much dopamine can create a manic state, whereas too little dopamine can cause a person to become depressed or apathetic. Although dopamine is generated from limited areas of the brain, dopamine receptors are widely distributed throughout the brain. In the frontal cortex, dopamine is involved in executive functions like attention. It's not unusual for someone with tinnitus to also have a low level of dopamine. It's no wonder that people with tinnitus complain of difficulty concentrating. It's not just the phantom sound that's interfering with their focus; the depleted dopamine is also a factor.

Tinnitus often causes depression, which in turn can cause one to focus obsessively on their tinnitus. There is speculation that increasing dopamine levels is one way to lessen the perception of tinnitus. Unfortunately, excessive tampering with dopamine supplementation can result in long-term alteration of the body's natural dopamine regulation. This can lead to pleasurable events feeling less pleasurable, and unpleasant events having less emotional impact than would be experienced by someone with a healthy dopamine system. Apathy is the loss of emotional highs and lows, to the point of not caring about anything at all. That's a fairly accurate way of describing a dysfunctional dopamine system. On the other hand, for someone who has a medical condition that is tied to persistent low dopamine levels, ADHD for example, studies have shown that drugs which increase dopamine levels can be helpful both short-term and long-term. However, the research is inconclusive on how much to tamper with supplementation, and for how long.

Just as dopamine is called the "feel good" chemical, alpha waves are known as the "feel good" brain waves. Low dopamine levels are linked to sub-normal alpha brain wave activity. People who perceive their tinnitus as loud or severe have been shown to have abnormally low alpha brain wave activity. As an alternative to taking prescription medications, an excellent way to naturally increase your dopamine levels is through exercise. Many people with tinnitus report that they feel better after exercise, whether it be riding a bike, running a few miles, or a session at the gym. Another method to naturally increase your dopamine level is to practice mindfulness meditation. Exercise and meditation enhance alpha wave activity, which in turn releases dopamine, serotonin, and endorphins in the body. Unless you are in a critical state of depression requiring professional intervention, try alternative remedies first to see if naturally raising your dopamine level and/or your alpha brain waves helps you to cope with tinnitus or lessen its intrusiveness. If your healthcare practitioner recommends raising your dopamine levels with medication, be sure to ask about long-term effects and how that medication might affect your tinnitus.

The neurotransmitter serotonin is an inhibitory neurotransmitter. Serotonin helps to keep your mood stable and is responsible for balancing the excitatory neurotransmitters. Serotonin is manufactured in the brain, but 90% of our body's serotonin supply is in the digestive tract and blood platelets.

Most people have heard of SSRIs, selective serotonin re-uptake inhibitors. These are antidepressants which block receptors in the brain from reabsorbing serotonin. This means there is more serotonin available to communicate between brain cells. More serotonin promotes relaxation and a calmer mood. If you're always on edge or feeling anxious, there's a chance your serotonin level is too low and so it's affecting your sense of well-being. Because anxiety is a factor in tinnitus perception, it's important to do what you can to keep a calm mood when you have tinnitus. This will help you to not engage in catastrophic thinking, an anxiety disorder in which your thoughts become fixated on worst-case scenarios. Two examples of catastrophic thinking are, "My life is ruined by tinnitus," and, "I can't live like this." It's perfectly natural to feel despondent in the initial weeks of dealing with intrusive tinnitus, but if those thoughts continue or you're thinking of harming yourself, you should seek professional help. It isn't a character deficiency to look for assistance if you feel defeated when you're confronted day after day with loud tinnitus. Chronic stress can be responsible for depleting serotonin levels, and it's very possible that a lack of sufficient serotonin is one reason you can't envision living a happy life despite having tinnitus. In other words, it's a vicious cycle that needs to be broken in order for you to move forward and deal realistically with the condition of tinnitus.

If you want to increase your serotonin level without resorting to prescription medications, you can first try getting more sunlight. People who are depressed are often told, "Get out and walk, you'll feel better." It isn't just the exercise that's helping, it's the exposure to sunlight, a natural way of promoting the release of serotonin. One study at the Center for Addiction and Health at the University of Toronto has shown that sunlight is responsible for the control of serotonin transporters. These are proteins that block nerves from receiving serotonin. The less sunlight a person receives, the more likely they are to have a higher level of serotonin transporters in the brain, and therefore less available serotonin for emotional health. Natural sunlight boosts serotonin in your brain, but light therapy can also help. Light therapy involves basking in a specific spectrum of artificial light for a certain amount of time each day. WebMD has a good explanation about light therapy and its benefits, at www.webmd.com/a-to-z-guides/light-therapy. More info on how to use light therapy is covered in Chapter 35, "Methods for Better Sleep."

Maintaining a healthy level of serotonin helps to prevent hardening of the arteries. It also helps to combat the effects of cortisol, otherwise known as the stress hormone. If you begin to exercise regularly, you'll gain the benefit of a healthier body, an uplifted mood, and hopefully a noticeable improvement in your tinnitus.

Glutamate, also called l-glutamate, is the major excitatory neurotransmitter in the central nervous system, accounting for approximately 40% of nerve signals in the brain. Glutamate is extremely important for its function in synaptic transmissions, but it also plays a role in brain plasticity and higher cognitive functions. The problem with glutamate is that there can be too much of a good thing. When glutamate levels exceed the body's ability to properly handle them, nerve cell damage and death can result. For example, when acoustic trauma occurs, the hair cells in the cochlea become stressed and release excessive glutamate. Without sufficient inhibitory neurotransmitters like GABA to counteract this excess, both the outer hair cells and inner hair cells of the cochlea are at risk of being damaged or destroyed. This in turn leads to faulty transmission of nerve impulses to the auditory cortex, with the end result being hearing loss and possibly tinnitus as well. Ototoxic drugs can also stress the hair cells, causing excess glutamate to be released.

When glutamate levels rise above the body's ability to handle them, then the glutamate is no longer simply an excitatory neurotransmitter. It has become an *excitotoxin*, meaning it is toxic to nerve cells. A nerve cell in a hyperexcited state fires uncontrollably. In very simple terms, glutamate excitotoxicity allows too many calcium ions to enter nerve cells, triggering an enzymatic reaction that causes destruction of cell structures. The brain cells in the hypothalamus are particularly sensitive to excitotoxicity. The hypothalamus is the part of the limbic system which receives signals from the amygdala and initiates the fight-or-flight response. Another important role of the hypothalamus is controlling the pituitary gland, which in turn helps to regulate the adrenal glands. When the adrenal glands are not functioning in a healthy manner, when they become either overactive or underactive, then the body's ability to handle stress is diminished. As mentioned earlier, stress has been identified as possibly a cause and most likely a contributor to both the onset and persistence of tinnitus. To make matters worse, chronic stress contributes to increased levels of cortisol, which in turn promotes the release of excess glutamate in the limbic and cortical regions of the brain, thereby increasing the risk of excitotoxicity.

You may be wondering if there's anything you can do about glutamate excess and its relationship to tinnitus, since glutamate is naturally produced by the body. Although you might not realize it, you could be unintentionally increasing glutamate in your system simply by ingesting certain foods and drinks. More than likely you are familiar with MSG, monosodium glutamate, which is used as a flavor enhancer in almost every processed food on your grocer's shelves. MSG, which is nothing more than the sodium salt of glutamic acid, was discovered by a Japanese biochemist who was seeking to replicate the flavor of kombu, an edible seaweed. Once the flavor-enhancing properties of MSG were revealed, food manufacturers rushed to add it to their products, and now it seems to be added to almost every processed food, despite its well-known excitotoxic properties. MSG does not cross the blood-brain barrier, but it has been shown to penetrate brain regions not protected by the barrier, in particular the hypothalamus. Monosodium glutamate therefore has the potential to negatively affect the functioning of the adrenal glands.

There is controversy surrounding just how safe the addition of MSG is in our food supply. The U.S. Food and Drug Administration has classified it as Generally Recognized As Safe (GRAS), and the European Union classifies it as a permissible food additive up to a certain limit. Many consumers and consumer advocacy groups have voiced strong opposition to its use as a food ingredient. There are countless websites decrying the effects of MSG. They link its consumption to everything from the rise in asthma deaths (which the FDA admits that asthmatics are more sensitive to MSG), to the increased incidence of bipolar disorder in the general population following the addition of MSG to the food supply. To support the bipolar disorder connection, they point out that Lamictal, a glutamate blocker, is used in the treatment of manic depression.

The interesting thing about MSG is that we have receptors on our tongue for glutamate. In other words, our taste buds not only detect sweet, sour, salty, and bitter, they also detect umami. Umami means "pleasant savory taste," and is used to describe the specific taste imparted by glutamate. Many of our foods contain a natural amount of glutamate, such as chicken, peas, walnuts, tomatoes, corn, and mushrooms, to name just a few. The difference is that monosodium glutamate is "free" glutamic acid, whereas glutamate in food is mostly "bound" glutamic acid. (One notable exception is cheese, which technically is a processed food, and contains high amounts of "free" glutamate.) Our bodies were designed to absorb and utilize the glutamic acid found in food, thereby helping to keep a proper balance between glutamate and GABA. I believe that ingesting excess glutamate in the form of MSG, simply for the sake of fooling our taste buds, is not healthy. It leads to unnatural cravings for processed foods, and may well tip the scales to excitotoxicity. With tinnitus, you need to do everything you can to maintain a healthy brain and be vigilant to prevent further damage to your hair cells. It's better to err on the side of caution and avoid MSG whenever possible.

Russell L. Blaylock, M.D., a board-certified neurosurgeon, is the author of the book, *Excitotoxins: The Taste That Kills*. It covers the subject of MSG and other excitotoxins in our food supply, including aspartame, cysteine, and hydrolyzed protein. If you're interested in exploring this subject further, the book appears to be out of print, but used copies can still be found online. You can also watch his presentation on YouTube, "Dr. Russell Blaylock: Excitotoxins - The Taste That Kills."

Now that you have a better understanding of how important neurotransmitters are in tinnitus, let's take a look at one of the biological wonders of the world: the human ear.

22
HOW WE HEAR SOUND

Until something goes wrong, we usually don't give our ability to hear and our enjoyment of silence a lot of thought. Most of us take for granted that we'll be able to focus on what we want to hear, such as conversation with friends and family, the songs of birds in springtime, the gentle tapping of rain against the window, and the soothing sound of wind in the trees. We learn to accept that our ability to hear higher frequencies will gradually diminish with age, but it's a shock when what we hear is suddenly cut through with a loud high-pitched tone, a constant buzzing, a sizzling, a roaring, a whooshing, a hissing, or any number of the strange sounds of tinnitus.

Tinnitus is most often caused by noise exposure, so it's important to understand the process of hearing and how our auditory system can become damaged. When you understand the most likely cause of damage, it's possible to prevent further harm. Even if your tinnitus is associated with presbycusis, the medical term for age-related hearing loss, it makes sense to do everything you can to give your ears proper care and protection.

I remember being fascinated by drawings of the human ear when I was in school. The ear isn't a solo organ like the heart or dual organs like the lungs. The ear is comprised of the outer ear, a middle ear, and an inner ear, an increasingly complicated network of interrelated parts designed for the crucial task of helping us navigate in the world. The outer ear, also known as the pinna, is made of ridged cartilage covered with skin. It collects sound waves and directs them into the ear canal. The ear canal ends at the tympanic membrane, commonly known as the eardrum, which is connected to tiny bones in the middle ear. These tiny bones are the ossicles, usually referred to as the hammer, anvil, and stirrup. When sound waves hit the eardrum, it causes the eardrum and those tiny bones to vibrate. The vibrations are conducted to the cochlea, the snail-shaped organ located in the inner ear. The cochlea's job is to transform sound into nerve impulses that travel to the brain. In other words, the inner ear is where the serious job of collecting sound begins for further processing by the brain.

Our auditory system features an incredible level of sophisticated biological engineering. Within the cochlea is the organ of Corti, a structure which contains the 16,000 to 20,000 hair cells essential to our sense of hearing. The hair cells are sensory cells which resemble stiff standing hairs; thus their name. The organ of Corti is situated on the basilar membrane, which follows the spiral of the cochlea. When the energy of an incoming sound wave is strong enough, the hair cells move and send raw data in the form of electrical impulses to the auditory cortex. The auditory cortex is the final destination in the auditory system communication highway. It interprets the raw data as a particular sound, as well as the volume of that sound, so you'll know the difference between a bird singing and a police siren wailing. When hair cells are damaged or dead, they are no longer capable of sending useful data. This may result in hearing loss, tinnitus, or both.

Hair cells are as sensitive as they are complex. They can be temporarily or permanently damaged by various things that happen to us in life, such as acoustic trauma, infection, fever, ototoxic medications, and of course the aging process. Constant loud noise can literally flatten hair cells to where they no longer function properly. Think of someone walking across grass. The blades of grass will flatten, and then slowly spring back up. However, if someone walks on those blades of grass over and over, eventually they weaken and die. We can plant seeds in a damaged lawn and grow new grass, but human hair cells cannot be replaced. This is why it's so critical to convince people who still have good hearing and no tinnitus to protect themselves from either sustained or extreme noise that the human auditory system isn't designed to tolerate. If hearing loss or tinnitus has already occurred, it's just as important to avoid further exposure to loud sounds.

Adult birds and amphibians are able to regenerate their hair cells. Humans and all other mammals are unable to do so, but researchers continue to look for a way. Scientists have been able to regenerate hair cells in laboratory mice with growth-promoting molecules, but we're still a long way from being able to do the same in humans. In 2013, in a breakthrough in hearing research, scientists stimulated resident cells in an adult mouse to become new hair cells. The experiments were conducted on an adult mouse with noise-induced hearing loss. There will be countless more studies and clinical trials done before the procedure can be proven to be safe, effective, and widely available for humans, but it does offer hope to those who have hearing loss and/or tinnitus. It takes many years for medical science to travel from a theoretical treatment to actually seeing it arrive on the market and be available to patients in need. In this respect, time is on the side of younger age groups.

The next chapter covers the amygdala and the limbic system, with emphasis on their roles in both the perception and persistence of tinnitus.

23
THE AMYGDALA AND LIMBIC SYSTEM

You're likely familiar with the phrase, "fight or flight." That's our survival instinct, fueled by adrenalin, that tells us to stay where we are and fight against danger, or run away if we believe we don't have the strength or the resources to overcome whatever we perceive is trying to harm us. But what initiates that fight or flight response?

It actually begins in a small almond-shaped organ called the amygdala, which is important to how we process the emotion of fear. You have one amygdala in each hemisphere of your brain. The amygdala reacts without thinking, as its primary responsibility is to protect you from danger. When a dangerous stimulus arises in your environment, information about that stimulus is instantly sent to the amygdala, whereupon the amygdala immediately transmits signals to the hypothalamus, which in turn triggers the fight or flight response. As mentioned previously, the hypothalamus is particularly sensitive to excitotoxicity. Perhaps hyperexcited neurons in the hypothalamus contribute to an increased perception of the tinnitus signal.

The fight-or-flight response is automatic, it's out of your control, and it doesn't stop to think whether the danger is real or imaginary. You have the same physical reaction in either instance. When someone silently approaches you from behind, grabs you and yells "Boo!," your body reacts as if an actual danger existed. When you're driving and an oncoming car suddenly veers into your lane, your body reacts to that very real danger. You're startled, your heart rate goes up, and you breathe faster, trying to take in more oxygen. You're instantly on high alert so you can execute whatever maneuvers are necessary to get out of the path of the oncoming car. This chain of events taking place in your brain is intended to protect us, because in primitive days, it likely wasn't a person sneaking up to grab us and shout "Boo!" Instead, it may very well may have been a tiger that would leap out from the brush and roar, prompting most of us to flee for our lives, except for the unfortunate few who experience temporary paralysis in the face of extreme danger.

The amygdala has another interesting feature. In addition to transmitting fight-or-flight signals to the hypothalamus, it's also responsible for aggression. Have you ever noticed that when some people feel threatened, they also become extremely angry and hostile? That's their amygdala taking over.

The amygdala is an emotional center and thus incapable of being swayed by the cerebral cortex of the brain, which is the seat of complex thought. Why is this important if you have tinnitus? Recent clinical studies are pointing to an intriguing connection between the role of the amygdala and the level of distress that people experience with their tinnitus, independent of perceived volume. The researchers discovered that those who experienced more distress from their tinnitus also engaged their amygdala more when processing emotional sounds. Those who claimed a lower level of distress from their tinnitus were more likely to rely upon the executive processing region of their brain, the cerebral cortex. They were either naturally inclined or had somehow adapted and found a way to react to their tinnitus by diminishing their emotional involvement with it. Over time, their reaction to tinnitus became less dependent on using the amygdala pathway and instead used the pathway of the frontal lobe, located in the cerebral cortex. Researchers theorize that actively engaging the frontal lobe is helpful in controlling the processing and expression of emotions. Allowing the frontal lobe to handle strong emotions could therefore change how one responds to tinnitus and thereby reduce the distress.

One ironic component regarding this altered pathway is that extroverts and risk-takers have a more active limbic system, but research indicates that introverts are more likely to be negatively affected by their tinnitus. What's interesting about this is that a 2012 study at Harvard University revealed that introverts tend to have more grey matter in their prefrontal cortex. Despite that seeming advantage, it appears that introverts tend to react to their tinnitus in an emotional manner via the limbic system. It would be far better if they could find a way to rely instead upon the executive functions of the prefrontal cortex to help them cope, rather than allowing the limbic system to gain the upper hand with an emotional response. As mentioned before, though, it's a matter of how we're wired that tends to determine the primary basis of our response to stressors, including tinnitus.

There is another very important reason why the amygdala has such a grip on our tinnitus. The limbic system has a powerful role in how we form memories. **The limbic system integrates our emotional states with our stored memories of physical sensations.** Tinnitus is a phantom sound, but we perceive it to be real and we usually react both physically and emotionally as if it were. The critical first reaction to tinnitus can set the stage for a cascade of negative effects to follow. If we panic, if we experience anxiety attacks, if we become depressed, angry, frustrated, any number of strong emotional responses can create a corresponding physical reaction. Even though we don't intend for it to happen and certainly don't *want* it to happen, if we react with strong and basically negative emotions, it only serves to lock the experience of tinnitus more firmly within the limbic system and dig deeper grooves in the amygdala pathway.

Incidentally, the amygdala is increasingly being shown not only to be the "fear center" of the brain, it's also linked to generating anxiety. That's a double whammy for people with both tinnitus and anxiety problems. It may also help to explain why people who have experienced anxiety issues for most of their lives, or for an extended period of time, appear to be more susceptible to developing idiopathic tinnitus.

As hard as it may be to understand, it's important to accept that loudness of tinnitus is not a factor in one's level of emotional distress. What matters is your reaction. That seems like a ridiculous thing to say, doesn't it? It's very difficult to believe that loudness isn't a factor when you have something blaring in your head or in your ears. I don't blame anyone for digging in their heels and saying, "It's so loud, of course I'm upset!" That's exactly what I did. And whenever I had a rare mild day and wasn't bothered by my tinnitus, it only served to prove me right, at least in my way of thinking. But carefully designed studies and extensive research have shown that loudness simply is not a factor in the level of emotional distress. The sooner you can accept that as true, no matter how counter-intuitive or illogical it seems, the sooner you can free yourself from the tyranny of your tinnitus.

Don't be hard on yourself if it takes a while; it took me almost two years to accept it, and I still struggle with the concept. For now, your amygdala is interfering with your ability to cope with tinnitus. Does this mean that you're overemotional or hysterical if you're distressed by tinnitus? No, it doesn't, because neither you nor anyone else has control over their limbic system. It processes things automatically, and has been doing a pretty good job at keeping you safe when danger arises. Unfortunately, it seems to be stuck on believing that you're in danger from the sound of your tinnitus, so it continues to transmit warning signals to your brain. The brain responds by keeping your auditory system on high alert.

We are genetically programmed for higher hearing sensitivity when in danger. It's been passed down from our primitive ancestors who needed to hear every soft footstep, the tiniest crackling of a twig, anything that would alert them to the presence of a predator when they were away from safe shelter. Dr. William Sedley of the Institute of Neuroscience at Newcastle has theorized that this high alert stage stays on and becomes entrenched because it accesses a wide network in the brain. As long as the limbic system is in control, you will perceive your tinnitus as being louder because the brain is turning up the gain. It can take time to reduce the influence of the limbic system, particularly if you're an emotionally reactive or sensitive person, but it's a critical step in lessening the perception of tinnitus loudness.

You may not feel like you have control now, but it is possible to gain control. With time and effort, you can gradually bypass the amygdala's influence. Chapter 65, "Train the Brain - Exercises," covers in more detail what you can do to positively affect the tinnitus reaction pathway.

The next chapter discusses what research has revealed regarding how the brain creates tinnitus.

24
THE BRAIN CREATES TINNITUS

No one really understands the aberration of tinnitus. Scientists continue to offer theories as to why the brain generates these annoying phantom sounds. These theories include the most basic explanation that acoustic trauma results in damage or death of hair cells, which in turn disrupts nerve impulses going to the auditory cortex. There are also evolving theories about maladaptive brain plasticity, whereby hyperactive neurons become a permanent rather than a temporary state. Brain plasticity, also referred to as neuroplasticity, refers to neural connections changing their structure or function either in response to a new experience and/or to adapt to loss of function. There is plenty of evidence which points to cochlear damage having negative repercussions throughout the auditory system, including neurochemical and physiological changes. To make matters worse, these negative effects are thought to extend beyond the auditory system and into other brain regions. This was clearly demonstrated when a unique patient allowed doctors to map his brain.

A 50-year-old man with epilepsy had electrodes implanted in the left hemisphere of his brain two weeks ahead of surgery intended to eliminate the source of his seizures. In an experiment conducted by Dr. William Sedley, this courageous patient gave permission to Dr. Sedley and his colleagues to implant 164 electrodes across the left hemisphere of his brain. Over a period of two weeks, the researchers tracked neural activity while the patient listened to white noise. Studies have shown that when many neurons are firing in synchrony, it creates specific oscillations in brain waves. The presence of those oscillations is an indicator of tinnitus. The mapping in the Sedley study revealed that the tinnitus signals were not limited to the auditory cortex; rather, they were found throughout much of the brain that was being sampled with the electrodes. There was heightened brain activity not only in the primary auditory cortex, which was expected, but also in the areas of the brain associated with memory, emotions, and attention. The website www.sciencedaily.com has published an article about this experiment, "In search of tinnitus, that phantom ringing in the ears." Their mapping illustration clearly shows the remarkable extent to which the tinnitus signals penetrated other regions of the brain.

This was a unique experiment, and it's unknown whether tinnitus signals are generated in a similar pattern throughout the brain in everyone with tinnitus. It's also unclear whether the widespread distribution of tinnitus signals is something which develops over a long period of time, that is, when tinnitus is considered chronic, or whether this distribution is specific to someone who has both epilepsy and tinnitus. Implanting electrodes in the brain is an invasive procedure which carries significant risks. It would be unethical to perform this mapping experiment on people with varying degrees of tinnitus severity in order to draw any evidence-based conclusions. However, the pervasive nature of tinnitus signaling within the brain may be one reason why people hear tinnitus in different areas of their head, and that sometimes the perception of where the sound is coming from actually moves around inside the head.

What I have learned from reading countless online articles and research abstracts is that the hippocampus plays a major role in tinnitus. Many studies point to a significant reduction in hippocampal volume that is linked to tinnitus. This same volume reduction can be seen in response to traumatic situations, depression, and anxiety. Traumatic situations are based on individual personality and background, and so what one person perceives as traumatic may be brushed off as insignificant by another. An event which might cause one person years of emotional turmoil may affect someone else to a much lesser degree. It's possible that our individual reactions to stress are coded into our genes, and then either reinforced or modified by our surrounding environment as we grow from infancy to adulthood. As noted in Chapter 12, "Why Me," a predisposition to anxiety appears to increase the odds of acquiring tinnitus. If that anxiety is contributing to a decrease in hippocampal volume, it might be setting the stage for tinnitus.

What does research tell us about what's causing this reduction in hippocampal volume? One significant study points to the excessive secretion of cortisol when a person undergoes long-term stress. The hippocampus is the major site of neurogenesis in the brain. That's where most of our new neurons are born, so to speak. You will recall that neurons are nerve cells that transmit messages between the brain and body. When high cortisol levels are sustained for a long period of time, neurogenesis decreases. Without new neurons to replenish dead or damaged nerve cells, the hippocampus loses volume. Less volume means less function and possibly impaired function. A shrinking hippocampus is a classic marker of Alzheimer's. Because the hippocampus is in effect the GPS of the brain, a severe loss of hippocampal function can result in a sense of disorientation, even in a familiar landscape. One of the first signs of Alzheimer's is a decreasing ability to navigate in what was once a well-known and recognized area.

Scientists are also looking at the cerebellum and its role in how tinnitus is perceived. Richard Salvi of the University of Buffalo has conducted studies on tinnitus and its relationship with various parts of the brain. He and his team have studied the network of tinnitus within structures of the brain. Like many other researchers, they identified involvement of the amygdala and hippocampus, but were surprised to discover that the cerebellum may also play a role. The cerebellum is not considered part of the emotional or auditory systems. Instead, it's responsible for letting us know where a part of our body is in space and time. It's the motor planning part of the brain that helps you pick up a glass of water from the table, or catch a ball that someone tosses your way. Initial speculation is that the cerebellum might be the gateway to perception of tinnitus. In other words, something has gone wrong and, instead of blocking the tinnitus signals, the cerebellum fails to stop them and so a person hears the phantom sounds.

Another theory why the brain fails to block the perception of tinnitus is based on evidence that damaged cochlear hair cells become hyperactive as they try to fill in the missing frequencies. This hyperactivity is thought to be responsible for the phantom noise of tinnitus. There is a feedback loop between the limbic system and the thalamus, which regulates sensory information. One of the jobs of this feedback loop is to suppress the phantom noise before it reaches the cerebral cortex. The cerebral cortex is where we experience consciousness of our senses. Somehow the feedback loop fails to suppress the phantom noise and it continues to the cerebral cortex. At that point the phantom sound is experienced as an actual sound to the person with tinnitus. Incidentally, phantom limb pain, which is experienced by 70 to 80% of amputees, is also created by thalamic dysfunction. Phantom limb pain is very real to the person who experiences it, despite the fact that the amputated limb no longer exists. However, the imprint of the limb continues to exist in the brain and the thalamus fails to stop the pain signals, just as it fails to stop the phantom sounds of tinnitus.

It's encouraging that medical science is getting closer to a definitive answer as to what causes or contributes to tinnitus, but as you can see, it's a very complex relationship between the auditory system and various regions of the brain. When you factor in the role of neurotransmitters, neurogenesis, diet, family history, emotional and mental health, stress level, and quite possibly other factors still yet unknown, you can see why this is such a vexing condition that as yet has no cure. And even with the knowledge available, it still doesn't address why people hear such an incredible variety of sounds, or why some people have mild tinnitus and others experience excruciatingly severe tinnitus. No one yet knows why tinnitus volume follows an ebb and flow pattern in some people, whereas in others it's a constant never-changing volume. In the meantime, now that you know the significant role of your brain in creating and perpetuating tinnitus, it's important that you do whatever you can to achieve emotional well-being and to nourish your brain. Section VII, "Coping Techniques," and "Section VIII, "Treatments," address those issues in depth.

25
THE BASICS OF BRAIN WAVES

Brain waves are the measurable patterns of electrical impulses generated by neural activity in the brain. EEGs (electroencephalograms) can precisely measure the activity of your brain by monitoring its brain waves. By learning about brain wave activity, it will help you to understand how tinnitus affects the brain, which in turn affects your moods, your sleep patterns, and even your ability to think and concentrate.

There are five major patterns of brain wave activity. Theta and delta are the brain waves during sleep, and are pretty much out of our control. Gamma, beta, and alpha are the dominant brain waves while we're conscious and awake. They can change depending on our state of alertness and level of activity. There is also a sixth brain wave pattern, known as mu, which has similar patterns to the alpha waves but is located in another part of the brain. Mu brain waves are of particular interest to scientists who study autism spectrum disorder.

Brain waves are measured in terms of amplitude and frequency. Think of amplitude as waves with peaks and valleys. The greater the amplitude, the higher the peaks will be and the lower the valleys. Frequency, expressed as hertz (cycles per second), is a measurement of how many times per second each wave will peak. Sound is also measured in amplitude and frequency, with frequency being the more important factor. As frequency increases, pitch becomes higher. For example, the bark of a Chihuahua has a higher frequency than the deeper robust bark of a German Shepherd. I think it's safe to say that most people would rather hear a German Shepherd bark for 10 minutes than listen to a Chihuahua bark for five. This is because bursts of sound composed of higher pitched frequencies are generally perceived as more annoying than frequencies in the lower range.

Each human brain wave pattern has its own amplitude and frequency that correspond to our different states of consciousness and are clearly evident on EEG readings. The assigned bandwidths and definitions of each brain wave vary amongst different sources, but they generally fall within the following parameters:

- Gamma (40 - 100 Hz), the waves related to learning, information processing, and cognitive functioning. If the level is too high, it results in anxiety and heightened stress. Too low a level correlates with ADHD, learning disabilities, and depression;
- Beta (12 - 40 Hz), your awake and active state. The higher the frequency, the more likely you'll go from a state of high functioning to a state of feeling stressed and anxious. Too low a level is characteristic of ADHD, depression, and poor cognition;
- Alpha (8 - 12 Hz), when you're feeling relaxed or in a meditative state. Alpha waves can be induced by daydreaming with your eyes open, or by closing your eyes and envisioning pleasant images. Guided meditation, also called mindfulness meditation, is noted as being particularly helpful for promoting alpha waves. Too high a level of alpha waves indicates an inability to focus and concentrate on the task at hand. Too low a level may result in anxiety, insomnia, a high stress level, and obsessive compulsive disorder (OCD);
- Mu (8 - 13Hz), which arises from large groups of neurons in the brain, are activated when we watch another person doing something, such as playing a sport. It is thought that the mu waves play a role in helping us to learn something through imitation;
- Theta (4 - 8 Hz), the brain waves of sleep and daydreaming. Restorative sleep is associated with theta waves, as well as enhanced intuition and creativity. Too low a level is associated with high stress, depression, and being out of touch with one's emotions;
- Delta (0 - 4 Hz), dominant in infants and young children, and decreasing as we get older except in periods of deep sleep or profound relaxation. In our normal waking state, too much delta wave activity results in an inability to concentrate, difficulty learning, and ADHD. Brain damage can show up on EEGs as too much delta wave activity.

We may be unconscious while we sleep, but there's still a lot of mental activity going on during this time. Our brain is busy with performing tasks in the background while our bodies rest, and our brain waves are a reflection of the level of activity. Sleep is measured in five stages:

- Stage I is the transition stage between wakefulness and sleeping, lasting between five and 10 minutes. Brain activity is a mix of beta and theta waves;
- Stage II is a deeper transitional stage, lasting between 15 and 20 minutes. Theta waves increase and become more consistent;
- Stage III lasts 15 to 30 minutes. Delta waves begin, but they are less than 50 percent of brain wave activity. Stage III is non rapid eye movement (NREM) sleep;
- Stage IV is very similar to Stage III, except delta waves now comprise over 50 percent of brain wave activity. Stage IV is your deepest stage of sleep, sometimes referred to as slow wave sleep because delta waves dominate. Like Stage III, it is also dreamless sleep;
- Stage V is rapid eye movement (REM) sleep, the dreaming stage, accounting for 20 to 30 percent of our total sleep time. In this stage beta waves dominate. Although we are asleep, the brain waves are very similar to conscious brain activity.

The varying cycles of brain wave activity during sleep may explain why people with tinnitus tend to wake up one or more times in the night. Brain waves shift from deep sleep to lighter sleep. During this process, tinnitus signals in the brain gradually rise to the surface of conscious awareness and can then break through and awaken the sleeper. For those who have never had problems with staying asleep through the night, this breakthrough phase can be a very difficult thing to deal with. And for those who were already experiencing difficulty with getting enough sleep, acquiring tinnitus can make it immeasurably worse. For more information on how tinnitus affects sleep and what you can do about it, see Chapter 34, "Sleeping."

26
BRAIN WAVES AND TINNITUS

All mammals have brain wave activity, some of which is remarkably similar to our own. Scientists compared the electroencephalogram (EEG) measurement of sleeping dogs in the rapid eye movement (REM) stage to the EEG measurement of humans. What they discovered is that dogs and humans in REM stage create basically the same erratic brain wave patterns. Based on these studies, researchers are fairly confident that the twitching, running motions, growling, whining, and other vocalizations of dogs while asleep are in fact indicators of a dreaming dog.

An unusual aspect of delta wave activity is that adult females tend to have more delta wave activity, not just in humans but in most mammals as well. The reason for this isn't understood, but perhaps it partially accounts for "women's intuition," since intuition is considered to be a function of delta wave activity. It's also recognized that children tend to be more intuitive than adults, and their delta wave activity is correspondingly higher than that of adults.

Brain wave measurements of adults with tinnitus indicate lower than normal alpha brain wave activity, and abnormally elevated delta and gamma brain wave activity. Interestingly enough, higher than average levels of delta wave activity while awake are associated with brain damage, as well as with ADHD (Attention Deficit Hyperactivity Disorder), which among other symptoms includes a pronounced inability to focus. ADHD and tinnitus share several characteristics, including this unusual brain wave activity. It would be nice if these abnormally high delta wave levels significantly enhanced one's intuitive ability, but apparently no one has reported that as a side effect nor has anyone done a study on it. More than likely, the distress or annoyance of hearing tinnitus would interfere with one's ability to hear what is often referred to as the voice of intuition.

Delta wave increase is associated with a meditative state. It may seem illogical that an activity which raises your delta wave levels can help with tinnitus. However, it's acknowledged by the medical community that meditation is in fact a beneficial long-term coping mechanism for tinnitus. This is more likely due to the fact that meditation, practiced regularly, has been proven to increase grey matter in the hippocampus. The hippocampus, located in the limbic region, has been shown to exhibit a decrease in grey matter in tinnitus subjects. It's possible that restoring some of that grey matter is partially responsible for reducing tinnitus perception in those who practice regular meditation. Dominant delta wave activity is seen in states of transcendental meditation, usually accompanied by a sense of emotional detachment. This is something to aspire to in reducing negative reactions to hearing your tinnitus.

Although meditation temporarily raises delta wave activity, that heightened delta wave activity is probably not the reason for the eventual increase of grey matter in the hippocampus. More than likely it's because anxiety adversely affects neurogenesis, the process by which new brain cells are created. When we're anxious or stressed for long enough periods of time, neurogenesis slows down. That means less brain cells and therefore less grey matter. Meditation tends to soothe the entire nervous system, which in turn reduces anxiety, promotes neurogenesis, and has the additional positive side effect of decreasing perception of tinnitus. I would suggest that you avoid increasing delta wave activity through methods such as listening to binaural beats audio for delta waves. It's unknown how elevated delta waves affect tinnitus long-term when induced by methods other than meditation. If you don't want to meditate, then look into coping activities that decrease rather than increase delta wave activity.

A very pleasant way to reduce delta wave activity is through aromatherapy massage. As explained in the article, "Modulatory effects of aromatherapy massage intervention," on the www.sciencedirect.com website, aromatherapy massage can reduce delta wave activity in as little as one treatment session. Not only does the delta wave activity go down, but the alpha wave activity goes up. This is precisely the outcome that someone with tinnitus needs. If you don't have the funds to pay for a professional massage, there are books on self-massage available on Amazon and at your local bookstore, and perhaps even your local library. Information on which aromatherapy oils to use is included in Chapter 41, "Aromatherapy."

Studies conducted on subjects experiencing residual inhibition have shown a corresponding decrease in delta wave activity. Residual inhibition is a known phenomenon wherein the perception of tinnitus volume can be temporarily suppressed in tinnitus subjects by listening to sounds which match their tinnitus in frequency or characteristics. In other words, someone with tinnitus that sounds like a tea kettle may experience temporary suppression of tinnitus if they listen to an actual tea kettle sound, whereas someone whose tinnitus sounds like cicadas may experience residual inhibition by listening to a recording of buzzing insects. There are people with tinnitus who can take a shower and not only get the benefit of temporarily masking their tinnitus, but they also experience residual inhibition that lasts several hours.

One study of residual inhibition showed changes in the oscillating patterns of neural networks in the cortex. This suggests that perception of tinnitus is related to imbalanced neuronal activity on a large scale, as evidenced by the elevated delta waves. In order to stop the perception of tinnitus, one would need to permanently interrupt the underlying oscillatory pattern. At this time, medical science does not have a reliable and safe technique or drug capable of doing that. Residual inhibition and its application to tinnitus is covered in greater detail in Chapter 61, "Residual Inhibition."

As mentioned earlier, adults with tinnitus show abnormally elevated gamma brain wave activity. Remember that high gamma waves are correlated with anxiety and heightened stress. Gamma waves are a little easier to consciously influence than delta wave activity, but it does require a serious commitment to change one's emotional reactions to stressors. You need to refrain from any activities that increase anxiety, elevate stress, and raise your arousal state. For example, if you play sports and you have strong reactions to your team losing, instead of yelling and becoming agitated and letting your anger reach the point where you want to punch somebody, step back and take some deep breaths. Keep your system calm. There may have been a time when you could indulge your emotional reaction, but it certainly isn't helpful to your tinnitus condition now. If you're a parent, and your child does something that in the past would make you lose your temper, count to 10, cool down, and remember that this kind of outburst is a negative physical arousal which is harmful to you. If you're a workaholic and are constantly bringing work home from the office, or if you're an entrepreneur who consistently works long hours, you need to stop stressing your body to the breaking point. Remember that tinnitus is not a disease, it is a symptom of something going wrong in the auditory system and/or the brain. Give yourself a timeout from whatever is stressing you, and let your brain waves normalize as much as possible. Many experts will tell you that stress increases perception of tinnitus. It certainly goes without saying that stressful situations make it more difficult to cope with tinnitus, because it can feel like the straw that's breaking the camel's back. It's very important that you learn to be aware of your body's rising stress levels and stop them in their tracks whenever possible.

If the above paragraph isn't enough to convince you to reduce stress in your life, consider this: stress depletes glutathione, the most important antioxidant molecule in your body. Lower levels of glutathione lead to a weaker defense against free radicals, those destructive molecules which are to blame for aging and tissue degeneration. Glutathione depletion goes beyond affecting the tissues of our skin, muscles, and organs. It can also cause neurodegeneration. One of the most important things that someone with tinnitus needs to do is to protect all their neurons from further damage. If your circumstances are such that you're constantly feeling stressed but you have little to no control of your current situation, be sure to get some daily exercise. Glutathione levels are boosted by exercise, so that's another good reason to walk or jog for 30 minutes every day, in addition to the well-known cardiovascular benefits. If walking or running is out of the question, you can achieve the same effect by strength training three to four days a week. For more information on glutathione and how you can increase your glutathione levels, see the article, "Essential Glutathione: The Mother of All Anti-Oxidants," by Mark Hyman, M.D., on http://drhyman.com.

There has been a tremendous amount of interest in the last two decades about alpha waves and how to raise them. This is in response to the need for a drug-free solution to the relentless stress and pressure of our society. It would not be far-fetched to say that we are a society where beta waves dominate. As such, we are lacking a proper balance of alpha waves to counter the beta influence. If you search on Google for "increase alpha brain waves," you will get over 2 million results. Many of the proposed solutions rely on an audio-based therapy called binaural beats. A specially composed audio file is played through headphones, whereby one frequency is played in one ear and a slightly modified but similar frequency is played in the other ear. This causes your brain to combine the two and create a third frequency, which is said to result in a pleasant state of altered consciousness. This altered state purportedly increases relaxation, reduces stress, improves focus, and promotes better sleep. If you're interested in trying this technique, you can sign up for a trial basis at www.OmHarmonics.com. I haven't used any OmHarmonics products and cannot attest to how effective they are, but their methods are aligned with the prevailing theories of binaural beats therapy. In addition, YouTube has many binaural beats videos available that you can listen to and find out if they work for you. Be sure to wear headphones or the third frequency will not be generated. Remember to keep the volume at a comfortable and safe level.

An easy way to increase your alpha brain waves is by watching television, if you don't mind being in an unfocused state that's overly receptive to suggestion. Becoming engrossed in a television show or movie is very similar to being hypnotized. That is, your focus is narrowed to one subject and you are inattentive to your environment. One researcher remarked that a person watching television is "like a bird watching a snake." Unfortunately, the increase in alpha wave activity when you watch television is temporary and really isn't helpful in the long run as far as calming your nervous system down. However, it may explain why some people have a decreased perception of tinnitus when they watch television or videos, aside from the audio that might be masking their tinnitus. Any activity which intently holds your focus tends to diminish the perception of tinnitus. This diminished perception usually ends as soon as you turn off the television or stop doing whatever has your attention, and your brain waves resume the normal activity of your conscious, alert mind. In other words, alpha waves go down, beta waves go up.

Devoting time every day to the practice of yoga is an excellent way to increase alpha wave activity. By focusing on the poses, your alpha waves will begin to elevate during your session. Over time, with continued practice of yoga, the increase in alpha wave level is sustained. Yoga helps

SECTION VII

COPING TECHNIQUES

27
ALCOHOL AND MARIJUANA

Alcohol is a psychoactive sedative, so it's not unusual for people with tinnitus to consider whether it might help them to better handle the anxiety that often accompanies tinnitus. Some people report that in very moderate amounts, perhaps one to two beers, or a glass or two of wine, it seems to lessen the volume or perception of intrusiveness. However, anecdotal reports indicate that drinking an excess of alcohol in an effort to subdue tinnitus creates the opposite effect. It tends to raise the volume rather than lower it, and it also increases awareness of the tinnitus. It makes no difference what type of alcoholic drink they're consuming. Whether it's beer, wine, whiskey, or any other type of alcoholic beverage, too much of it generally results in negative and disappointing effects.

If you're taking any prescribed or over-the-counter sedative for anxiety or as a sleep aid, then you definitely should not be drinking alcohol. The synergistic combination can lead to severe harmful side effects. There's no way anyone can know what their individual tolerance level is on any given day, and it's complicated by factors such as how much food has been consumed, level of fatigue, and anything else relating to your physical well-being. If you are not taking any contraindicated medications, the generally accepted safe level of alcohol consumption is two drinks per day for a man, and one drink per day for a woman or anyone over 65. Some experts believe there is no such thing as a safe level, and that it doesn't matter if someone is only drinking one or two alcoholic beverages daily.

The risk, of course, is that if one glass of wine makes the tinnitus more bearable, then it's easy to get in the habit of drinking two glasses of wine to deal with it, or maybe three. Unfortunately, whether it's one glass or two, alcohol is likely to prevent you from getting a proper amount of sleep. Seven to nine hours of restful sleep every night is probably the most important thing to help you cope with your tinnitus until it either lessens in severity or you become habituated to it. It would be far better for you to take the money you would spend on alcoholic drinks and instead go to a qualified massage therapist once or twice a month. Having someone remove the knots of tension on a regular basis is certainly a healthier approach than trying to blunt your perception of tinnitus with alcohol.

One thing to be mindful of with alcohol is that it affects the balance of neurotransmitters. When alcohol enters your system, it triggers the release of endorphins. These endorphins then bind to the opiate receptors in your brain, which in turn stimulates the release of dopamine. This can produce feelings which range from casual indifference all the way to euphoria, depending on how much dopamine is released. As time goes on, increasing amounts of alcohol are needed to re-create those feelings. The end result is an imbalance in dopamine levels and other neurotransmitters, leading to altered neurological pathways. Most people with tinnitus likely already have neurotransmitter dysfunctions and need to be careful not to aggravate the situation further. If you can limit your alcohol to low or moderate consumption in social contexts, you'll probably be okay. However, it's best to avoid self-treating with alcohol in the hopes of either dulling your tinnitus or your reaction to it. This is at best a short-term solution, and at worst can lead to the dual problem of tinnitus and alcoholism.

By the way, if you enjoy alcoholic mixed drinks, you'll want to pay attention to the tonic being used in your drink. Many tonics contain quinine water, which is known to cause or aggravate tinnitus.

Marijuana is very intriguing as a treatment for tinnitus. Its effectiveness has been reported to depend on the amount of cannabinoid (CBD) in the marijuana. CBD is not psychoactive to the same level as tetrahydrocannabinol (THC), the euphoria-inducing component of marijuana. Instead, CBD has been shown to act as an anti-depressant, anxiolytic (reducing anxiety), as well as an anti-inflammatory and pain reliever.

Dr. Thanos Tzounopoulos is a leading expert on tinnitus. He discovered that there is plasticity in the brain's auditory brain stem. Part of his research focuses on the endocannabinoid system, which plays a significant role in brain plasticity and is the system which responds to inhalation or ingestion of medical marijuana. He believes there are similarities with how the brain handles chronic pain and addiction, and how it processes tinnitus. At this time there are no conclusive results, but

Dr. Tzounopoulos is attempting to determine if medical marijuana can indeed reduce the severity of tinnitus. Interestingly, endocannabinoids and their receptors have been found in the cochlear nucleus. The cochlear nucleus is located in the mid brain. Impulses carried by the auditory nerve are received by the cochlear nucleus. Those impulses are then transmitted to other pathways in the brain, with the auditory cortex as the final destination. To learn more about the fascinating biology of endocannabinoids, I recommend reading the www.leafly.com article, "What is the Endocannabinoid System and What is Its Role?"

One evening when my tinnitus was particularly intrusive and difficult to deal with, I tried smoking some low-THC marijuana to see if it would relieve my tinnitus. Unfortunately, it did nothing to relax me, but it did have the unfortunate effect of severely spiking my tinnitus for the next three days. Whether that was due to the marijuana itself or simply a coincidence, I don't know, but I'm not willing to repeat the experiment. Like any other drug, however, people have different reactions to marijuana that cannot be predicted. Some people use marijuana to soothe their nerves and ease their anxiety, which in turn decreases their perception of tinnitus. For others, marijuana turns down the volume regardless of their level of relaxation. Then there are those who experience a worsening of tinnitus, or no change whatsoever.

There are so many strains of marijuana that it would be counterproductive, and possibly misleading, to list them here with regard to their typical effects on tinnitus. If you're interested in learning more about user experiences from people who have tinnitus, visit the Leafly website and read what users have to say about it on the page, "The Best Strains for Tinnitus." Be mindful that if you wish to try marijuana to cope with your tinnitus, that certain strains can be extremely potent. Proceed with caution. Give yourself a couple minutes in between each toke or puff, so that you can gauge your reaction and avoid getting too much into your system. The goal here is to give you a break from tinnitus, not to become stoned as an escape mechanism. Treat it with the same caution as you would any other prescription medication. If you have never smoked marijuana before, you'll first want to read the Leafly article, "Cannabis Science 101: The Physics and Chemistry of the Joint."

It's a scientific fact that ingesting marijuana is more potent, and lasts longer in your system, than smoking marijuana. If you get a marijuana cookie or brownie, be sure to nibble sparingly and give yourself time between nibbles, until you learn how much it takes to achieve the effect you need. For more information, read the article, "Smoke vs. Snack: Why Edible Marijuana is Stronger Than Smoking," at www.thedailybeast.com.

As of 2017, the following states allow both medicinal and recreational use of marijuana: Alaska, Colorado, Oregon, California, Nevada, and Washington. Laws regarding marijuana continue to change across the United States. The State Marijuana Laws in 2017 Map at www.governing.com contains updated information. If your state does not allow medicinal and/or recreational use, marijuana possession may be treated as a misdemeanor or felony. There also may be specific restrictions regarding the use or possession of marijuana. If in doubt, be sure to do some research on the laws in your state.

28
HABITUATION

Habituation is the process by which a person becomes accustomed to a stimulus in their environment after repeated exposure. As a coping mechanism for tinnitus, habituation is a gradual ongoing transformation whereby a person eventually adapts to their tinnitus and no longer notices or reacts to it. Habituation can evolve to the degree where you don't consciously hear the tinnitus at all unless you actively listen for it. Even if that level cannot be achieved, habituation can occur to the point where you still hear it at the same volume and intensity, but, unlike before, it does not trigger a negative emotional response. One incredible example of habituation that I read about is an incident where a woman's neighbors had to knock on her apartment door to get her out of the building because of a fire. Although the other residents of the apartment complex easily heard the fire alarm, this woman was totally unaware of it. Her tinnitus was a high-pitched siren. Over time, she had adapted to it and gradually tuned it out, to the point where an actual fire alarm going off in her vicinity simply did not register with her. It may seem impossible that someone could adapt to something so intrusive, but the human brain can be taught to disregard signals if we persistently refuse to acknowledge those signals. It's critical that you accept and believe in the possibility that you can establish control over whether or not you hear the phantom sounds of tinnitus.

For habituation to occur, it's very important to regard your tinnitus as a neutral stimulus. This of course is easier said than done, particularly with loud tinnitus or tinnitus with irritating characteristics. People who value silence and tranquil surroundings generally have a much more difficult time viewing tinnitus as neutral. They can't help but perceive it as an unwelcome force disrupting their peace and quiet. For them, it's worse than a baby wailing nonstop in the seat behind you on an airplane. You know what a challenge it can be to tune that out, even when you put on your headphones and listen to music. No matter what you tell yourself, it's very hard not to react with annoyance, even if you keep your frustrations to yourself. That airplane ride doesn't last as long as tinnitus, though. When you reach your destination, you can leave the crying baby, but you don't have the comfort of knowing that you can go elsewhere and leave the tinnitus behind. The odds are that it's always going to be with you at some level, which is why you need to step back and begin to objectively view it not as a threat, but simply as a new part of who you are.

This is not to suggest that you should just wave a white flag of surrender to tinnitus without considering any treatment options. That would mean you see it as something stronger, more powerful than you. Instead, you want to neutralize it by accepting its presence without resentment, fear, or anger. Strive to adopt an attitude that even though you would prefer that tinnitus not be part of your life, you can learn to ignore it in time. The natural tendency of humans is to adapt to unpleasant conditions, whether it be a bodily condition or an environmental condition. Keep in mind that habituation is just another form of learning. By tuning out stimuli that isn't essential to survival or dealing with the tasks of your day, habituation allows you to focus on things that really matter. If an annoying sound isn't essential to your survival, it has no value. When you hear your tinnitus, tell yourself, "This sound isn't important, I have things to do that need my attention." If necessary, repeat that a hundred or a thousand times a day, until it becomes an automatic mental and emotional response.

In Section VIII, "Treatments," I review some treatments that can be used both as tinnitus therapy and as a means to promote habituation. Among these are audio notch therapy and Acoustic Coordinated Reset® Neuromodulation (ACRN). These treatments require you to listen to audio files that are uniquely constructed to remap and calm the hyperactive neurons in the auditory cortex. One interesting aspect of ACRN is that as time goes on, you will find the tones fade away from your conscious awareness. Even though the ACRN sound is external, whereas tinnitus often feels like you're hearing it in your head, it's still validation that anything can be tuned out once you are exposed to it long enough and don't view it as a threat. If you can habituate to ACRN, or if you use sound enrichment therapy to mask your tinnitus and discover that after a while you're not noticing the masking sounds, then you can habituate to the tinnitus as well. It doesn't happen overnight. It's a slow and steady process with occasional setbacks, but some level of habituation does occur for the vast majority of people with tinnitus.

People who move from the calm of the country to the bustle of the city can be initially overwhelmed by all the new sounds, but then gradually become accustomed to them. Oddly enough, people who move from the city likewise need an adjustment period until they adapt to an environment without the constant sounds of city life around them. Again, it's a brain thing. Your brain really likes whatever it's used to and generally does not want imposed change, especially in its sound environment. Give your brain enough time, be consistent and persistent with non-emotional responses, and your brain will likely adapt to the new environment.

It doesn't seem possible to habituate to a sound that's in your head, but remember that your brain is causing you to hear the sound. Your brain wants you to pay attention to the tinnitus sound because it's programmed to alert you to unusual and possibly dangerous things in your environment. It also places a higher priority on anything you're focusing on. As you go about your daily activities, do your best to distract yourself from paying attention to your tinnitus. In doing so, you will be essentially instructing your brain that tinnitus is a low priority and you aren't interested in paying attention to it. In time, you may notice that the tinnitus signal becomes weaker and less intrusive, and that you are able to go about your daily life without tinnitus controlling what you do and how you feel.

The power of distraction is very important in the habituation process. A focused distraction can affect any of our five senses. For example, there is a phenomenon known as inattentional blindness. This is when you literally don't see something happening despite it occurring in plain sight. A famous experiment was conducted by Daniel Simons of the University of Illinois at Urbana-Champaign and Christopher Chablis of Harvard University. The test consisted of subjects watching a video which showed a basketball being passed back and forth between members of a team wearing white shirts and members of a team wearing black shirts. The test subjects were asked to report how many times the players in white shirts passed the basketball back and forth. During the video, a person dressed in a gorilla suit strolls onto the court amongst the players, faces the camera, beats his chest, and then ambles off the court. Astonishingly, nearly half of the test subjects said there was nothing unusual that happened in the video. Their minds were so focused on counting the number of times the basketball was passed from player to player that their brain simply did not register the gorilla on the court. The video, "selective attention test," is available on the Daniel Simons channel on YouTube.

If it seems impossible to believe that people could look right at something and not see it, there is a modern phenomenon called "banner blindness." This refers to Internet users who have become so accustomed to seeing banner ads on websites, that they don't even notice them anymore. Think about all the ads you see every day; how many do you actually *notice?*

Inattentional blindness is also referred to as selective attention, which is probably a better description. With time and determination, you can teach your brain to shift its attention from the tinnitus and to select something else in the environment to keep your brain occupied. This can be done by watching a movie and paying close attention to the dialogue and action, by listening to music and immersing yourself in the arrangement of the notes and the creativity of the lyrics, going out for coffee with friends and intently listening to what each one of them has to say in the conversation, or reading a book with vivid scenes that capture your imagination and transport you to another time and place. I personally have discovered that when I'm on a hike with my dog, my tinnitus seems to momentarily subside whenever we encounter someone else with a dog. My attention shifts to watching the interaction between the dogs and being alert to signs of either friendliness or aggression from the other dog. Whether it's a case of selective attention, or whether my protective instinct overrides the tinnitus signal, I don't know. However, as soon as the meet and greet is over and my dog and I resume our hike, my tinnitus returns to whatever level it was at before the encounter. I've heard of instances where someone completely forgets about their severe tinnitus when a loved one has an emergency situation. As long as there's something in your environment which demands high priority attention, the more likely it is that your tinnitus will recede into the background of your consciousness.

There are plenty of opportunities in everyday life to practice selective attention. You might walk through your neighborhood and become enchanted by someone's flower garden with its variety of colors and fragrance, and it isn't until you move on that you realize you didn't notice your tinnitus at all while you were admiring the garden. Or perhaps you go window shopping where you can get caught up in fantasizing what it would be like to own whatever is on display, and for a while you just don't hear the tinnitus. Whatever it is that takes your mind away from tinnitus, make a note of what you were doing or what you were thinking just before it dawned on you that your tinnitus momentarily vanished. Relive that event in your mind and embellish it with your imagination, making it better than it was in reality. Closing your eyes and reliving pleasant memories stimulates the alpha brain waves, shifts your focus, and helps to lessen the perception of tinnitus. The same thing happens when you close your eyes and daydream, when you envision pleasant things that you would like to happen.

It's been proven that humans have the ability to override incoming signals of sight, sound, and touch. That should give you some hope that you can live a good, productive life, even if at this moment you're struggling with moderate to severe tinnitus. Do your best every chance you can to ignore it and shift your attention elsewhere. It may take weeks or it may take months or a year or longer, but one day you'll experience the tinnitus momentarily disappearing from your awareness for a minute. The next time it may be for several minutes, then an hour, and eventually you won't notice it at all for several hours or an entire day. The phantom sounds continue to be generated by your brain; they simply don't break through to conscious awareness until you shift your focus and deliberately listen for your tinnitus. The challenge at that stage is to not listen for it, and to let go of the natural compulsion to monitor it. The point is, if it doesn't intrude for a short period of time, then it's possible for it to not intrude for an extended period of time.

29
HEARING LOSS

Hearing aids can help you with your tinnitus. Generally speaking, this applies more when tinnitus is associated with age-related hearing loss (ARHL) or sensorineural hearing loss (SNHL). Before discussing how hearing aids might help and what to look for if you decide to use them, it's helpful to understand the basics of ARHL and SNHL.

Age-related hearing loss is called presbycusis, (sometimes spelled "presbyacusis"). It is the natural irreversible decline of hearing acuity that occurs in everyone as they get older, and is most pronounced in the higher frequencies. One-third of adults between 65 and 75 have hearing loss. After the age of 75, hearing loss affects up to 50 percent of adults.

You may believe there is nothing wrong with your hearing, but the change can be so gradual that you never notice the loss of upper frequencies. The average frequency of human speech is between 80 to 260 hertz. The average man's voice is between 85 to 155 hertz, whereas the average woman's voice is between 165 to 255 hertz. Children's voices are typically between 250 to 300 hertz and higher. This is why some people first become aware of the onset of hearing loss when they begin to experience difficulty understanding the higher-pitched speech of women and children and yet have no problem understanding men when they speak.

Another marker of hearing loss is when the lower and higher-pitched sounds in ordinary speech are difficult to understand. High-pitched consonant sounds are d, t, sh, s, f and th. Low-pitched consonant sounds are o, a, ah, i and e. For reasons unknown, women with age-related hearing loss tend to have difficulty hearing lower-pitched sounds, whereas men have difficulty hearing higher-pitched sounds. The meaning of speech relies heavily on higher-pitched sounds, which explains why men with hearing loss have more difficulty understanding speech. This difficulty tends to become more pronounced in environments with background noise. Because women and children have naturally higher-pitched voices, people with hearing loss may find it easier to understand men when they speak. When certain higher-pitched consonants and diphthongs such as "s" and "th" become muddled, clarity of hearing is diminished. What many people with hearing loss complain about is not that they can't hear what is being said, it's that they can't *understand* what's being said. This is often due to the muffling of those higher-pitched consonants and diphthongs. To make things worse, a puzzling development is that certain sounds which never bothered them before may now become uncomfortably loud or annoying.

Why do we lose the higher frequencies first? Remember that the inner ear, the cochlea, is where our hair cells are located. These hair cells convert sound waves into electrical signals, which travel to the brain via the auditory nerve. The brain interprets the signals into volume and pitch of sound. The hair cells which detect higher frequencies are located at the base of the cochlea. As one goes deeper into the cochlea, the hair cells are designed to detect increasingly lower frequencies. All sound waves hit the higher frequency hair cells first. When the hair cells match the actual frequency of the incoming sound, the sound wave stops at that point and the signal is sent to the brain. Therefore, outer hair cells are exposed to every sound frequency, while inner hair cells are exposed to lower frequency sounds. The common experience of losing higher frequency hearing may simply be due to outer hair cells becoming worn out over time because all sound waves must travel through them first.

Damage to the cochlea or to the nerve pathways that transmit signals from the cochlea to the brain can cause or contribute to acquired sensorineural hearing loss (SNHL), which means one is not born with it, but develops it over time. Age-related hearing loss is a common form of SNHL, but it can also be caused by ototoxic drugs, diseases, tumors, trauma to the head, and extreme noise exposure. With sensorineural hearing loss, one simply cannot hear as well, and the general consensus is that the damage cannot be reversed. Most cases of hearing loss fall into the category of acquired sensorineural hearing loss, but congenital sensorineural hearing loss develops in the womb or during birth. In addition to hereditary factors and abnormal development of the auditory system itself, congenital SNHL can occur when the mother transmits a disease such as rubella (German measles) to her unborn child. If a pregnant woman has diabetes, there is a risk of the baby developing sensorineural hearing loss. It can also occur when the baby is born prematurely, or is deprived of sufficient oxygen during birth.

Sudden sensorineural hearing loss (SSNHL or SSHL) can happen over the course of a few hours or several days, but it can also be quite sudden and very dramatic in its onset. Although it usually occurs between the ages of 30 and 60, anyone can wake up one morning to find that they have become completely deaf in one or both ears. Older adults are more likely to experience SSNHL. In almost 98% of cases, only one ear is affected, and most of those involve the left ear, although there is no explanation for that phenomenon. Sudden sensorineural hearing loss is a medical emergency which requires immediate treatment.

Tinnitus without hearing loss is bad enough, but when hearing loss accompanies the tinnitus, it usually makes the tinnitus much more difficult to deal with. It's even worse with profound hearing loss. Ambient noise and everyday background sounds become muted and the tinnitus takes center stage. Almost everyone has had the experience of being in an environment such as a restaurant or club where the background noise is so loud that you can barely hear what your companions are saying. Now imagine that your ears are stuffed with cotton but still the background noise pierces through every other sound. It becomes difficult to concentrate and understand what people are saying in your everyday conversations. The subtle nuances of your favorite music may be lost, so that you longer appreciate music as you once did. You may struggle to hear the dialogue in a movie, and it gets worse if the musical score is ramped up for certain scenes. If you have severe tinnitus and muffled hearing, you need to have your hearing tested to see whether restoring your ability to hear normal ambient sounds can reduce the perceived intrusion of tinnitus.

Although tinnitus in senior adults is usually attributed to hearing loss, it's well-known that people can have significant hearing loss yet have no tinnitus whatsoever. On the other hand, there are plenty of people with test results showing normal hearing yet they have moderate to severe tinnitus. As noted previously, we all eventually experience hearing loss in the upper frequencies. The theory used to be that tinnitus is the result of our auditory system trying to fill in the missing frequencies. The current prevailing belief is that the auditory pathway undergoes changes that correlate with the missing frequencies, a process referred to as neuroplasticity. Because of neuroplasticity, the brain attempts to adapt as it tries to compensate for the loss of functioning hair cells at certain frequencies, with the result being hyperactive neurons firing randomly and generating the phantom sounds of tinnitus. Why the neuroplastic changes in some people's brains result in tinnitus but not in others is a mystery that medical science is still trying to unravel. And of course, this is only one possible reason for tinnitus associated with hearing loss. It is more likely the result of several contributing factors that add up to a disruption and eventual breakdown in the normal auditory processing of the brain.

There are hearing tests online to help you determine if you do have hearing loss. An excellent Online Hearing Test has been developed by Dr. Stéphane Pigeon, the developer of the myNoise website, which is discussed in Chapter 31, "Masking." The hearing test isn't difficult, but please read the instructions thoroughly before proceeding. It will even give you a personalized audiogram once your test is complete, something that I have not seen offered anywhere else. Starkey, a well-known manufacturer of hearing aids, also offers an online hearing test, along with other helpful information. You can access it at www.starkey.com/online-hearing-test.

Obviously you will obtain the most precise results if you are tested by an audiologist. However, starting with an online test will give you time to emotionally process the situation, so that you can do some research into what treatment options are available. If you have significant or bothersome hearing loss, you will eventually need to have your hearing tested by a trained professional. When you understand the reason and extent of your hearing loss, it will be easier for you and your audiologist to decide on the best course of action. It's possible that not only will you improve your hearing, but your tinnitus symptoms may reduce as well.

No matter what your age, you have plenty of company with regard to hearing loss. Visit www.Pinterest.com and search for "Famous People with Hearing Loss and Tinnitus." It may give you some comfort to know that many celebrities and other famous people have one or both afflictions, but they still lead satisfying, productive lives.

30
HEARING AIDS

It may surprise you to learn that hearing aids can be useful as a treatment for tinnitus. If you have hearing loss at one or more frequencies, particularly in the upper range, your auditory system may respond to that loss by turning up the gain and trying to capture and process those frequencies. Because the hair cells that are attuned to those frequencies are damaged or dead, the result is hyperactive neurons expressed as tinnitus. It's been shown that people with hearing loss and tinnitus can sometimes reduce and potentially eliminate their tinnitus with hearing aids. This occurs because the hearing aids restore balance to your auditory system. It can now process those previously missing frequencies. As a result, the hyperactive neurons calm down, and then the tinnitus calms down as well.

Hearing aids don't help everyone with tinnitus. If they did, tinnitus would not be such a troublesome issue for so many people. Hearing aids tend to be of more benefit to people who have tinnitus due to age-related hearing loss (ARHL), also known as presbycusis, and sensorineural hearing loss (SNHL). It's possible for hearing aids to be tailored to your specific hearing loss frequency. If your tinnitus frequency matches the frequency of your hearing loss, there is a stronger likelihood that using hearing aids will noticeably reduce your tinnitus.

People with hearing loss and tinnitus have the option of choosing hearing aids that include a masking accessory. These dual-purpose hearing aids make it easier for someone to hear what's going on around them, with the option of generating either white noise or gentle tones to distract the brain from focusing on the tinnitus. The effectiveness of dual-purpose hearing aids in coping with tinnitus may be related to the type of tinnitus sound a person hears. Generally speaking, if you can listen to white noise or soothing audio tones and it reduces your perception of tinnitus, these kind of hearing aids will likely work well for you. If your tinnitus is not easily masked by white noise or gentle tones, or if these types of sounds irritate rather than soothe you, you would be better off with a traditional hearing aid.

Neuromonics and Widex Zen are two of the better-known tinnitus relief devices. Neuromonics claims that its device uses "spectrally modified" music which takes advantage of brain plasticity. As the brain changes in response to the neural stimulus contained in the music or sounds, eventually the brain learns to filter out the tinnitus, thereby providing relief to the user. The Neuromonics device uses a custom hearing profile obtained by an audiologist, as well as providing counseling sessions. The device must be worn for two or more hours every day, for at least six months. This device is FDA approved and clinical trials show that improvement is experienced by most people who use it. However, that being said, studies show that the majority of people will experience improvement with any sort of sound generator therapy. For example, consistently using masking with a simple MP3 or similar playback device has been shown to reduce tinnitus distress over a consistent period of use of six months or more. If finances are a consideration, please note that the Neuromonics device is generally considered to be one of the more expensive options for tinnitus treatment. You can learn more by visiting their website at www.neuromonics.com.

The Widex Zen offers the combination of a hearing aid with therapeutic sounds. Instead of music, the Widex device plays random harmonic tones. Because the tones are not predictable, the brain doesn't learn any specific pattern of tones and instead trains itself to listen for the next tone. It's similar to listening to wind chimes on a day when a slight breeze randomly stirs them into motion. As the chimes move, you tend to focus on listening for the next pleasant tones that will play, while assigning lesser importance to other sound stimuli in your environment. Instead of Bluetooth, Widex uses Widexlink. It's a wireless technology which they promote as being superior to Bluetooth in speed, battery savings, and streaming consistency. In general, Widex costs less than Neuromonics, but special features may cost more. If you don't like white noise or listening to programmed music for hours at a time, Widex may be a good choice. Like Neuromonics, counseling is also part of the program. This is necessary in order to reshape one's beliefs and assumptions about tinnitus and to reduce its emotional significance and impact. The website for Widex Zen and other specialized hearing aids is www.widex.com.

I have no affiliation with Neuromonics or Widex, and have only summarized the information that I learned about both companies from their websites, as well as reviews from people with tinnitus who have used either or both technologies. There are other hearing aid manufacturers that offer similar devices. Among these are Muse, Halo2 and SoundLens from Starkey, and Tinnitus Balance from Phonak. A list of the better-known hearing aid manufacturers is on the www.HearIt.org website. You can search the manufacturer websites to see whether or not they include tinnitus remedies in their devices. This will give you a good idea of what options are available that will fit your unique situation and budget. You can also ask your personal audiologist or ENT for a recommendation.

There are hearing aids which do not include a built-in masker or programmed sound therapy, but are still Bluetooth compatible. These allow you to stream the masking or relaxation sound you prefer into your hearing aid via a Bluetooth connection to your computer or smartphone. You can choose from nature sounds, gentle instrumental music, or some other form of music to distract your brain's attention away from the tinnitus. A wonderful online source for audio streaming of realistic and soothing sound generators is www.myNoise.net, designed and maintained by Dr. Stéphane Pigeon. There are many grateful testimonials on that site by people with severe tinnitus. When you visit the site, click on the heart icon. The sound generators for tinnitus and hyperacusis will then be highlighted in green so you can quickly see the best choices. Of course, there are also sound generators that aren't necessarily indicated for tinnitus but which can still provide helpful sound enrichment. The Waterfall generator is a good place to start.

It wasn't that long ago that wearing a hearing aid was a source of embarrassment for many people. Hearing aids carried the false stigma of being associated with old age or even feebleness, and many people preferred to adapt as best they could to hearing loss rather than wear a hearing aid. Just a few decades ago it was also considered a stigma if you wore glasses, and particularly if you were a woman. Now it's a fashion statement and no one looks at anyone who wears glasses as somehow being defective. I would like to see the same positive attitude develop towards hearing aids. Hearing aid manufacturers are now paying as much attention to the cosmetic impact of hearing aids as they do to the functionality. The truth is, hearing loss affects people of all ages. Modern youth are particularly vulnerable to losing hearing acuity because they don't understand the danger of extremely loud music and also because our social environment is increasingly immersed in sound. It's quite possible that they will need to wear a hearing aid at an earlier age than their parents or grandparents, maybe in their forties or fifties instead of in their sixties or seventies.

Back in the early 19th century, a hearing aid was basically a large funnel you aimed at the source of sound. Attached to the funnel was a tapering tube, the end of which was inserted into one's ear. It was a very rudimentary and clumsy method to amplify sound. In 1876, before the advent of more modern-day hearing aids, Alexander Graham Bell invented the telephone. The carbon microphone and a battery were essential for amplifying sound in this groundbreaking invention. Then in 1886, Thomas Edison invented the carbon transmitter, whereby sound could be converted to electrical signals, carried through a wire and converted back to sound again. Hearing aid manufacturers adopted the concept of combining Bell's carbon microphone and battery, along with Edison's carbon transmitter. These changes represented major steps in electronic technology, and were used in the first manufactured hearing aids.

Fast forward to the 21st century, and you have what seems to be a limitless selection of hearing aids. You have more than just a choice of which hearing aid is best for your type of hearing loss or tinnitus. You can also decide whether you want it to be a discreet, inconspicuous device, or be bold and trendy with a bright and colorful hearing aid that makes it clear you want to hear everything going on in your world and you're proud of it. You can see some of these innovative designs, including decorative hearing aid embellishments, on the "Pretty Hearing Aids" page of Pinterest. Some are discreet, some are bold, but all of them show a creative trend developing with hearing aids as a fashion accessory.

Hearing aids are manufactured as either analog or digital. Analog hearing aids basically make all sounds louder, similar to cupping your hand behind your ear to hear better. Analog hearing aids can be equipped with a microchip programmed for different settings so the user is able to select how much amplification they need according to their current sound environment. When moving from a quiet environment such as a library to a noisier environment like a restaurant, the user presses a button to change the setting accordingly. It's a somewhat awkward way of modulating incoming sound, but the advantage is that analog is generally less expensive than digital.

Digital hearing aids, also known as digital signal processor (DSP), are a giant step up from analog. A DSP hearing aid converts sound waves to digital signals, resulting in an accurate duplication of sound rather than simple amplification. Computer chips within the DSP hearing aid precisely analyze the sound before amplifying it. It's a complex process which results in the user being able to more clearly hear important sounds like speech and music. Noise reduction algorithms may be included which filter out obtrusive background sounds. The DSP hearing aid usually has a wide array of program settings that allow it to be fine-tuned to a user's specific hearing loss and/or typical sound environment.

There are six basic designs of hearing aids:

- Hearing aid positioned behind the ear;
- Hearing aid receiver inserted into ear canal;
- Hearing aid itself inserted into ear canal;
- Hearing aid inserted deep within ear canal;
- Hearing aid worn on the body; and,
- Hearing aid affixed to arms of eyeglasses.

Most of us are familiar with seeing the hearing aid positioned behind the ear (BTE). A plastic casing encloses the electronic components, and a thin tube with a small dome at the end leads from the casing and inserts into the ear canal. The electronic components are the microphone, amplifier, and receiver. The microphone picks up sound waves from the environment which are then converted into electrical signals. The amplifier increases the strength of the signals, as well as including sophisticated filters designed to keep the focus only on relevant sound. In other words, the volume of someone speaking to you is amplified, whereas the rumbling sound of a truck driving by is not. The receiver converts the electric signals into audio sounds that the user can hear and understand. Many people prefer the BTE design because the sound processed by the hearing aid blends with the natural sound coming in from the environment. BTE hearing aids are rather inconspicuous, and are usually comfortable to wear for long periods of time.

Next is the receiver in the canal design (RIC). It's very similar to the BTE, except that the amplifier (loudspeaker) is not located in the casing behind the ear. Instead, it's at the end of a thin tubing which inserts into the ear canal. The part of the RIC that rests behind the ear is therefore smaller than the BTE design, making it even more inconspicuous and easier to hide. One drawback of this design is the greater likelihood of ear wax buildup which can interfere with its function. If your ears tend to build wax quickly, this may not be a good choice.

An in-the-canal hearing aid (ITC) is a hearing aid that is inserted directly into the ear canal. There are no wires or additional casings. These devices are good for people who wear glasses, as some people feel like the BTE or RIC designs interfere with the arms of their eyeglasses. Generally the shell of an ITC hearing aid is molded to conform to the individual ear. When the entire hearing aid is inserted into the ear canal, it's fairly inconspicuous, but it can cause a somewhat "blocked" feeling for incoming sound, similar to wearing an earplug. Like the RIC design, the function of an in-the-canal hearing aid can be affected by ear wax buildup and must be kept meticulously clean for it to function properly.

If your hearing loss is not severe, if you don't mind having less programming options, and if cosmetic appeal is important to you, then consider a hearing aid that is inserted completely into the ear canal (CIC). These devices are small, so amplification is limited and battery life is not as robust as the other designs. Because it's inserted deep into the canal, this type of hearing aid must be custom manufactured and fitted.

When hearing loss is profound, there is the option of wearing a body-worn hearing aid. This is essentially a box with a microphone to pick up sound, which is transmitted through a wire. At the end of the wire is an amplifier encased in a small dome, (somewhat like the receiver in the canal design), and the dome is inserted into the ear. This design has two advantages. First, it can significantly amplify sound; and, second, it runs on AA or AAA batteries rather than hearing aid batteries which tend to cost more. Some designs even offer solar power batteries for more savings. The disadvantages are the length of cord running from the box to the ear, the awkwardness of having to affix the box somewhere on your outer clothing so that the microphone is always exposed and able to pick up sound, and of course the device is clearly visible.

Least popular is the hearing aid that is attached to the arms of eyeglasses. This type of hearing aid works via conduction. That is, the amplifier of the hearing aid rests against the mastoid bone of the skull. Sound is basically conducted through that bone into the inner ear canal. This is the same principle behind the growing popularity of bone conduction headsets. People like this style of headset because they can listen to music or conversation and still be aware of sounds in their immediate environment. One obvious disadvantage to hearing aids on eyeglass arms is that the hearing aids are rendered ineffective once the user takes off the eyeglasses. However, this design is good for people with conductive hearing loss, where the outer and/or middle ear do not function well and therefore don't transmit sound to the inner ear.

By the way, if you've ever wondered why the noise of a dentist's drill is so loud inside your head, that's an example of bone conduction. It's a major reason why people with tinnitus dread going to the dentist. People with reactive tinnitus experience even greater anxiety. They fear the amplified volume of the drill will cause a spike in their tinnitus. It doesn't always happen, but it can. It's important to talk to your dentist ahead of time and let her know you have tinnitus and how severe it is. Some dentists reduce length of drilling times, for example, five seconds on and 10 seconds off, to give your tinnitus a break from the noise. Be sure before your dental appointment to take N-acetyl-L-cysteine supplements (NAC), which can protect your ears in advance. See Chapter 58, "Popular Supplements for Tinnitus," for more information on the protective benefits of NAC.

Hearing, like vision, doesn't improve with time once it begins to deteriorate. It usually takes about 10 years before hearing loss becomes so noticeable and disruptive to quality of life that it can no longer be ignored. If you suspect any hearing loss, don't delay in addressing it. One effect of the complex interaction between the auditory system and the brain is that you can actually lose the ability to understand sounds that you no longer hear. It's hard to believe that can happen, but the brain stores memories of sounds for only about three years following hearing loss. After seven years, the memory becomes progressively weaker. You may finally decide to get hearing aids, only to discover that there are sounds in your environment that you no longer recognize! If you wait too long, you'll need to relearn all the sounds your brain has forgotten. It would be a great disappointment to listen once again to your favorite music and not be able to appreciate it because your brain fails to recognize what you're hearing.

A note of caution: Beware of advertisements for really cheap hearing aids. They tend to be poorly manufactured and lacking in the proper components as offered by reliable manufacturers. You want to get the best hearing experience you can afford. The ideal situation is to be fitted by a trained audiologist who can guide you in selecting a hearing aid device that matches your needs as well as your budget. Consumer Reports online has a well-written article, "Hearing Aid Buying Guide," to help you get started. It includes buyer experiences and offers good advice for finding the best deal.

If you have a limited budget, you might consider an online seller of hearing aids such as www.HearingDirect.com. Their prices range from approximately $250 to $700 and up, depending on which device you choose. The website includes an online hearing test and buying guides to help you decide which product is best for you. They also indicate a willingness to discuss your personal hearing needs via email, chat or phone. Their hearing aids are preprogrammed for high frequency hearing loss. However, the website states that if you have an audiogram, they will personalize your device to match your hearing loss needs. At the bottom of each page is a contact email and phone number if you want more information. Please note that I am not affiliated with HearingDirect nor am I recommending them. This information is included only as a possible option for those on limited budgets or who simply prefer not to obtain hearing aids through an audiologist or other healthcare provider. HearingDirect also sells phones, alarm clocks and doorbells with amplification or visual alert features.

31
MASKING

For those who are unable to take their mind off tinnitus because the sound is too intrusive, masking is by far the most popular coping mechanism. Masking means listening to a neutral or pleasant sound at a level that is slightly below the volume of your tinnitus. This serves two purposes. First, it helps to cover the discordant sound of tinnitus, so that it isn't the only thing you're hearing. Second, by keeping the volume of the masking below the level of the tinnitus volume, it essentially forces your brain to work harder to hear the masking sound, thereby training it to tune out the tinnitus sound. That's the theory, anyway. Some people get the distinct impression that the tinnitus volume actually increases, as if the tinnitus is fighting to be heard as much as possible. Don't let this discourage you from trying it. For most people, masking is a blessing. They find it very difficult to cope without it for at least part of the day or night. Some people use masking full-time in the first few difficult months of adjusting to tinnitus. Those with chronic severe tinnitus that does not respond to treatment rely on masking to help them function, as it can be extremely useful if they work either in a quiet office or in an environment where there is too much background noise. For example, a busy workplace with people talking, doors being opened and closed, and the hum of numerous electronics can overwhelm someone with moderate to severe tinnitus unless they have a means of blocking out at least some of the sounds.

If you want to use masking without disturbing others who share your space, you can use earbuds or headphones. If your work environment allows you to play audio without affecting anyone else, then you can listen to the masking sounds through your regular speakers. Again, make sure you can hear your tinnitus above the masking. If the masking completely covers the tinnitus, then your brain will not learn to focus its attention away from the tinnitus and toward the masking sound. You'll want to be very careful to keep earbuds or headphones at a very low level, and only use them if you have to. Try to limit as much as possible the length of time you have sound playing directly into your ears. This advice applies to everyone, but even more so if you already have auditory system damage.

The type of tinnitus you have will make a difference in the masking sound you prefer. Whether it's high pitched, low pitched, a drone, a tonal sound, a hiss, a squeal, a ringing, low frequency, mid frequency, high frequency, all these characteristics can influence how effective masking is for you and how you react to it. Fortunately, you have plenty of choices. White noise is very popular, and can be extremely useful for tonal tinnitus that sounds like "eeeeeeeeeeeee." Pink noise is well-suited for tinnitus that sounds like sizzling, electronic hissing, or static. People with tinnitus at low frequencies, usually expressed as a drone or low hum, tend to prefer brown noise. The different noise colors are explained in more detail in Chapter 44, "The Colors of Noise."

An indoor water fountain can be very helpful, as most people find the sound of running water to not only help with masking the tinnitus, but it has an emotionally soothing quality as well. (The shower is a favorite masking method for people with tinnitus, but of course it isn't practical to stay in the shower all day.) YouTube has some wonderful 10-hour videos with a wide variety of water sounds that are excellent for masking in the daytime, and also as a sleep aid at night. You can start the video when you go to bed and it will play straight through to the morning. Go to www.YouTube.com and choose from the videos listed under "Relaxing White Noise" and "Texas High Def." Those are two extremely popular YouTube channels with 10-hour videos that are useful to mask tinnitus, and are especially helpful at night. They also offer very reasonably priced downloadable audio files from their websites if you would like to get a higher quality recording.

Of course, there are many other YouTube channels offering videos that are useful for masking. It's a matter of experimenting to find what you like best. Try using search terms like "white noise," "water fountain," "gentle rain," "seaside," "country meadow," and "crickets." There are thousands to choose from, and the most popular will be displayed first in the results. If one doesn't suit you, try another one. Some sounds are great in the daytime but not at night, and vice versa. Invest some time in listening to different videos until you find the right ones for you. One of my favorites is a bamboo fountain. It has a soft bubbly sound which I enjoy while working on tasks that require minimal concentration. However, I find that it's a bit too intrusive when I need to intensely concentrate. That's one example of why it's helpful to experiment with what kinds of masking sounds work best for different activities.

For superior quality streaming soundscapes, I encourage you to visit www.myNoise.net, which I covered in the previous chapter. It's also featured in the next chapter, "Sound Enrichment." myNoise is developed and maintained by research engineer and sound designer Dr. Stéphane Pigeon. His site is used by soundscape fans around the world. Their testimonials range from tinnitus sufferers who find relief, to people who play sound generators to help them concentrate on work or studies, and of course those who simply need to block out the intrusion of everyday noise. Some folks listen for the sheer enjoyment of hearing a cat purr, or maybe closing their eyes and feeling like they're being transported in a 1940s B-17 Flying Fortress. myNoise has many sound generators to help block out environmental noise, including those with unusual effects, such as Audio Jammer. Dr. Pigeon has written an overview of the usefulness of sound generators in different environments and why they're helpful for conditions such as tinnitus and hyperacusis, at https://mynoise.net/howToUseSoundMachines.php.

Keeping a fan on is another masking technique. A box fan is more likely to give you a white noise effect. Some people run a ceiling fan, as they find that the gentle whirr-whirr-whirr sound helps to cover their tinnitus. Soft music playing in the background can be helpful. Turning on a television set and keeping it at low volume is an excellent way to mask for people who like to feel that there's some kind of activity going on around them. The sound not only helps to mask their tinnitus, it also engages the brain in listening to conversation. It isn't unusual for people to completely forget about their tinnitus while watching television or movies, unless the tinnitus volume is loud. Even then it's helpful as a distraction, to turn your focus away from the tinnitus, if only for a little while.

Bluetooth headsets are a great choice when you want to mask your tinnitus with streaming soundscapes. You can listen to your own private audio without being encumbered by wires and without intruding on the personal hearing space of others around you. Plantronics manufactures an extensive variety of wireless headsets that are ideal for streaming music or sound generators. Their Voyager Focus UC headset has a useful "OpenMic" feature, giving you the option to hear your surroundings without removing the headset. Note that Plantronics has a reputation for manufacturing quality products, and it's reflected in their prices.

Some people have tinnitus that cannot be masked, no matter what level they set the masking volume at. If you have this type of tinnitus, please seek professional advice. Ask your healthcare provider to consider whether you might benefit from taking a medication that can calm your nervous system, which in turn should lead to at least a slight reduction in your perception of tinnitus volume. Xanax and clonazepam are commonly prescribed for daytime use, and Remeron for help in sleeping at night. These are serious medications and should not be taken long-term. However, they may be beneficial to help you clear the hurdle of the first few months, which is usually the most difficult time as far as perception of volume and intrusiveness. I review the most common prescription drugs for tinnitus in Chapter 59, "Prescription Drugs."

❖

Masking is based on the principle that tinnitus symptoms can be reduced by adding pleasant soundscapes to your environment. The next chapter reviews the concept of sound enrichment and the critical role it plays in helping you cope with tinnitus.

32
SOUND ENRICHMENT

Dr. Pawel Jastreboff, creator of tinnitus retraining therapy, theorized that the human auditory system abhors silence, just as nature abhors a vacuum. The eyes and ears of our primitive ancestors were constantly attuned to the smallest bits of sensory information around them because it was necessary for their survival. Those days are gone, but our auditory system still behaves as if danger lurks in silence. Think about those movies where a scene takes place deep in the jungle. The birds are cawing, the insects are buzzing, the jungle is alive with sounds. Suddenly, all sound stops, which is your cue that a dangerous predator has appeared somewhere on the scene. Every creature in the jungle and all the humans are on high alert, straining to hear the faintest sound of the stalking beast.

Most of us no longer worry about panthers and other predators, but our auditory system still equates silence with danger. It turns up the gain to hear the slightest sound whenever we're in an environment that is unnaturally quiet. Many people live their lives in relative quiet and never get tinnitus. Some, however, do develop tinnitus, and they soon learn that silence and increased intrusiveness of tinnitus go hand in hand. It isn't just the silent surroundings that are causing you to hear your tinnitus so clearly. It's the quiet combined with the built-in attentiveness of your auditory system as it searches for clues of impending danger. It simply is doing its job to protect you, and really isn't concerned whether you like peace and quiet or not. It wants to hear everything, so if you have tinnitus, it doesn't make a distinction between phantom sounds versus actual sounds in your environment.

When you deliberately include sound in your environment, your auditory system is no longer focused exclusively on your tinnitus. Sound enrichment reduces the contrast between the tinnitus and complete silence. This makes it harder for the brain to pay attention to the tinnitus. Think of tinnitus as red and silence as white. Place them next to each other and the red really pops. Now replace the white color of silence with sound enrichment. We'll color it brown. There is a lot less contrast between red and brown than there is between red and white. The result is that the brain still notices the red, but it's also paying nearly equal attention to the brown. Your perception of tinnitus will be reduced whenever you can divert all or part of your attention away from it.

Sound enrichment is not intended to completely cover the sound of your tinnitus. With moderate to severe tinnitus, that would create too much of a distraction because the volume would be uncomfortably loud. As with masking, keep it below the threshold of your tinnitus. This will cause your brain to seek out the softer sound with the lower volume. Sound enrichment that is below the threshold of your tinnitus will also contribute to the process of habituation. The goal is to create a safe stimulus that draws the attention of your brain away from tinnitus and toward another sound source.

For most people, their favorite sound enrichment mimics the sounds of nature. Streams, waterfalls, meadows with birdsong, wind in the trees, crickets, storms, and different patterns of rainfall are well suited to masking tinnitus and soothing frayed nerves. You may have noticed that I like to recommend YouTube videos for masking sounds. Unfortunately, to save bandwidth, YouTube compresses audio files. Therefore, if you're going to use sound enrichment, there is no substitute for superior quality audio rendering.

If you want sound enrichment that's easier for your auditory system to process, it's better to purchase CDs of nature tracks rather than relying on compressed audio files from video sharing sites like YouTube. For absolute highest quality, go to www.myNoise.net for masking and sound enrichment. The sound generators mimic nature with such exquisite detail that you won't believe your ears. myNoise offers free streaming audio that you can listen to as long as you like. Each sound is classified under different categories: noise blocker, healthcare, sound therapy, meditation, eerie, tonal, music, calibrated, and headphones. There is cross-over, as well. Sound generators can be included within several categories. For example, if you search for "rain," you will find it in Synthetic Noises, Traffic Noises, and Natural Noises. If you're familiar with binaural beats, there's no substitute for the binaural beats from myNoise. Wear quality headphones, not earbuds, for the binaural beats. It makes a world of difference. To get the most benefit and enjoyment, watch the myNoise Screencasts video tutorials at https://mynoise.net/screencasts.php.

iTunes offers a free myNoise app for iOS devices, with several sound generators on it. Currently they are White Noise, Rain Noise, Binaural Beats, Spring Walk, and Temple Bells. Rain Noise is wonderful when tinnitus is more intrusive at night, as the sound of falling raindrops shifts the focus of your listening to its random patterns. The free myNoise app for Android devices is available on Google Play. You can also purchase individual audio files and albums by myNoise through iTunes, Amazon, Google Play, Spotify, Deezer, and Rdio.

Beltone, a hearing aid company, offers a free Tinnitus Calmer app, which they describe as "a combination of Sound Therapy and relaxing exercises." It's available from both the App Store and Google Play.

Sound enrichment goes hand-in-hand with meditation. The next chapter covers the basics of meditation for tinnitus, including the scientific explanation for why meditation can help you cope with tinnitus and may actually in time lessen its severity.

33
MEDITATION

Meditation has become so widely accepted as a health benefit that it is no longer looked upon as incompatible with Western culture. In fact, meditation is precisely what the Western world needs, something to calm the nerves and slow down our hectic pace. People from all walks of life have discovered that 30 minutes of meditating is far more relaxing, and longer lasting, than a glass of wine or shot of whiskey. Everywhere in the world, people have trained themselves to wake up just a bit earlier than they used to. They use this extra sliver of time to meditate, calm their mind, and start the day refreshed and recharged. Meditation creates balance in your outlook, promotes a positive attitude, and increases your energy level. If you have tinnitus, you will gain even more benefit from meditating than the average person.

People with tinnitus tend to feel constantly stressed from dealing with the unwelcome sounds in their ears and head. Meditation is well-known for relieving stress. When you meditate, it lowers the level of cortisol in your blood serum. Cortisol is a stress hormone that has been nicknamed "public enemy number one" for its adverse and pervasive effects on the human body. There has been speculation that as cortisol levels fluctuate throughout the day, the volume of tinnitus changes. This makes sense, as tinnitus perception tends to increase when one feels stressful and anxious. Many people with tinnitus state that their tinnitus is highest in the morning, then gradually tapers off. This correlates with studies that indicate cortisol levels in the morning are higher in approximately 77% of adults. This is thought to be related to the adrenals preparing the body for the upcoming activities of the day. The cortisol level reaches its highest point about half an hour after awakening. Wouldn't it be nice to suppress that rise by beginning your day with meditation instead of rushing around to get ready for the world outside? Incidentally, an extra benefit of lower cortisol is less accumulation of fat in your body. High cortisol levels have been shown to be responsible for the body creating extra fat. This is likely due to stress mimicking the same responses in the body that the survival instinct creates.

You might be saying, "I would love to try this, but how can I possibly meditate when the tinnitus is so intrusive that it's driving me crazy?" It may be difficult when you first begin, then it becomes easier as time goes on and it becomes a part of your natural routine. The important thing to remember is that the purpose of meditation isn't to train your mind to run away from something. Instead, meditation helps you to observe something in a detached manner, free of emotion. If you've ever practiced meditation before, you already know the basics of doing this. If you haven't, read up on it before beginning. Basically, as you sit still and try to clear your mind, thoughts will intrude. Acknowledge each thought and let it go. By doing so, you shift your reaction to the frontal lobe and away from the limbic system, as discussed in Chapter 65, "Train the Brain - Exercises."

Learning to be detached from your obsessive thoughts about tinnitus is something that comes with the passage of time. Devoting daily time to the practice of meditation helps with that gradual process of emotional detachment. If you have a busy life and feel like you just can't set aside 30 minutes a day to meditate, which is what most practitioners recommend, then set aside 10 minutes a day. Spend less time on the Internet, read one less chapter in a book, curtail your phone time by 10 minutes, and do something that will make a positive difference in how tinnitus affects you. Try it for 21 days, which is the generally recognized time it takes to form a habit, or at least give it solid momentum. Once you've invested 21 days, there is a natural inclination to continue, especially if you're beginning to notice some benefits.

Pick the same time every day, as both the body and mind thrive on regular habits. For example, after a shower is a good opportunity for a meditation session. Wrap yourself in a soft robe and bask in the sensation of not being restricted by garments. As has been noted, taking a shower masks tinnitus completely in many people. Even if it's only temporary, that can be enough to set the stage for a positive outlook. Moving water has the added benefit of producing negative ions, which naturally makes us feel better. That's why people gravitate to fountains and waterfalls. It's why the air feels wonderfully charged after a powerful thunderstorm, due to the high concentration of negative ions released into the air. There has been a lot of hype about miraculous cures from negative ions, but the science is sound as far as proving that people do feel better when there is a concentration of negative ions in the air. Take advantage of the privacy and the atmosphere after having taken a shower, and spend at least 10 minutes in meditation before venturing back into the reality of day-to-day life.

The great thing about meditation is that once you feel comfortable with it, you can do it whenever and wherever you get the chance. If you go for a walk in the woods and find a large rock to sit on, take a break from your walk to meditate for five minutes, appreciating the beauty of nature around you. If you're at an event and the commotion becomes too intense, step outside or into an unoccupied room and take a two-minute meditation break. As time goes on, it will be easier for you to quickly slip into a meditative state and calm your mind.

In researching meditation as it relates to tinnitus, I discovered that two forms of meditation are generally preferred: guided meditation, also known as mindfulness meditation, and Vipassana meditation. Silence isn't required for meditation. If your tinnitus is intrusive and you feel like you just can't ignore it, you might want to play some calming music while you meditate. Choose background music that helps to mask the tinnitus but doesn't grab your attention. Meditation is so popular that there's no shortage of peaceful music to choose from, either locally or online. Find something that resonates with you and helps you to remain still and focused.

Vyanah is a popular YouTube channel for calming music, whether for meditating or simply to play in the background while working on tasks. Some of his videos are designed to enhance delta brain wave activity, the brain waves most associated with relaxation and soothing of hyperactive brain neurons. Tinnitus is more likely to fade into the background when the body is calm and the brain is producing more delta wave activity. Vyanah describes his channel as "Music for Meditation and Inner Balance."

Some people choose to meditate in the evening, usually just before bedtime. With the day behind you, it's the ideal time to set aside any thoughts of things you need to do. Light a lavender-scented candle, and allow yourself to completely relax your body as well as your mind.

34
SLEEPING

I mentioned in an earlier chapter about how tinnitus can fade into the background when you're busy and keeping your focus on something which is important to you. The opposite is also true. When you don't have something to distract you and instead you're only paying attention to your tinnitus, especially if you become anxious about its volume, your brain is going to ramp up the sound. This is why tinnitus tends to bother people most at night. Think about your own current nightly routine. You're lying in bed, ready to sleep. You've probably turned off the television or set aside the book you've been reading. There's nothing external for you to focus on, and so here comes tinnitus to center stage. You want to sleep, but you're hearing eeeeeeeeeee, or tssss tssss tssss, or cicadas, or some kind of ringing or bells shimmering or maybe even train brakes screeching on rails. The tinnitus brain can really act up when your mind isn't engaged in a distracting activity, which is why it's so common for tinnitus to interfere with falling asleep.

There's another reason for tinnitus volume increasing at night. It has to do with your body's built-in defense system. Our primitive ancestors relied heavily on two very important senses to survive: vision, and hearing. Have you ever closed your eyes while listening to a song to enjoy it more? Have you ever turned down the radio when driving through an unfamiliar area so you could pay closer attention to signs and landmarks? If so, you understand that whenever one very important sense is reduced, the other one heightens. Humans have evolved so that when vision is effectively turned off during sleep, the brain compensates by increasing your sense of hearing. Thus, the volume of your tinnitus seems to go up at night. The sense of hearing is so important to our survival that we cannot shut it off anatomically, the same way we can close our eyes and shut off our vision. This is what makes tinnitus incredibly frustrating, that we feel like we can never get away from it, except during sleep.

Tinnitus actually doesn't stop when you go to sleep. You may not consciously hear it while you're asleep, but it's there, it can wake you up, and it can be louder than normal. If this happens to you, do your best not to react emotionally. Take slow, deep breaths, and the tinnitus should calm down fairly soon and return to baseline.

Tinnitus is most likely to awaken you after a dream. Sleep takes place in five stages, one of which is the dreaming stage, also called the Rapid Eye Movement (REM) stage. In the REM stage, your brain activity increases. In fact, it's been proven with electroencephalogram (EEG) studies that your brain is almost as active when you're dreaming as when you're awake. No wonder the sound of tinnitus can break through and wake you up. Some unfortunate folks hear tinnitus in their dreams, but most do not. If it breaks through and becomes too pronounced in your dream, it's quite possible that you will wake up, just as you would awaken to the sound of an alarm clock.

Going to sleep, and staying asleep, is a major issue for a lot of people who suffer from intrusive tinnitus. This tends to be more of an issue in the first few months, but the problem can linger for years if not addressed. Getting enough sleep can be difficult even under ordinary circumstances. However, when you have a constant sound in your ears or your head, it may become a real challenge. It's well known that the quality and quantity of your sleep can affect how you perceive your tinnitus when you're awake, just as quality and quantity of sleep can affect how you perceive pain during your waking hours. It also seems to be true for many people that the volume of tinnitus improves with sufficient sleep and worsens with lack of sleep, probably because resistance to stress is lower. It's ironic that the one thing we need most to help us deal with tinnitus is disrupted because of our tinnitus.

A helpful device for masking tinnitus at night is a sound generator which creates pleasing sounds designed for relaxation. They are often called sleep machines because so many people find them useful to help them go to sleep in noisy environments. These devices have become increasingly sophisticated in their ability to replicate the sounds of nature and everyday life. One sleep machine I looked at online, Ecotone, has 10 different sound categories: waterfall, fireplace, ocean, meadow, train, city, rainfall, brook, meditation, and white noise. Each sound category allows you to make adjustments by adding different elements. For example, in the meadows selection, you can add the buzzing of bees, flapping of wings, birds singing, and other nature sounds. I was pleasantly surprised to discover that the white noise is not just restricted to a choice of only white noise. You can change it to a low-pitched brown noise, a medium-pitched pink noise, or even a higher-pitched white noise. This is excellent for people with tinnitus, who often find that one sound frequency is irritating but another is easy to listen to. If you search online for "sleep sound machines," you'll find plenty of manufacturers who offer different features to suit your preferences.

In Chapter 32, "Sound Enrichment," I explained the importance to the auditory system of avoiding absolute quiet if you have tinnitus. For almost two years I deliberately kept my surroundings quiet whenever I could, including at night. Even if my brain was manufacturing tinnitus, I still wanted to go to sleep in the same way as I always had, in a dark and quiet environment. That is, quiet except for the sounds in my head. I used various methods of deep breathing techniques and even self-hypnosis to fall asleep, despite the tinnitus hissing and oscillating. Now that I've researched sound enrichment and the importance of avoiding quiet if you have tinnitus, I make sure that some level of sound is generated throughout the night. There are people who prefer not to do this, believing that their ears need to rest during the night, but the truth is that your auditory system never rests anyway. Whether your bedroom is quiet or whether you're playing an audio with soft sounds to lull you to sleep, your auditory system is working at listening to everything going on. The rustle of your bedsheets as you change positions, the sound of your slow breaths while in deep sleep, the tapping of rain against the window or the soft padding sounds of your dog going to its water bowl for a drink, all of these sounds are noted by your brain and classified as harmless, so you continue to sleep. But if anything creaks, if the doorknob turns in the middle of the night, you're up in a flash because your brain recognizes that as out of the ordinary and awakens you to tend to it. So, don't worry about giving your ears a rest. They'll be fine.

There are supporting reasons for sound enrichment at night. First, by keeping the volume just below the threshold of your tinnitus volume, you will continue the process of habituation. When you give your ears something to focus on other than tinnitus, it tells your brain that the tinnitus is not important. In other words, it's not the only player in the game; it's got competition.

Second, it's very common for someone with tinnitus to wake up one or more times during the night. If you wake up and all you hear is your tinnitus, it can be difficult to go back to sleep. Unfortunately, it's not unusual for tinnitus to actually be louder when you wake up in the night than it is during the day, which adds to the difficulty. However, if you wake up and you have soothing sound enrichment in your bedroom, you can turn your attention to that, making it easier to calm your nerves and return to sleep. The rain sound generators on the myNoise website are relaxing and a good choice if you want to drift back into sleep. Rain Noise is a favorite of people who are calmed by the sound of rain. You can either use one of the myNoise apps mentioned in Chapter 32, "Sound Enrichment," or you can connect your smartphone or computer via Bluetooth to a mini speaker on your nightstand, visit the website, and stream whichever sound generator helps you to feel calm and relaxed. Do your best to avoid focusing on your tinnitus and turn your attention instead to the gentle flow of the soundscape. Another favorite is the Distant Thunder soundscape. It has no thunderclaps which can startle you, but for those who love the sound of rain and thunder, it's remarkably peaceful and may be just what you need to lull you into sleep.

If you use sound enrichment at night and it helps you fall asleep but then it wakes you up during the night, try playing the sounds for only a set amount of time. You can do this by playing a CD in a device that turns off when it's finished, or with a sound machine that includes a timer function. Set the timer so that you have enough time to go to sleep plus another half hour or so. That way you won't feel like you have to "hurry up and go to sleep." myNoise sound generators have a timer function, located beneath the slider settings. This is very useful for falling asleep without worrying that the sound will awaken you before morning.

If nighttime sound enrichment doesn't help you to fall asleep, or if it seems to make the perception of your tinnitus worse, you'll need to consider other ways to help you relax. However, do continue to use sound enrichment during the day when you're up and about.

I mentioned in Chapter 14, "How It Begins," that tinnitus is linked with the sleep cycle. The intensity of tinnitus can change drastically, for better or worse, after a night's sleep. This seems to be most noticeable in those who have cycling tinnitus. People who have constant tinnitus tend to experience a softening of their tinnitus upon awakening if they've had a deep and restful sleep the night before. That isn't always the case, but at the very least a good night's sleep will decrease stress and help you to cope with your tinnitus better. You probably know from personal experience that even the slightest irritation becomes magnified when you're suffering from sleep deprivation. Lack of sleep also downgrades dopamine receptors in the brain, meaning they don't operate as efficiently as they should. People with tinnitus need to be especially careful to maintain a healthy dopamine level.

Taking a short nap reduces the intensity of tinnitus for some folks, but for others it will almost certainly make it much worse, at least temporarily. There are many people with tinnitus who dare not take a nap, because it's almost guaranteed that upon awakening their tinnitus will be high volume, regardless whether it was mild, moderate, or severe just prior to the nap. They often decide that having loud tinnitus that lasts for hours afterwards isn't worth the short nap. Starting up the tinnitus is part of the brain's coming to consciousness routine now, whether you're waking up in the morning with an alarm clock, waking up from a nap, or waking up during the night. Some people will have their tinnitus kick into high gear if they doze off for even a few seconds. It's an unfortunate and upsetting side effect of this affliction.

Neuroimaging studies have revealed that otherwise healthy adults who experience persistent sleep deprivation show increased activity in the amygdala (located in the limbic system), and decreased volume in the frontal, temporal, and parietal lobes. Remember that the frontal lobe is the executive center of the brain where higher thinking processes take place; the temporal lobe is where the auditory cortex is located; and the parietal lobe processes sensory information such as touch, taste, and temperature. The frontal lobe is crucial for taking control away from the limbic system in regards to how one perceives and reacts to their tinnitus. Researchers haven't determined if sleep loss causes these changes in brain volume, or if the changes in volume occurred first and that's what triggered the sleep loss. There is also a reduction of volume in the frontal lobe of people with long-term chronic tinnitus. Again, researchers aren't sure whether the tinnitus itself is responsible for the loss of volume in the frontal lobe, or whether a loss of volume in the frontal lobe contributes to causation of tinnitus. Perhaps it's tied to the disrupted sleep patterns of people with moderate to severe tinnitus. It's interesting to note that seniors are more often afflicted with tinnitus than any other age group, and that is also the time of life when it becomes increasingly difficult for many of them to get a good night's sleep.

Functional magnetic resonance imaging studies have also shown that sleep loss negatively affects the connection between the amygdala and the medial prefrontal cortex (MPC). The MPC is the part of your brain that helps you to regulate feelings, such as keeping you calm in stressful situations and tamping down your anger when provoked. When this connection is disrupted or cut off from lack of sleep, the amygdala asserts its dominance and makes it more of a challenge to control your emotions. From a primitive point of view, this makes sense. If you're awakened by an immediate threat, you have to react instinctively and aggressively. You can't stand there and weigh your options and consider possible consequences, or you might not survive an attack. The amygdala does its job very well, but it can be harmful to your emotional well-being when you're sleep deprived, especially during those times when it's difficult for you to control your emotional reactions to tinnitus. It's not your fault if you become enraged, feel panicky, or cry in frustration. That's your amygdala talking, so be patient and forgiving with yourself when that happens. If you find yourself consistently losing emotional control because you're unable to sleep by using natural means and methods, it may be wise to talk to your healthcare provider about an over-the-counter or prescription strength sleep aid to help you stabilize your sleep patterns so you can regain your emotional balance.

If you're interested in learning more about how lack of sleep affects your health and everyday life, visit www.BrainHQ.com. Their blog features a detailed Sleep Loss Infographic. Click on the image to expand it for easier reading. You might be surprised to learn the many different ways that chronic sleep deprivation can harm your brain. For example, "Sleeping Disorder Statistics" on www.StatisticBrain.com reveals some sobering facts, such as 40,000 nonfatal vehicular accidents every year are caused by sleep deprivation, and 1,550 fatalities. You'll be helping yourself and others if you do your best to make sure you're as well-rested as possible every day.

Before tinnitus, except for an occasional restless episode, it was always easy for me to fall asleep and then sleep through the night. Even in the first few months after acquiring tinnitus, by using self-hypnosis techniques to relax and fall asleep, I slept pretty much through the night. As time went on, however, nothing was helping, and it often took one or two hours to fall asleep. I would also awaken two to five times each night with the tinnitus blaring in my head, like an alarm clock with its own schedule. By the end of the first year, I was becoming seriously sleep deprived, averaging four and a half to five hours per night. This lasted through February of 2016. I was consistently sleep deprived for a year and a half, and it was really taking a toll on my health. Then came a particularly bad night when the tinnitus was roaring in waves in my head until 3:00 a.m. The next day I was determined to find something to help me sleep, something that would knock me out so I could escape the tinnitus when it became unbearable. Like many people, I resist taking any sort of medication, but sometimes the body needs extra help.

I researched online, read hundreds of reviews, and narrowed it down to two choices: diphenhydramine, the active ingredient in Benadryl; and doxylamine succinate, the active ingredient in Unisom. The local pharmacist suggested that the doxylamine succinate was the better choice for restful sleep. I bought the product, and read more reviews when I came home. Each pill is 25mg, but there were many reviewers who said they took only half a pill and were pleased with the results. That night I took half a pill of generic doxylamine succinate, and slept through the night for the first time in over a year. I continue to take 12.5mg regularly, it still works just as well, and I think it's having a positive effect on my tinnitus. At the very least, on the days when the tinnitus is more intrusive, I'm better able to cope with it if I've had seven or eight hours of sleep instead of only five or six, and I no longer wake up several times a night. When I do wake up in the middle of the night, it's fairly easy to fall asleep again.

One more thing on the subject of sleep. For severely disrupted sleep, there is a possibility that sleep apnea is the problem. Sleep apnea can cause hearing loss, and is sometimes linked to tinnitus as well. CPAP therapy (Continuous Positive Airway Pressure) is an effective method of treating obstructive sleep apnea. This could in turn reduce the severity of

35
METHODS FOR BETTER SLEEP

Sleep deprivation is an epidemic in modern society. Industrialization has interfered with our natural biological rhythms to the point where approximately 40 percent of the adult population and close to 25 percent of the adolescent population do not get sufficient sleep on a regular basis. The reasons for lack of sleep are numerous. However, four typical reasons are (1) cutting back on sleep due to a desire to be regarded as a productive human being in an overly competitive society; (2) school and work schedules that conflict with our natural sleep-and-wake cycles; (3) a physical or mental condition which interferes with sleep; and, (4) technology devices for information and entertainment that keep us artificially alert when we should be settling in and preparing for a restful night's sleep.

Moderate to severe tinnitus can be disruptive to the sleep cycle, as it not only makes going to sleep more difficult, it can also disturb the natural phases of sleep by waking you up two or more times during the night. The closer to your normal waking time the tinnitus disrupts your sleep, the harder it is to get back to sleep. It's not unusual for people with severe tinnitus to only get five hours of sleep a night. This mean they have a continuing deficit of anywhere from one to four hours of sleep night after night. There's no making up for lost sleep on the weekends either. Tinnitus doesn't allow it.

You'll remember from the prior chapter that long-term sleep deprivation is associated with loss of volume in the prefrontal cortex and excess activity of the amygdala, and that people with chronic tinnitus display similar findings on neuroimaging studies. If you have tinnitus, it's very important to get sufficient sleep, not just for the sake of your overall health, but to help you cope with tinnitus and function in your work and personal life. It isn't a hopeless situation. There are things you can do in your waking hours that will make a difference, as well as things to avoid doing as your bedtime hour approaches. Most of the following recommendations are common sense advice that you've probably heard before, but are included here in the context of helping you to cope with tinnitus and possibly helping to improve the tinnitus condition itself.

If you stay inside most of the day with nothing but artificial light surrounding you, it's important for you to get outside and enjoy some natural direct sunlight. Not only do you need sunlight to help your body manufacture vitamin D, but sunlight entering the eye and reaching the retina helps to maintain a natural circadian rhythm. (The circadian rhythm is your biological cycle that occurs once every approximately 24 hours.) If tinnitus has caused you to constantly have problems falling asleep until long past midnight, followed by difficulty waking up in the morning, your sleep phase rhythm may have become irregular. This is known as delayed sleep phase disorder. It's common in adolescents because school schedules are incompatible with the unique circadian rhythms of youth, and it develops in people who work swing shifts or whose personal life situations interfere with their ability to sleep. Older adults have the opposite problem, in that they find themselves becoming fatigued and going to bed much earlier than in years past. They wake up long before dawn, unable to return to sleep. This is known as advanced sleep phase disorder.

If you find yourself struggling with either disorder, an hour dose of sunlight every day may help you to reset your internal clock so that you can fall asleep and wake up in a healthier pattern, making it easier to function in your work and home life. It's best to get that one hour dose of sunshine at the same time every day, because the time of day you expose yourself to sunlight matters when you're trying to reset your circadian rhythm to its natural state. If you're staying up too late and waking up much later than you want, get the sunshine in as soon as possible after awakening. If you're going to bed too early and waking up in the wee hours of the morning, unable to return to sleep, take in some sunshine as late in the day as possible.

It isn't always practical to stay outside for an hour at the same time every day. The sun isn't always shining, you may have long working hours with demanding deadlines and unreliable schedules, and the weather doesn't always cooperate, particularly in rainy climes. Luckily, a light box or light visor can achieve the same effect by mimicking natural sunlight. This is the same type of device that's used to treat seasonal affective disorder, also known as SAD. These devices have become increasingly sophisticated, including being able to produce powerful therapeutic light without the damaging UV rays. This means you can set them nearby and enjoy the light without worrying about damage to your eyes or skin that UV rays can cause. You can find these devices locally or online at budget-friendly prices. Look for one with at least 10,000 lumens at 12 inches. The distance from the light is important, as the further away you set the light, the more time you will need to be exposed to it. Follow the instructions that come with it to ensure you're using it correctly to obtain the best benefit. Be sure to pay attention to any safety precautions included in the instructions.

If you have delayed sleep phase disorder where it's hard to fall asleep at night and difficult to wake up in the morning, you'll want to begin your light therapy treatment by setting your alarm so that you awaken one hour before your usual rise time. For example, if you're regularly falling asleep at 2 a.m. and sleeping until 10 a.m., set your alarm for 9 a.m. Use the light therapy as soon as you awaken, for 30 minutes to as long as two hours, depending on how much time you have available. After several days of treatment, it should feel more natural for you to awaken at 9 a.m., and you may even begin waking before the alarm goes off. Now set your alarm to 8 a.m., and once again use the light therapy upon awakening for 30 minutes up to two hours. Repeat the light therapy for several days. When you're waking easily at 8 a.m. but would still like to get up earlier in the day, set your alarm for 7 a.m., and repeat the light therapy routine until you're comfortably waking up at that time, feeling alert and able to function well. If you want to establish an earlier waking time, keep repeating the steps until you're easily waking up at the desired time. When you begin arising with ease earlier in the morning, it should naturally follow that you become sleepier earlier in the night. Instead of feeling the need for sleep at midnight or 1 a.m. or 2 a.m., you will probably begin to feel sleepy enough for bedtime at 10 p.m. or 11 p.m. As time goes by, if you find yourself slipping back into delayed sleep phase disorder, repeat the process again.

For advanced sleep phase disorder, that is, going to bed too early and waking up too early, you will be using the light therapy in the evening. If you have been overcome with drowsiness at 8 p.m. and find yourself waking up at 4 a.m. the next morning, use the light therapy at 6 p.m. for one hour. Do this several days in a row and see if your drowsiness is delayed until 9 p.m., with awakening at 5 a.m. Many people really enjoy getting up that early in the morning, as long as they feel alert and ready to face the day. If that's still too early for you, use the light therapy at 7 p.m. for one hour. This should delay your drowsiness until 10 p.m., and allowing you to awaken at 6 a.m. If that doesn't suit you and you want to move your bedtime up even further, use one hour of light therapy at 8 p.m. for several days, and see if you start becoming sleepy at 11 p.m. and waking at 7 a.m.

Generally speaking, to treat advanced sleep phase disorder, use the light therapy three hours before you want to fall asleep. That's one hour of light therapy, with the goal being that you will become drowsy enough to fall asleep two hours after the session ends. The schedules given here assume sleeping for eight hours a night, so you'll need to adjust the light therapy schedule if you want less or more sleep.

Light therapy, or phototherapy as it's sometimes called, is basically the reorganization of a disrupted circadian rhythm and should not be performed without first discussing the procedure with your healthcare practitioner. A rare side effect may occur from using phototherapy to treat delayed sleep phase disorder, in which your circadian rhythm becomes longer; for example, 25 hours. In time, as the extra hour accumulates, this 25-hour cycle leads to a need for sleep in the daytime with alertness at night for part of the month, and then sleeping at night with alertness occurring during the day for the remainder of the month. For most people, this would result in being out of sync with their personal and work relationships.

Please keep in mind that phototherapy, for whatever use it's being applied, can cause the following side effects: headache, particularly in people who are prone to migraines; photophobia, literally "fear of light," which is a condition of increased sensitivity to light; hypomania, an exaggerated elevation of mood; and irritability or mood swings. If you experience any of these side effects, you are not a good candidate for phototherapy. You and your healthcare practitioner will need to discuss an alternate method of establishing a healthy sleep pattern.

I mentioned technology as a sleep disruptor. The temptation of being able to instantly access information and entertainment can be overwhelming, particularly for someone with tinnitus who is trying to distract themselves by focusing on something interesting. If you have tinnitus and ADHD, you have the dual challenge of trying to stay focused on a single distraction, but you're also dealing with a lower threshold of resistance to multiple distractions. When you go to bed and take your Kindle Fire, your iPad, or other tablet with you, it's easy for one, two, or three hours to quickly pass by as you go from website to website or from game to game. Instead of allowing your mind to settle down, you're keeping it alert and engaged, which is extremely counterproductive for falling into a relaxing sleep. Note that this is less of an issue with E-ink readers, like the Kindle Paperwhite, as their function is limited to reading.

It isn't just the mental stimulation that keeps you awake after you've set aside the Kindle Fire or other tablet. A lot of research has been conducted on the effects that device screens have on our brains at night, and the results are discouraging. The problem is the excess blue light emission from the screens, which suppresses the natural level of melatonin production. In Chapter 58, "Popular Supplements for Tinnitus," I discuss melatonin, the hormone secreted by the pineal gland and helpful for promoting sleep. As we get older, melatonin production naturally decreases. Exposing yourself before bedtime to any kind of light interferes with the body's natural sleep process, whether it's the illumination of a light bulb or the glowing light from your television. Incidentally, if you've been using those curly-shaped energy-saving light bulbs, be aware that they emit more blue light than incandescent light bulbs.

The best thing you can do is to stay away from all your electronic devices at least an hour before bedtime, but that might be asking too much of anyone who is addicted to technology. Some of the newer devices feature a blue light blocking option, which may or may not switch on automatically at night. Check your device to see if it offers this feature as an option, and be sure to use it at night if it does. There are apps which will automatically adjust the screen to match your environment lighting. One of these is f.lux, which is available for Windows, iPhone, iPad, Mac, Linux, and Android devices.

You can buy blue light blocking screen protectors for your electronic devices if they don't have that built-in option. You can also purchase blue light blocking glasses to wear in the daytime and at night. Their purpose is to ease the eyestrain that comes from spending hours in front of a computer screen, but they serve double duty by blocking UV light, including blue light. The more popular blue light blocking glasses are made with reader glasses strength and are also available without magnification. One of these is the Gamma Ray Flexlite brand. They are very reasonably priced, and have an overall fairly high rating in Amazon customer reviews.

To avoid excess blue light at night, use alternative illumination in your home. Make the switch to warmer colors like amber and red. They interfere the least with your melatonin production that's necessary for sleep and other biological functions. Dedicate one lamp in the living room and each bedroom to either amber or red light, and switch to that lighting a couple hours before bedtime. Amber light in particular casts a warm and comforting glow, and as a bonus it's wonderful for flattering skin tones. If any member of your household needs a night light for comfort or safety, there are amber night lights available to help them see in the darkness without activating the waking response that even a low wattage typical night light can cause.

Being sedentary isn't good for you, for many reasons. But when you have tinnitus, it becomes even more important to become physically active and as fit as possible, depending on your circumstances. With a healthy body, you will be better able to cope with your tinnitus. Getting regular exercise during the day has been proven to result in better quality of sleep at night. This doesn't mean you need to have the athletic level of a marathon runner. Any exercise, including a simple cardiovascular workout like walking every day, will elevate the levels of the neurotransmitter GABA in your brain. This in turn will help to inhibit the hyperexcited neurons that play a role in your tinnitus. If you haven't exercised in a long time or if you have any restrictive medical conditions, ask your healthcare practitioner for guidance on how to begin. If you don't like outdoor exercise, there are plenty of indoor exercise equipment products on the market. One which is fairly easy to use is a mini stair-stepper. It doesn't take up much space, so you can watch television to pass the time while you're on it. The mini stair-stepper products usually include rubber cords to add an upper body workout, and you can track your progress with the built-in digital meter. When you first start using the stepper, keep a high-backed chair close by in case you need to hold on to something for balance until you become accustomed to it.

One thing that sleep experts agree on is that your bedroom should be devoted only to sleeping and intimacy with your partner. There should be no televisions and no computers in your bedroom. Draw the drapes to block any glaring porch lights or street lights shining into your bedroom. For illumination, use a lamp with an amber bulb. If you and your partner like aromatherapy, lavender is very conducive to relaxation. Your sheets need to be clean and comfortable. If your mattress is getting old and doesn't support your back as it should, consider replacing it or buying a memory foam topper. There are many choices for memory foam toppers, from sink-down-into-it soft to very firm. Not only will your bed be more comfortable for your back, these toppers can extend the useful life of your mattress. You'll find a wide selection on www.overstock.com, with plenty of customer reviews as a helpful guide for deciding which one to buy.

To promote sleep, conventional wisdom says it's good to keep the room temperature on the cooler side, but evidence now suggests that this isn't always the case. What's comfortably cool for one person may be uncomfortably chilly for another. Experiment with adjusting the thermostat and see if you begin sleeping for longer periods of time. If you've been keeping it cool, turn up the heat a bit, and vice versa. As already noted, any tech devices with screens need to have a blue light blocking shield, or you can wear blue light blocking glasses while using them at night. However, it's much better if you abandon using such devices altogether in your bedroom. If you like to read, visit your local library or bookstore and get some books for your bedroom. You can rediscover the joy of reading the old-fashioned way, turning actual pages and reading words on paper. A 60-watt amber light works just as well for reading at night as the traditional white incandescent light bulb.

There are other things you can do to create a good night's sleep. Half an hour of meditation before bedtime, even if it's nothing more than closing your eyes, listening to soothing music, and imagining peaceful scenery, tells your brain that it's time to relax. Remember that closing the eyes increases alpha waves, which promotes a sense of calm. If you prefer to take a bath or shower at night instead of in the morning, do so two hours before bedtime and not just before. Immersion in warm water raises your body temperature a degree or two. If you wait a couple hours before bedtime, the gradual drop in body temperature afterwards is more likely to put you into a deep sleep. Another thing you can do is to set out your clothes and accessories for the next day, giving you the freedom of one less task to take care of the next morning. Nightly writing in a journal, whether it's two or three sentences or several paragraphs, is an excellent way to clear your head of any troubling thoughts or to end the day with pleasant memories. The point here is that you want to establish a regular comfortable routine that your mind and body recognize as a reliable signal that you're preparing yourself for sleep.

If you're familiar with the concept of biofeedback, you may want to consider 2breathe, an FDA-approved device available from www.2breathe.com. Worn around your torso, it measures your respiration and uses gentle tones to guide your breathing, and provides visual feedback through your smartphone. You can watch a demonstration on the 2Breathe Sleep inducer YouTube video. The cost is a reasonable $180 for this sophisticated device. They offer a 60-day guarantee, as well as online and phone support.

A simple but apparently effective approach to feeling more rested is to wake up when you're in your lightest sleep phase. As the saying goes, there's an app for that. The Sleep Cycle alarm clock app is highly rated on both Google Play and the App Store, in free and premium versions. You can learn more about this app on their "How it works" page, at https://www.sleepcycle.com/how-it-works/.

36
SUPPLEMENTS TO HELP YOU SLEEP

Sometimes you need a little extra help to ease your mind and body into a relaxed and drowsy state. Even if you do everything right, such as maintaining a healthy lifestyle and adopting a regular pre-bedtime routine, tinnitus can still turn your bed into a nightly struggle to fall asleep. In that case, there are online supplements and over-the-counter remedies that can help. I'll focus on seven which are generally recognized as safe by the medical establishment. They also have a solid reputation amongst consumers, as well as scientifically-based evidence to support the claims of being reliable sleep aids. These seven favorites are passionflower, magnolia bark, tart cherry juice, hops, lemon balm, chamomile, and valerian.

Passionflower, also known as Sign of the Cross, is a plant with a unique and beautiful flower. It has traditionally been used for treating anxiety and insomnia, but has also been used in the treatment of seizures, ADHD, symptoms of menopause, and high blood pressure, to name a few. It is considered to be a mild sedative which works by increasing the level of GABA in the brain. In earlier chapters I noted that hyperactive brain neurons have been linked to tinnitus. Increasing the level of GABA lowers that hyperactivity. Anxiety is often a component of tinnitus, and passionflower has been shown to be as effective as oxazepam (Serax) in the treatment of generalized anxiety disorder. Studies have shown that it takes longer to achieve results with passionflower, but produces less impairment in job functions. You can choose to buy passionflower extract in capsules, teas, and tinctures. Do not take passionflower if you are pregnant. It is absolutely not safe for pregnant women because some of its chemical compounds can cause the uterus to contract. Also, do not use passionflower for at least two weeks before any scheduled surgery, as it does affect the central nervous system and might strengthen the effects of anesthesia and other medications.

Magnolia bark is growing in popularity as a sleep aid because it has the dual effects of inducing relaxation and lowering cortisol. You'll recall from prior chapters that high cortisol levels are thought to contribute to increased tinnitus volume. It's also possible for cortisol to spike during the night, which can cause you to awaken and be unable to fall back asleep. If you fall asleep fairly easily but wake up during the night, you might try taking 200 to 300mg of magnolia bark at bedtime to see if that resolves the problem of interrupted sleep.

Magnolia bark is discussed more thoroughly in Chapter 58, "Popular Supplements for Tinnitus," because it has additional potential benefits for people with tinnitus, including its anti-inflammatory and neuroprotective properties.

Tart cherry extract and tart cherry juice have become increasingly popular as a sleep remedy. One study reported that drinking one to two cups of tart cherry juice every day reduces insomnia. The likely reason for its ability to induce sleep is its high melatonin content. Another contributor is its high proanthocyanidin content, which gives the cherries their brilliant ruby color. The proanthocyanidin slows down the breakdown of tryptophan in the body, which makes it effective for a longer period of time. Tryptophan is an amino acid which, when combined with vitamin B6, transforms into niacin and the inhibitory neurotransmitter serotonin, helping to promote a relaxed state.

Drinking tart cherry juice regularly can be somewhat costly, but you will get the same benefit from tart cherry extract in capsule form. Solgar has a reputation for high quality supplements. You can read the reviews for their product on Amazon. Many of the reviews address the anti-inflammatory benefits of tart cherry, as well as using it for a sleep aid. If you have aches and pains that are keeping you awake along with your tinnitus, tart cherry juice may deliver double benefits.

Hops is the common name for the female flowers of *Humulus lupulus*. Most people are familiar with hops being used in beer. Hop tea is a natural sedative due to the bitter resins in the hop leaves. Like passionflower, one of the pharmacological effects of hops is to increase the activity of GABA. People have been using hops for centuries as a natural sedative, but research has indicated that it's most likely to be effective when combined with valerian. Hops by itself and hops with valerian are available in extract form in capsules or as a tincture. Keep in mind that hops is a phytoestrogen, meaning a plant with estrogen-mimicking properties. Although it's sometimes used as an herbal medicine to treat menopausal symptoms, do not take hops if you have thyroid disease or any condition which can be worsened with additional estrogen in your system.

Lemon balm, *Melissa officinalis*, is an herb in the mint family. It contains terpenes, a natural chemical thought to be responsible for its relaxing effects. Lemon balm can be an effective sleep aid if anxiety is keeping you awake. In teas, it is often combined with other relaxation herbs, such as chamomile, passionflower, and most often valerian. Lemon balm extract, when taken by itself in 600 mg doses, has been shown to elevate mood and increase calmness. One study of patients with mild to moderate Alzheimer's showed less agitation in the patients taking lemon balm than in the control group which only received a placebo. Agitation is a state of emotional disturbance when someone feels tense, restless, or irritable. If your tinnitus causes you to feel these types of emotions, try some lemon balm to see if it relaxes you emotionally as well as physically. Some reports indicate that lemon balm can produce enough of a sedated effect that it reduces one's mental sharpness, so keep that in mind and don't take it when you need to remain alert.

No sleep aid list is complete without including Sleepytime Extra from Celestial Seasonings, a delightfully fragrant and soul-soothing tea that is ideal for bedtime. The box features an illustration of a charming nightgown-clad bear, snoozing happily beneath a quarter moon. It's like an open invitation for you to join him and do the same. Sleepytime Extra is an extraordinary blend of chamomile, valerian, spearmint, and other herbs. Chamomile has been used for centuries as a botanical sleep aid. Some researchers believe chamomile is a natural sedative because it contains antigenin, an antioxidant compound which affects brain chemicals involved in sleep. Valerian is a flowering perennial, with sweetly scented pink or white flowers that bloom in summer. The fragrance is so appealing that valerian flower extracts were used as a perfume in the 16th century. When you make a tea with the aroma of valerian at bedtime, you're combining a natural sleep aid with a form of aromatherapy, making it easier to feel relaxed and calm.

Although supplements may be relatively inexpensive and easier to obtain than prescription meds, they do affect your body chemistry and should be considered as serious medicine. The information I've listed is just a summary of some helpful herbs and compounds that are known to be mild sedatives when used according to package directions. If you decide to take any of these supplements to help you sleep better, please research the particular herb or supplement. This will give you a good idea of the possible side effects, contraindications, and manufacturer's warnings associated with the product. Any herbal supplement, no matter how safe you think it may be, should be taken under the supervision of a healthcare practitioner Having a chronic medical condition requires a greater degree of caution. This is even more important if you are currently taking any prescription medication.

Sedative-type herbs, because they can sometimes affect serotonin levels, should never be used if you are taking a selective serotonin reuptake inhibitor, commonly referred to as an SSRI. The most commonly prescribed SSRIs include citalopram (Celexa), escitalopram (Lexapro), fluoxetine (Prozac), paroxetine (Paxil, Pexeva), sertraline (Zoloft), vilazodone (Viibryd), and fluvoxamine (Luvox, Luvox CR). This is not a complete list, so please check with your doctor to find out if any medication you're taking is an SSRI. They are usually prescribed for depression or anxiety.

Pregnant and lactating women should not take herbal supplements unless approved by their treating physician. A developing fetus, or a breastfeeding infant, cannot metabolize the chemical compounds in herbs at the same rate as an adult.

Alcohol intensifies the effect of any type of sedative, whether prescription, over-the-counter, synthetic or natural, and can lead to unexpected and harmful side effects. Reduce or avoid consumption of alcoholic beverages during the day if you're taking any sedative at night, and never take them at the same time. Follow the recommendations of the manufacturer. If you've been taking a supplement for a long time, taper off gradually, just like you would with a prescription drug.

37
YOGA

Like most of the general population, it isn't unusual for people with tinnitus to also have poor posture habits. Remember your mother telling you to sit up straight whenever she caught you slouching? We seem to have a lot of difficulty doing that. Those of us who spend most of our day in front of a computer screen are more likely to have poor working posture. Take note of your posture now. Are your shoulders hunched? Is your head craned forward of your body? Is the screen too close to your eyes? Not only do we allow our posture to deteriorate at our desktop computer, we go home and use our laptop computers and tablets in awkward positions when we're sitting at the dining table, reclining on the couch, or relaxing in bed. Our increasing reliance on smartphones for text messaging is reflected in the numbers of people you see walking in public with their head bent downward, looking (or squinting) at a small screen, and thumb-typing messages to co-workers or friends. In decades past, those same people would most likely be walking with their eyes straight ahead and their head held erect. It was a healthier time where posture is concerned.

Poor posture contributes to poor circulation, which in turn can affect tinnitus. To establish and maintain good posture when we're immersed in a world of computers and tech gadgets requires conscious attention to how we sit and stand. Practicing good posture isn't simply a matter of walking back and forth in a room with a book balanced on your head, which is how many of us were taught in the past. There are specially-designed braces you can wear under your clothes to essentially force your shoulders back, but they don't address how you hold your neck and head. They aren't sufficient to improve the alignment of your spine. Such devices do nothing to strengthen your core muscles, an essential component of good posture. To obtain a genuine and lasting improvement in posture, it's hard to find anything better than yoga. You can begin with easy poses, advance at your own pace, and, best of all, you're never too old to start.

What is yoga? The word "yoga" is from Sanskrit, a language of ancient India and Nepal. It derives from the word "yuj," which means to yoke, as one would yoke together a team of oxen. The modern interpretation is that it means "union," to represent the uniting of mind, body, and spirit. When most people think of yoga, they think of stretching and precise poses, but it's more than that. It's really all about balance, achieved through strength and flexibility. This takes time and patience, but the effort pays off. Yoga is an excellent way to calm the mind, relieve stress, increase flexibility, and improve the alignment of the body. People with somatic tinnitus may be more likely to obtain benefit as their body begins to return to its natural symmetry.

Yoga's popularity has grown over the last few decades in the Western world, but its basics have remained unchanged for centuries. Even if your local library only carries yoga books from the 1970s, the asanas (poses) that it describes are the same as those published in modern texts. There is of course a wide selection of yoga books available online and in retail bookstores. If you're interested in pursuing this seriously, I recommend you skim through a few books to find one that you believe will best suit your lifestyle and current physical condition. You can also take online classes in yoga, learning the poses at home at your convenience. For example, www.yogisanonymous.com is one such online class. They offer a 15-day free trial. That's enough time for you to decide whether you think yoga is something you can stick with for the long term, or if you're just not that attuned to it. The subscription cost for Yogis Anonymous is $15 a month, a reasonable price for being able to attend class whenever you want in the comfort and privacy of your home.

The word "asana" is the Sanskrit word for "posture" or "seat." An asana is typically understood to mean a specific yoga pose or position. The following poses are recommended if you have tinnitus. They are not strenuous, and you can complete them in 10 to 15-minute sessions. Take two to three full breaths with each rep, starting with two to three reps for each asana and building up to 20 or 30 as you become more comfortable with them. These are basic poses which are usually included in any yoga book for beginners. Detailed instructions and photo illustrations can be found at www.yogajournal.com, www.verywell.com, and www.wikihow.com. See page 415 in the Resources section of this book for the website links to each pose.

Sphinx asana - beginner
Cat asana - beginner
Cow Face asana - intermediate.
If you're a beginner, substitute Balancing Table pose or Downward
Facing Dog for Cow Face asana
Plank asana - beginner
Warrior asana - beginner

Be sure to read any accompanying information about
contraindications as well as benefits before attempting any pose for the
first time. If it's difficult for you to understand the sequence of
movements in a pose, YouTube is an excellent online source for yoga
tutorials; for example, the "Sphinx Pose Explained" tutorial on the
Ekhart Yoga channel.

Yoga is an activity which helps to release endorphins. These are the
neurotransmitters which bind to opiate receptors in your brain.
Endorphins give you a natural "high" that helps to lessen anxiety and
fear. Yoga also increases GABA in the brain, which you'll recall is a
calming neurotransmitter that is vital for helping to tamp down
hyperactive neurons in the brain. MRIs of yoga practitioners have shown
increased GABA levels in the thalamus of the brain after only 12 weeks
of yoga, with one-hour sessions three days a week. The thalamus is the
part of the brain where incoming sensory information is regulated. There
is a feedback loop between the limbic system and the thalamus. With
tinnitus, something goes wrong in that feedback loop and the phantom
sounds of tinnitus reach the cerebral cortex and conscious awareness.
Anecdotal evidence indicates that yoga dampens the negative emotional
reactions associated with tinnitus. Perhaps that is partly due to the
increase of GABA in the thalamus, along with the physically relaxing
routine of doing asanas on a regular basis.

As with all exercise programs, if you have any medical problems,
physical limitations, persistent aches or pains in any joints or muscles, or
if you have led a sedentary lifestyle with very little daily exercise, please
check with your healthcare practitioner before beginning yoga.

38
REALISTIC BUT POSITIVE ATTITUDE

It's a natural human tendency to dwell on the negative, but now more than ever you need to emphasize the positive in your life. Keep a daily journal of the good things that happen, no matter how simple they are. A hike with a friend, a wagging tail from a friendly dog that's glad to see you, a wonderful meal, a favorite song that you hear on the radio, the smile or laughter of someone you love, all these joyful moments add up and make a difference in how you perceive what makes life worth living. Keep a journal and write down the pleasant things which you experience during the day. Your mind cannot reconstruct true sound within a memory, only a faint reproduction of it. As time goes by, you'll read your journal and smile at the memories, as if the tinnitus never existed while those memories were being made.

You can also keep a dark journal to express your anger, fear, frustration, and sorrow. You have two choices with this type of journal. Either wait a month to read what you have written to see how things have improved, or simply tear the pages from the journal once they're written and either shred them or burn them. The process of writing your thoughts down is productive therapy, whereas the act of destroying what you've written is cathartic, a way of releasing anger towards the problem that is causing you pain or anguish. Avoid reliving the pain by reading the words over and over, as this just activates and reinforces memories that are better left alone.

It's the rare person who can stay upbeat day after day when dealing with something like tinnitus. There will likely be times when it feels like the tinnitus is overwhelming your ability to cope with it. There may be days when extraordinary stressful events of life make the burden of tinnitus that much harder to bear. Do your best to avoid sinking into a pit of despair. Look for something to distract yourself and lighten your mood, even if it's as simple as taking 10 deep relaxing breaths while telling yourself, "It's going to be all right, it's going to be all right." If your tinnitus is chronic, accept the reality that it's part of who you are, just like the color of your eyes or size of your feet. That might seem like too much to accept in the early stages, but it's an important step in letting go of the internal struggle and accompanying misery that tinnitus can cause. Keep a positive outlook that either the tinnitus will improve or you will habituate to it so that it no longer dominates your thoughts or your life. Even the world-renowned Mayo Clinic agrees that thinking positively is good for your overall health, such as reducing the effects of stress and maintaining better coping skills. You can read about it in their online article, "Positive thinking: stop negative self-talk to reduce stress."

Remember that video of Letterman and Shatner that I brought up earlier? As they share the history of their tinnitus with one another, they sometimes make light of the subject. Any time you can find humor in a situation, it helps to promote a positive attitude, which is a step in the right direction towards learning to live with tinnitus. Because they're professionals, Letterman and Shatner don't want to bring down the good mood of their audience, but the sincerity of their discussion highlights how serious an issue it has been for both of them. Although I'm sure they would prefer not to have tinnitus at all, it's no longer the obstacle it once was in their lives. They have learned through knowledge and therapy how to cope with their tinnitus. Just imagine how difficult it must have been for Shatner to memorize his lines with a constant sound in his head, or for Letterman to stay upbeat and informed so he and his guests could entertain audiences night after night. Using their lives as an example, you can feel confident that the odds are on your side. If you stay positive and work towards keeping your body and mind healthy, you'll be able to get back into your life and function as well as you always have, even if it does take more effort than before tinnitus arrived.

39
STAY BUSY

One of the best things you can do to push tinnitus into the background of your mind is to stay busy and keep your focus on other things going on in your life. The more your mind is engaged in mental or emotional activities, the less attention it's going to pay to the sounds your brain is making. A member of Tinnitus Talk put it this way: "If someone threw a cobra on your keyboard, you would forget all about your tinnitus, even if it was only for a few moments." Obviously it would be foolish to expose yourself to danger so you can focus on that rather than your tinnitus, but he makes a good point. When confronted with an emergency or when dealing with an overwhelming emotion, tinnitus usually takes a back seat. Why? It's because tinnitus retreats when you are intensely focused on what's right in front of you, something which demands your full attention. In that moment, your mind discards everything that isn't essential to your survival, and so the tinnitus temporarily disappears from your awareness. Many people with tinnitus will tell you that once in a while it will dawn on them that they haven't heard their tinnitus for a few minutes or even hours, but as soon as they notice they aren't hearing it, they instantly become aware of it again.

Everybody has something they are passionate about. If you have tinnitus to the degree that you feel so depressed that nothing arouses your sense of passion anymore, take small steps to bring that joy back into your life. If you were a hiker and no longer feel like going out, watch programs of faraway places that intrigue you, choosing those with terrain that's challenging to hikers. You might find yourself longing to be back in nature again, and from there it's just a few more steps to putting on your hiking boots and hitting the trails. If you've developed poor eating habits, take the time to watch videos of how to prepare quick and easy nutritious meals. Websites featuring recipes and cooking videos are available for every culinary interest, from beginner to expert. Perhaps you've always wanted to paint. What better time to start than now? Immerse your imagination in the colors on the canvas. If you love animals, especially dogs and cats, there are endless opportunities to become involved.

If you've always wanted to write a book, don't put it off because of your tinnitus. Almost every page in this book has been written to the accompaniment of buzzing, hissing, or whistling in my head. One source of inspiration for would-be writers is Sam Harris, author of the best-selling books *The End of Faith*, *The Moral Landscape*, *Free Will*, *Lying*, *Waking Up*, and more. He rates his "endless whistle" tinnitus as being somewhere between scarcely consequential and life-wrecking, and that it is maskable only in environments such as loud restaurants. Like many people with tinnitus, it's the first thing he notices every morning. Despite this, he continues to write prolifically. His books are not fluff. They cover serious subjects requiring extensive research and contemplation. If Sam Harris can thrive while burdened with tinnitus, you can, too. Ironically, Sam Harris has a Ph.D. in neuroscience from UCLA. Even though he has the education to understand more about tinnitus than the average layperson, he has struggled to adapt to it just like almost everyone else who has moderate to severe tinnitus. He shares his story in his blog article, "Adventures in the Land of Illness."

Maybe you don't know what your passion is because you've been mired in the responsibilities of everyday life for so long that you've forgotten what motivates and inspires you. There are plenty of books and website articles, such as "Five Steps to Finding Your Passion" on www.PsychologyToday.com, which will help you clear away the brambles and discover a renewed sense of purpose. Remember that anything which captures your attention and focuses your mind is a tool to convince the brain that the sound of tinnitus is not high priority. This is especially true if you have an emotional attachment to the object of your focus, because then the limbic system gets into the act. It's great to be busy, but it's much better if you're busy doing something you love.

Generally speaking, if you have a hobby, it's usually connected to a personal passion. All you need to do is figure out what it is about that hobby that captivates you, and take it to the next level. Don't let your tinnitus hold you back or deprive you from doing something you love, something you've always wanted to do. Be like Zoe Cartwright, the artist with both deafness and tinnitus. View your tinnitus as a challenge instead of a disability, and prove to yourself that you can accomplish what you want to accomplish in life. Be in the moment when pursuing your passion. When you hear your tinnitus, get in the habit of saying, "I hear you, but I'm busy now, I don't have time for you." Believe it or not, sometimes your brain will obey your instruction and the tinnitus will recede into the background. As much as you can, don't let your attention wander back to your tinnitus. Keep it focused on doing what you love, on what motivates and inspires you.

If you don't have a hobby or anything you feel particularly passionate about, consider enrolling in some online courses to keep you mentally stimulated. One great place to start is www.Udemy.com, with many courses being either free or priced at $10 or less. If you sign up for their emails, they will send out special offers for reduced prices on courses that are similar to subjects you've shown an interest in. Udemy offers a money-back guarantee, and you can take as long as you want to complete any course you buy. Udemy isn't the only online education portal. Just do a search for "online learning courses" and you'll have plenty to choose from.

SECTION VIII

TREATMENTS

40
ALLOPATHIC PROVIDERS

The word "allopathic" refers to healthcare practitioners who customarily treat and/or cure disorders and diseases through the use of conservative physical therapy, drugs, and/or surgery. For instance, someone with an "M.D." (Doctor of Medicine) after her name is an allopathic physician. This distinguishes her from a colleague who might be a Doctor of Osteopathic Medicine (D.O.), Doctor of Naturopathy (D.N.), or Doctor of Homeopathic Medicine (D.H.M.). Because most people will generally first go to a medical doctor for treatment of tinnitus, you can assume that if I use the term "doctor" in this chapter that I'm referring to an M.D. However, I take no position on whether one approach to treatment is better for you than another. If you're more comfortable with an osteopathic physician, a naturopath, or even a homeopathic specialist, you should consult with the practitioner of your choice and determine if they are best suited to help you. As common as tinnitus is, there are over 200 possible causes for it, and of course there are so many variations amongst individuals that a one-size-fits-all approach does not work for tinnitus. No matter which practitioner you eventually choose, if you can review your long-term or recent history and try to pinpoint the most likely cause, you will be better able to select a healthcare provider who can help you during the critical first days and weeks of tinnitus.

One major advantage of seeing a medical or osteopathic doctor is that in general they have easier access to a broader range of medical tests and equipment. This is important in the initial stages of tinnitus, particularly when it's of unknown origin. Tinnitus itself is not a disease or disorder, it is a symptom of something that's gone wrong. You'll want to know if there is a physical-based reason for your tinnitus; for example, fluid in the ear, excess ear wax pressing against the eardrum, muscle spasms of the tiny muscles in the ear, or more serious disorders like otosclerosis or acoustic neuroma.

Tinnitus is most often linked to disorders that originate from the ear, but can also be caused by problems with your bite, teeth grinding (bruxism), misalignment of your jaw, a temporomandibular joint (TMJ) problem, and other oral-related dysfunctions. If you or your healthcare provider suspects any of those as the cause of your tinnitus, you will need to consult with a Doctor of Dental Surgery (D.D.S.), otherwise known as a dentist. If the problem is extensive or complicated, you will likely be referred to an oral surgeon (D.D.S., M.D.) for treatment.

With that foundation, let's cover the experts who are medically trained to help you with your tinnitus.

If you have a sudden and severe onset of tinnitus, something that sounds like a freight train with screeching brakes or the Liberty Bell clanging in your head, there's a good chance you'll go to the closest emergency room or outpatient clinic. It can be extremely frightening to experience tinnitus at such a catastrophic level. It's wise to seek treatment as soon as possible when the sound makes your head feel like it's going to explode. Tinnitus typically doesn't begin in such a dramatic fashion, but it can and does happen. Visiting an ER with mild or moderate tinnitus isn't unusual, either. People with recent onset tinnitus sometimes visit the emergency room or an outpatient clinic because they can't get in right away to see the doctor they want. Not being willing to wait for treatment, they look for the next best opportunity to ease their symptoms, or at least get an explanation of what's going on.

Emergency rooms are so varied from city to city, with different specialties rotating on day shift and night shift, it's impossible to say what kind of experience you'll have once you get there, but there are some common procedures that you can expect. There will be routine questions about your medical history and what drugs you're currently taking or have recently taken, including illegal substances. Be sure to tell them if you're taking illegal substances of any kind, and when the last time was you took that substance. You don't want any nasty surprises if they give you a medication in the ER and it clashes with something already in your system. They will probably ask if you're taking any over-the-counter remedies and supplements, but even if they don't, tell them about those, too. The definition of a drug is basically any medicine or substance that affects the function of your body or mind. That includes aspirin, St. John's Wort, caffeine, alcohol, marijuana, or any similar products. To prevent adverse effects from contraindications, healthcare providers need to know everything you're taking that could be altering your body chemistry, no matter how mild or insignificant you may think it is.

The ER physician will check your vital signs and look in your ears for any signs of inflammation that might indicate an infection. They'll check to see if you have excess ear wax. They'll ask you whether you've recently experienced acoustic trauma, such as standing too close to a gunshot or firecracker, going to an extremely loud concert or nightclub, someone shouting in your ear, a fire alarm or siren too close nearby, or any event that might have triggered the tinnitus. If you've had any dizziness lately, a sore jaw, head trauma, exposure to an air bag deploying, severe headaches, anything unusual at all in your recent history, be sure to mention it. The smallest clue can be helpful not only in determining why you have tinnitus, but also how to treat it to get the best result. In the absence of obvious physical trauma to your head or ears, it's likely that the ER doctor will refer you to another physician for follow-up consultation and treatment. If you are suffering from severe anxiety or depression, don't put on a brave front. Tell the doctor what you're going through. He or she may write a prescription to help ease those symptoms until you can be further evaluated.

Depending upon the severity of your symptoms, the next physician you see will likely be your own family doctor, or you may be referred to an otolaryngologist. An "otolaryngologist" is the professional term for an ENT, an ear, nose and throat doctor. ENTs are specialists in ear and hearing disorders and usually have some experience in examining and treating tinnitus patients.

With sudden onset tinnitus, you may wish to seek out a physician who can start you on a course of steroids. However, there are three criteria that generally must be met for the best chance of having a good outcome with this type of treatment:

- Your tinnitus is due to acoustic trauma;
- You have demonstrable hearing loss associated with the acoustic trauma; and,
- Your tinnitus is of very recent onset, that is, within 24 to 48 hours.

The window of opportunity for steroids to be effective is extremely narrow. You may also have difficulty convincing a physician that your recent-onset tinnitus might respond to this treatment, especially if they have little to no experience with treating tinnitus. My personal opinion is that even if your tinnitus is as recent as within the past 10 days, it's worth attempting a course of steroids to see if the tinnitus can be reduced, and hopefully eliminated. Steroid treatment, and in particular prednisone, is discussed in Chapter 59, "Prescription Drugs."

Tinnitus is a very peculiar disorder, with so many variables that it can be a challenge for even the most knowledgeable doctor. Before you make an appointment, be sure to ask what their experience is in treating tinnitus and what treatment methods they generally recommend. It doesn't hurt to ask if they have tinnitus as well, and to what degree. A healthcare provider who has personal experience with tinnitus is more likely to understand the frustration, anxiety, panic, or depression that can arise in someone with recently acquired tinnitus. He or she may also be more flexible when it comes to trying a new form of treatment, or be willing to try different things to help you. Additionally, ask if they keep up with the latest clinical trials in tinnitus research and would they be willing to discuss you becoming a participant in those trials, if this is something you wish to pursue.

When it comes to tinnitus and healthcare providers, consider all possible options. I'm not saying you should run down every rabbit trail you come across, in a desperate attempt to find relief or a cure. I'm saying follow a logical path of treatment. If one thing doesn't work for you, try something else. Even with new treatments, there are usually enough people who have tried it that you'll have a good idea what sort of results can be reasonably expected. Because tinnitus is unique to every individual in how it originates and how it is perceived, what works for one person may not work for another. It can be a long process of trial and error, requiring both persistence and patience. However, if you do find something to ease the symptoms and it helps you to adjust to living with tinnitus, you will appreciate that you devoted the time and effort instead of simply "learning to live with it."

41
AROMATHERAPY

As you can guess, the word "aroma" means scent, and "therapy" means treatment. From as long ago as 3500 BC, aromatherapy has been used to soothe human ailments and create pleasant living conditions. Over the centuries, people have found countless ways of bringing desired scents into their lives. We go walking in the woods because the natural smell of trees and blossoming plants is so intoxicating and invigorating. We plant flowers for their heavenly fragrance as much as for their beauty. We burn scented candles and incense in our homes and hang air fresheners in our vehicles. We wear perfumes that have been meticulously synthesized to evoke specific responses. The perfume industry has scents to cater to every male or female preference. When it comes to our sense of smell, we are naturally drawn to what pleases us and repelled by what offends us.

We are so accustomed to fragrance all around us, many of us never notice how large a role scents play in our environment. The next time you go to a department store and visit the personal products aisle, walk a bit more slowly and inhale deeply. You might be surprised by the intensity of the scents in the air. In response to perceived consumer demand, companies add fragrance to our soaps, shampoos, conditioners, bath oils, body lotions, even toilet paper, as well as many other personal and home products. If you wash dishes by hand, you'll notice three popular scents for dish detergent: citrus, lavender, and vanilla. Lavender is the scent most often added to laundry detergent and fabric softener. The main reason for this is to draw consumers to a product with a favorite scent. The other reason is to associate a pleasing scent with a chore most of us would rather not do, thus making the chore seem a bit less tedious. We live in an environment saturated with scents designed to entice us, whether we are consciously aware of it or not. There are people with sensitive olfactory systems and people who simply prefer fragrance-free products. Manufacturers understand this need and accommodate them as well.

Aromatherapy, along with soothing music, is commonly used by massage therapists to set up a tranquil atmosphere for their patients.

Although there are many professions that would benefit from easing the troubled nerves of their clients and patients with aromatherapy, massage therapists by far are more likely to do so. Health spas also incorporate aromatherapy, as well as some doctors' and dentists' offices. Aromatherapy is more of an art than a science, but scientific studies do support the belief that aromatherapy can provide benefits when properly used. From those studies we have now learned which essential oils are most likely to produce the greatest benefit for a number of conditions.

Now that we've had a quick review of scents in our environment, let's take a closer look at how aromatherapy can offer calm and comfort when tinnitus is making you miserable. I'll be covering aromatherapy with essential oils because oils have been extensively studied for therapeutic uses. They are also readily available in local stores or online, and are easy to measure for different application methods. This helps you to control how much or how little oil is used, depending on your basic level of sensitivity, as well as your mood and what you are trying to achieve.

One side effect of tinnitus can be a constant feeling of underlying tension. This can produce a variety of unpleasant secondary effects such as a stiff neck, sore muscles in the shoulders, or an aching back. Teeth can become damaged from unconsciously gritting or grinding them. Tension can express itself in the body in all sorts of ways, most of which are detrimental over the long term. To ease tension, it's important to induce calm in both the mind and body. If a problem has you in its grip, you need to take away its power and regain your sense of well-being. The following essential oils have special properties that will help:

- Lavender
- Frankincense
- Orange
- Lemon
- Bergamot

As mentioned earlier, the scent of lavender is so popular that it's added to many home and personal products. Flower lovers everywhere plant lavender in their gardens and along their walkways and fence lines. It's a romantic flower, reminding us of the long-ago past, when life moved at a slower and more gentle pace. The scent of lavender reaches the emotional center of our brain through both our memories and scent receptors, a powerful combination. If you have difficulty going to sleep, try placing a drop or two of lavender essential oil on a cotton ball and place it on your nightstand or beside your pillow. You can also add a few drops to a warm bath before bedtime. Let your muscles relax, lean back in the tub, close your eyes and take in the delicate scent.

Frankincense is nicknamed "the king of oils." It has a fresh and woodsy scent, with a delicate overtone of spice and fruit. Frankincense is derived from the resin of Asian and African trees. It is also called olibanum, from the tree of the same name. The Bible mentions frankincense as a gift brought by the Magi to the baby Jesus. In ancient times, frankincense was used by the Greeks, Romans, and Israelites in religious ceremonies. Frankincense is considered to be most beneficial for easing anxious feelings and promoting a sense of wellness and relaxation. If you're unsure about which essential oil is best for you, choose frankincense.

Orange, being a citrus scent, lifts your mood. If you're feeling panicky, stressed, irritable, or angry, mix one or two drops with an ounce of carrier oil (almond would be ideal), and apply a few drops of the mixture to the back of your neck. Rub it in gently and feel the tension ease as the orange scent uplifts your spirit. Blending this oil with frankincense is a great anti-anxiety combination. Keep in mind that orange essential oil is photosensitive. Do not expose any oil-treated skin to sunlight for at least 24 to 48 hours.

Lemon, another citrus scent, has basically the same properties as orange essential oil. Its scent is unmistakable, sharp and clean. With higher quality lemon essential oil, the scent is less crisp and has a smoother property. Like orange, it is an uplifting essential oil, with the added sensation of promoting feelings of trust and security. An ideal word to describe lemon essential oil is "radiant." In the same way that sunlight clears away fog, lemon essential oil clears the mind of confusion and lifts your mood.

If you're familiar with the aroma of Earl Grey Tea, then you know the aroma of bergamot, also known as bee balm. Bergamot is a citrus fruit. In aromatherapy, it is both an uplifting and relaxing scent. It is said to help release locked-up emotions and is therefore useful for relieving depression and anxiety. Blending bergamot with frankincense and lavender is a wonderful combination for relaxing. This essential oil, like lemon and orange, is photosensitive.

We experience pleasure when inhaling certain scents, and may even close our eyes to intensify the sensation. This is why people close their eyes when they smell flowers, to better appreciate the fragrance. We do the same thing when inhaling the appetizing aroma of fresh bread when it first comes out of the oven. We do this for two reasons. First, shutting off the sense of vision enhances our other senses. People who work with deaf and/or blind children will tell you that those children have an exceedingly sharp sense of smell to help them navigate their environment and identify people and objects within that environment. Second, closing our eyes is an unconscious action which stimulates alpha wave activity in our brain. Increased alpha wave activity leads to a sense of well-being, which makes inhaling the scent that much more pleasurable. Our olfactory system sends messages to the neo-cortex, the higher thought center of the brain, but it also sends messages directly to the limbic system. This is the part of our brain where smells and memories join together to evoke emotions.

With the advent of neuroimaging and increasingly sophisticated measurements of human responses, aromatherapy has moved beyond the realm of being regarded as merely feel-good remedies. Aromatherapy is now increasingly being studied and acknowledged for its unique ability to influence how we feel mentally, emotionally, and physically. For example, it has been proven that essential oils can affect brain wave activity in a positive way. In particular, lavender and rose produce more alpha and theta brain waves. Keep in mind that people with tinnitus have lower than average levels of alpha waves. Whatever you can do to raise your alpha waves may also help to calm your tinnitus. (Brain wave activity and how to influence it is covered in Chapter 26, "Brain Waves and Tinnitus.")

The search for the right essential oil can be overwhelming. There are hundreds of essential oils and essential oil blends. I recommend you visit a store which sells high grade essential oils, and ask to smell the different varieties to see which one resonates with you. You may only be able to smell a few before your olfactory senses become confused with too much sensory input. Take your time, starting with the fragrances of lavender, frankincense, orange, lemon, and bergamot. It can sometimes be hard to remember what scents evoke particular feelings, so be prepared to make notes to help you in reaching a final decision.

There are many knowledgeable sellers of essential oils online, so that's a good starting place to narrow down which ones you think will do you the most good. www.MountainRoseHerbs.com is a very reputable and environmentally friendly company, with an extensive selection of essential oils to choose from. They also sell other products that you may find helpful in coping with tinnitus, such as teas, herbs, and spices.

When buying essential oils, look for wording on the label that indicates it is certified therapeutic grade. Many oils on the market are synthesized rather than extracted from the plants for which they are named. These cheaper oils may smell nice, but their inherent properties simply do not offer the same benefit as genuine essential oils.

No matter which essential oils you choose, remember that they are for topical (on the skin) or diffusion use only. Some oils can burn the skin and must be diluted with carrier oils. A carrier oil is a base oil which dilutes the strength of the essential oil. Popular carrier oils are almond oil, coconut oil, jojoba oil, and grapeseed oil. Do not use mineral oil or baby oil as a carrier oil.

To be on the safe side, it's always best to test your sensitivity before using a new essential oil. Follow the instructions on "Essential Oil Skin Patch Testing," on www.AromaWeb.com. Never use essential oils in the eyes or on mucous membranes. Sometimes essential oils are included in oral products such as toothpaste and mouthwash, but these products are manufactured under strict guidelines. Do not ingest any essential oil except under the guidance of a healthcare practitioner who is trained in their use. Obviously, keep essential oils out of reach of children and pets. For more information on how to use essential oils in the safest manner possible, I encourage you to read the National Capital Poison Center's website article, "Essential Oils: Poisonous When Misused." They point out that children have thin skin and their livers have not yet matured, so they are more susceptible to toxic effects. The National Association for

Holistic Aromatherapy has published "Exploring Aromatherapy - Safety Information," an extensive guide for safely using essential oils. Their website is www.naha.org.

Incidentally, there are essential oil products formulated as flea and tick repellents for pets. You can also find online formulas for do-it-yourself repellents. Please keep in mind how incredibly sensitive your pet's sense of smell is. What might be a light pleasant scent to you could be far too powerful for them. Use sparingly, with plenty of carrier oil, and exercise caution when applying essential oil products on your pets and in their environment.

42
AUDIO NOTCH THERAPY

Audio notch therapy is a treatment which requires a commitment of at least 1.5 hours per day of listening to a notched audio file, over the course of several months. The process is exactly what it sounds like. That is, a frequency notch which matches your tinnitus frequency is applied to either a music or noise audio file, and so that specific frequency is removed from the file. If you audio notch a music file, it's sometimes referred to as "notched music therapy," or NMT. The noise file is usually white noise, but it also works with violet noise, pink noise, blue noise, brown noise, etc. Once the frequency notch is applied to the audio file, you listen to it for the recommended amount of time, with the goal that this will eventually reduce the severity of your tinnitus.

Audio notch therapy is claimed to reduce tinnitus that is caused by noise exposure, but not if it's caused by a disease or disorder; for example, Ménière's disease or hypertension. If your tinnitus is idiopathic, with no cause identified, you are as likely to benefit from audio notch therapy as someone with damage from noise exposure. This is because many cases of idiopathic tinnitus involve some higher frequency hearing loss. Most of the sounds we hear in our everyday life are not in the high frequency range anyway, so we often don't notice the frequency loss. This is why many people believe their hearing is still normal, even though they experience tinnitus.

How does audio notch therapy work? Let's briefly review how tinnitus is created, as explained before in Chapter 22, "How We Hear Sound," and Chapter 24, "The Brain Creates Tinnitus." Neurons in your auditory cortex are designed to receive and interpret signals from the hair cells in the cochlea of your inner ear. When the hair cells designated for a specific frequency become damaged or die, the corresponding neurons in your auditory cortex no longer receive the signal for that frequency. Without the frequency-specific signal to direct them, those signal-deprived neurons begin rewiring in a dysfunctional manner with their neighboring normal neurons. They begin to fire spontaneously and out of sync. The normal neurons are unable to stop the dysfunctional neurons from firing, so the tinnitus continues to be generated. This spontaneous constant misfiring is why it's common for tinnitus to be described in very basic terms as hyperactive neurons in the brain.

But, what if it were possible for the normal neurons to stop the dysfunctional neurons from firing? This is the theory behind audio notch therapy, that it is specifically designed to suppress the errant misfiring. As you listen to the notched audio file, the normal neurons become stimulated. They send inhibitory signals to the dysfunctional neurons via lateral connections. This normalizes the misfiring neurons through a process called lateral inhibition, which eventually leads to rewiring of the neurons to reduce or eliminate the tinnitus. When this lateral inhibition is sustained for long periods of time, cortical reorganization takes place. Cortical reorganization in this instance refers to the natural rewiring of the connections between the normal and the dysfunctional neurons. In time, the dysfunctional neurons calm down, they stop their persistent firing, and this results in the tinnitus itself calming down. If you would like to read a more scientific explanation, the National Center for Biotechnology Information (NCBI) has published the abstract, "Listening to tailor-made notched music reduces tinnitus loudness and tinnitus-related auditory cortex activity." It presents a detailed explanation of the research behind notched music therapy, including clear evidence of improvement in subjects who participated in clinical trials.

Audio notch therapy is supported by research and clinical trials, but it is still a relatively new development in the treatment of tinnitus. Therefore, although the positive effect can last as long as weeks or months, it's not known whether the lateral inhibition of the dysfunctional neurons is permanent. In other words, audio notch therapy is not something that once it works it can be discarded and forgotten about. The brain has plasticity, meaning it can change and adapt. If cortical reorganization takes place via audio notch therapy, there's always the possibility that stopping audio notch therapy will eventually result in a reversal of cortical reorganization, whereby the lateral inhibition ceases to work and the dysfunctional neurons begin firing again. If audio notch therapy works for you, plan on using it regularly, just as you would include walking or jogging in your regular cardio workout. As time goes by, you will be able to figure out if and when you need to resume listening to your notched audio files. Note that if you listen to your notched audio file at a volume slightly lower than your tinnitus, it will help the habituation process. Again, keep in mind that this isn't a quick fix. You will need to listen to the audio for at least 1.5 hours every day for several months, and it may take a while to notice improvement.

If you want a notched audio file created by professionals, one option is to visit www.AudioNotch.com. They state their purpose clearly on the website, that AudioNotch creates custom sound therapy as a treatment for tinnitus, not a cure. Their FAQ page covers how their program works. It's clearly written, easy to understand, and answers many basic questions about audio notch therapy. AudioNotch charges a reasonable fee for a two-month trial subscription, a full subscription of six months, or a 12-month annual subscription, all of which include a 30-day money back guarantee if you feel like the program isn't helping you.

For those on a limited budget, you can create your own audio notch files. If you are comfortable with downloading noise or music files from the Internet and modifying them with audio software such as the free Audacity program, the next chapter covers how you can make your own notched audio file. I will take you through it step-by-step, with illustrated instructions.

43
AUDIO NOTCH - DO IT YOURSELF GUIDE

The instructions for creating a notched audio file will assume you have the following basic skills, or are willing to learn them through online tutorials or local sources:

- Downloading and installing free Audacity audio editing software
- Downloading an audio file, or any noise file other than brown, pink, or white, which are already included in Audacity
- Following step-by-step illustrated and written instructions to create the notched audio
- Importing an audio file into your smartphone, MP3 player, or other playback device

With the countless combinations of various operating systems and playback devices on the market, it would be nearly impossible to cover all the potential questions that might arise in following this DIY method. However, if you have the four skills noted above, you should be able to make your first notched audio file within 20 minutes, which includes downloading and installing Audacity, as well as downloading a noise file if you choose not to use any of the brown, pink, or white noise files included with Audacity. If you want to create additional notched audio files, they will probably take five to 10 minutes from start to finish. Most people are comfortable listening to white noise, but there are good reasons for using other audio files. The different color noise files are explained in the next chapter, "The Colors of Noise."

If you're unfamiliar with frequency measurements, "Hz" stands for hertz, and "kHz" stands for kilohertz. 1 hertz equals 1 cycle per second. As the number of cycles per second increase, the pitch rises. In other words, a tinnitus frequency of 2,000 hertz is low pitched, whereas a tinnitus frequency of 9,000 hertz is high pitched. 1,000 hertz is equal to 1 kilohertz.

If your frequency is above 8,000 Hz, it is recommended that you listen to your notched audio file for no more than one hour at a time, up to three times a day. If it is below 8,000 Hz, listen to the audio for as long as it's comfortable for you. If you need to mask your tinnitus in order to fall asleep, this is an ideal way to get in some extra listening time in addition to the hours you spend with audio notch therapy during the day. You can let the audio play all night long, since your brain hears the audio and keeps working on the lateral inhibition process even while you're asleep. This is not recommended if your tinnitus frequency is above 8,000 Hz, since it would exceed the one-hour listening limit.

Audio notch therapy is most effective if you're listening to the notched audio file by itself; that is, no other music file or soundscape in the background. As you go about your tasks or work, you may well find that you completely forget that the audio is playing. You're not consciously aware of it while you're focused on something else, but your brain is aware and continues to work on repairing your neural connections. However, it's okay to keep listening while you're engaged in conversation, watching a movie, or attending a non-music event. Your mind will still be paying attention to the audio. When you want to listen to regular music, turn off your notched audio and listen to just that music. If you listen to both at the same time, there's a good chance that the non-notched music will fill in the notched frequency. That would cancel out any benefit you might otherwise get from the notched audio.

Notched audio files can either be noise files (white, pink, brown, etc.), a neutral soundscape such as rainfall (as long as it contains the correct frequency range), or you can also create notched audio with your favorite music. First, however, it's important to know how to do it with basic noise audio. Start your computer, and let's begin.

To create a notched audio file, you need to know your tinnitus frequency. Go to the frequency matcher tool, "Find your tinnitus tone," at www.audionotch.com/app/tune. You do not need to set up an account to do this. You can also access the frequency matcher from their home page. Go to www.AudioNotch.com, and click on the link under "Step 1: Tune," listed below "How Does AudioNotch Treat Tinnitus." (There is another frequency matcher tool at www.GeneralFuzz.com/acrn, which is covered in more detail in Chapter 46 for ACRN sound therapy.) Wear headphones to obtain the most accurate match, as well as to protect other people and pets from the sounds. Be sure to set the volume at a safe level before beginning.

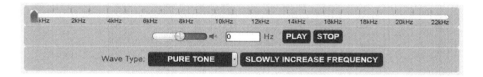

The frequency matcher app is easy to use. Leave the "Pure Tone" setting as-is, unless you're familiar with audio engineering terms and understand the differences between the settings. Click "Play," and then click "Slowly Increase Frequency." You'll see the blue marker at the left-hand side of the frequency level start moving to the right, and you should hear a tone playing. Click "Stop" to stop the tone and adjust the volume level if necessary. If you think your frequency is much higher and you don't want to wait for the blue marker to slowly move across, just click anywhere on the timeline, or click on the blue marker and drag it to the right, then click "Play" again. When the frequency that's being played matches your tinnitus frequency, click the "Stop" button. Each time you manually move the marker, you can fine-tune the frequency setting by using the keyboard left arrow and down arrow keys to decrease the frequency 2 hertz at a time, and the right arrow or up arrow keys to increase the frequency.

When you've determined your frequency, write down the number shown in the "Hz" box. You'll need it when you create the notch filter in Audacity. If you have trouble narrowing in on your frequency, ask a friend to move the marker for you while you close your eyes and concentrate on hearing the tone.

As an example, the next image shows what 7100 Hz looks like on the AudioNotch website tool.

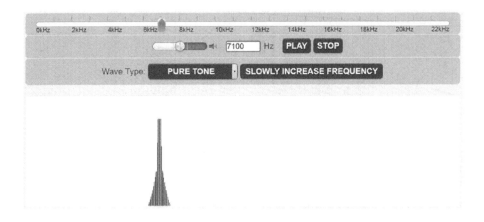

Now let's create a notched audio file. The screenshots in this tutorial were taken on a PC, but the steps for a Mac are the same.

Step 1. Download and install the free Audacity program from www.AudacityTeam.org. This is a March 2017 screenshot:

Audacity® is free, open source, cross-platform audio software for multi-track recording and editing.

Audacity is available for Windows®, Mac®, GNU/Linux® and other operating systems. Check our feature list, Wiki and Forum.

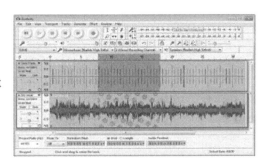

If you need help with installing the program, visit YouTube and type "install Audacity" into the Search bar. There, you can choose from tutorials which are specific for various operating systems.

Step 2. Open Audacity. Click "Generate" on the toolbar menu, then select "Noise."

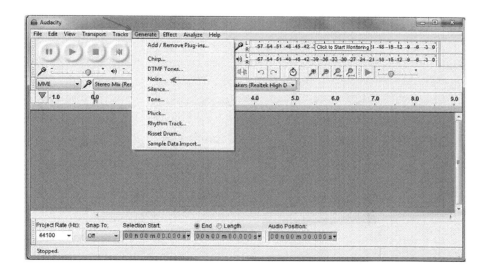

Step 3. A menu opens to input the Noise type, Amplitude, and Duration (file length). Start with white noise, and if you don't like it, try brownian (brown) noise or pink noise next. Keep 0.15 as the Amplitude default. I entered 30 minutes for the Duration, so I can import it into a smartphone and set it to loop (repeat) on playback.

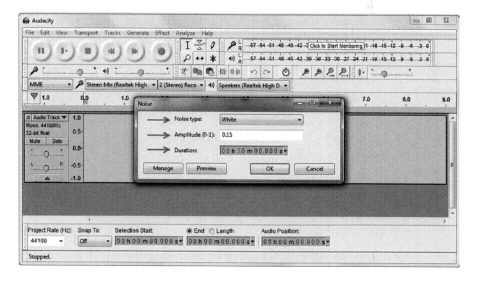

Click "OK" and let's go to the next step.

Step 4. After you click "OK," Audacity creates your white noise file. The next image shows how it will appear on your screen. At this point the dark borders have smooth edges. That will change after Step 5.

Before going to Step 5, you can test the sound by clicking the green triangle button to begin playing the audio file, and click the tan/yellow square button to stop. Reduce the volume on your computer before you test the sound, especially if you're wearing headphones. Listen for a few minutes to see if you think it's something you can listen to for one to 1.5 hours at a time. If you don't like it, start again at Step 2 and choose brown or pink noise.

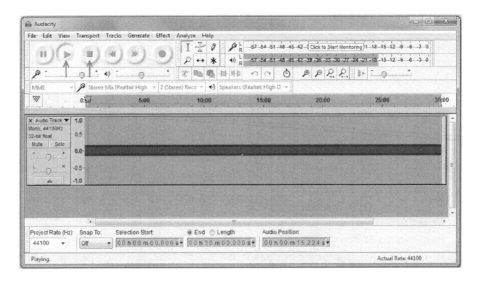

Step 5. Click "Effect" on the toolbar menu, then select "Notch Filter." There are more filters than those displayed in the next screenshot. I cropped the image to keep the focus on the main elements.

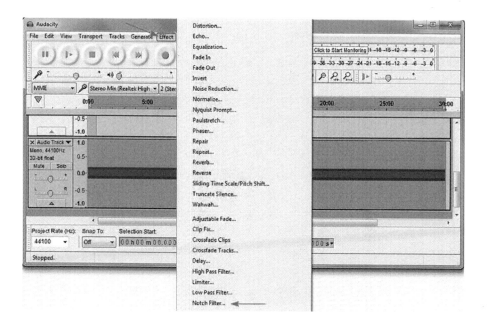

Step 6. A menu opens for you to input your frequency and the width of the notch. Enter the frequency you wrote down from the AudioNotch frequency matcher. Enter 0.3 for the Q value, which is a measurement of the width of the frequency range. A Q of 1 encompasses basically one entire octave, which would be a rather wide filter.

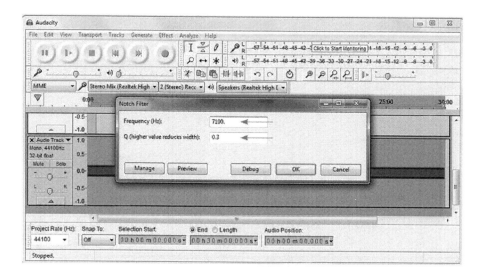

Clicking on "Preview" lets you listen to what the final audio will sound like. The Preview function at this stage really isn't helpful for a notched audio file because it's unlikely you'll notice any difference in the audio with the notch filter applied. Just go ahead and click "OK," and you'll see the bar graph progress as Audacity processes the notch filter into the audio.

Step 7. After Audacity processes the notch filter, you will see in the screenshot below that the dark borders now have a slightly ragged look.

If you want, you can verify that the notch filter has been applied. Choose "Analyze" from the toolbar menu, then select "Plot Spectrum." You may get a popup message, "Too much audio was selected. Only the first 237.8 seconds will be analyzed." Go ahead and click "OK." Audacity then generates a graphic of the notch filter and its frequency range.

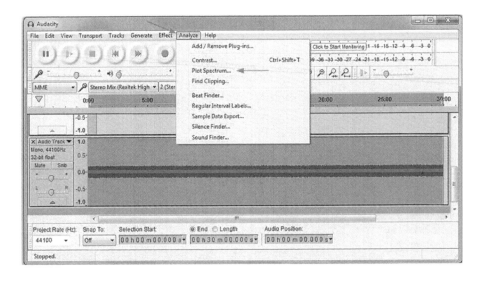

In the next screenshot, you can see how the Q value of 0.3 has notched out all frequencies from 6434 Hz to 7877 Hz. The beginning range of the notch is 6434 Hz, the upper range is 7877 Hz, and the tinnitus frequency of 7100 is approximately in the middle. You can view the precise Hz range by hovering your cursor over the beginning and ending margin of the notch filter. This is an example of the type of notch filter you want to see in your Plot Spectrum Analysis. It's difficult to precisely match a tinnitus frequency, so a notch filter with room for error on either side will give you the best chance of targeting your tinnitus frequency. Click "Close" and let's go to the next step, exporting the file.

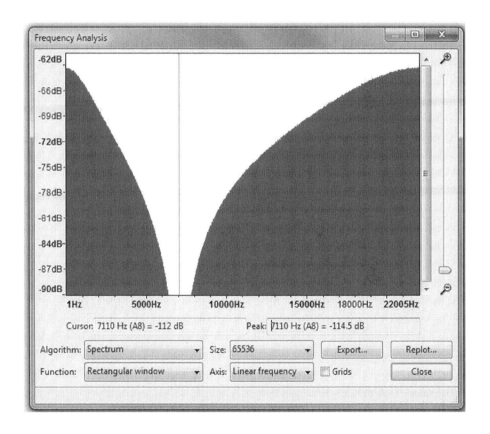

Step 8. Click "File" from the toolbar menu, then select "Export Audio."

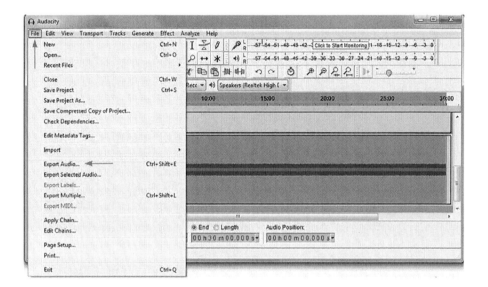

In the window that opens, choose a folder where you want to export the file. I created a folder in my Music Library and labeled it "Notch Filter." I named the file "WhiteNoise_7100_point3." This indicates that it's white noise, the notch filter frequency is 7100, and the notch filter width is 0.3. Naming your file in this manner makes it helpful if you decide to make several notched audio files. You'll be able to see instantly what kind of noise file has been used, the notch filter frequency, and how wide a notch filter has been applied.

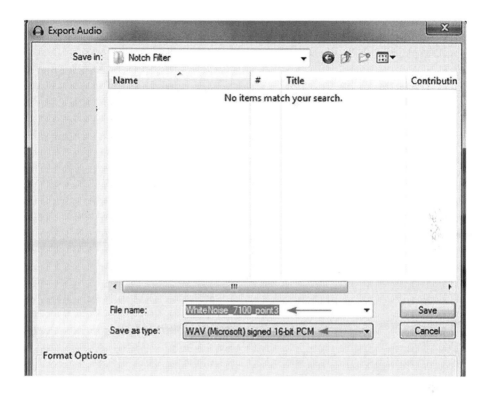

The file will be exported as a WAV file because this format has less data compression than an MP3 file. Data compression affects the quality and accuracy of frequency representation in audio. FLAC is an excellent choice for high quality encoding of frequencies, but some devices won't accept FLAC files. If your playback device accepts FLAC files, export your audio in that format. For a highly detailed explanation of the lossy quality of various audio file formats, visit www.SoundOnSound.com and read their article, "What Data Compression Does to Your Music." Keep in mind that choosing a higher quality audio export will increase the size of the file.

When you click "Save," you may get the message, "Your file will be mixed down to two stereo channels in the exported file." Just click "OK," because that's not a problem. Then a popup menu to insert metadata tags will appear, as shown in the next screenshot. You don't need to add metadata information, so just click the "OK" button. Your audio notch file will now be saved to the folder where you assigned it.

Step 9. Now that you've exported your file, you can import it into your playback device. It's basically the same procedure that you use to import any other audio file stored on your computer. If you don't know how, search for online tutorials or ask a tech-savvy friend to help you. Although it's more convenient to use a portable playback device, you can also play the audio file directly from your computer.

With audio notch therapy, it's important to remember that your frequency can change as your brain reorganizes the neural connections. Recheck your frequency every couple weeks, or at least once a month. If you have cycling tinnitus, where it fluctuates from mild to moderate or severe, choose a day to test your frequency when your tinnitus is loud enough that you can more accurately match its frequency.

How can audio notch therapy work when you have multiple sounds or tones in your head and/or ears? If that's the case, there is usually a dominant frequency that you can zero in on. If all the sounds seem to have the same level of volume and intrusiveness, find your matching frequencies one at a time and note their numbers. It will take you longer to create your custom audio notched file, but it isn't any more difficult than applying one notch filter.

The first step is to create an audio notch file with one matching frequency. Export that file into a folder or other location on your computer. Then, in Audacity, choose "File," select "Import," and import that same file back into Audacity. Make your second notch filter in that audio file, following the same steps as you did for creating the first notch filter. If you have more than two tinnitus frequencies, I recommend creating separate notched audio files. For example, if you have three tinnitus frequencies, put two notches on one file, and one on another. If you have four tinnitus frequencies, put two notches on one file, and two on another. I'm not a neurologist, but it's my opinion that more than two notches in the same audio file will give the brain too broad a range of neural connections to work on. Others may have a different opinion, and it's up to you to decide how you want to approach it.

Let's say you have tinnitus with four dominant frequencies. You have made two notched audio files, and each file contains two notched frequencies. You can approach your audio notch therapy two different ways:

1. Listen to the first notched audio file for a minimum of 1.5 hours, then listen to the second notched audio file for 1.5 hours, for a total of three hours. Do this every day for at least a month. If you think your tinnitus is improving, keep using this routine.

2. Listen to one of the notched audio files for a minimum of 1.5 hours every day until you're satisfied with the improvement in your tinnitus. Then switch to the second notched audio file. When you feel like you've reached maximum improvement from listening to the second notched audio file, you can listen to the first notched audio file again. Keep alternating the notched audio files for as long as you feel like you're getting some benefit. Again, if your tinnitus is over 8,000 Hz, restrict your listening time to one-hour sessions.

Whichever method you choose, remember to check your frequencies every couple of weeks or at least once a month.

Here's the summary of steps to create a notched audio file:

1. Go to www.AudioNotch.com;
2. Find your frequency/frequencies on their frequency matching tool and write down the Hz number(s);
3. Download and install the free Audacity program;
4. Open Audacity. Choose "Generate" on the toolbar menu, then select "Noise" from the dropdown menu;
5. Choose the color noise you want, leave the Amplitude at default setting, and set the file length;
6. Click "Effect" on the toolbar menu, then select "Notch Filter";
7. Input your frequency and the width of the notch (0.3 is a good width);
8. Choose "Analyze" on the toolbar menu, then select "Plot Spectrum" to verify the notch;
9. Choose "File" from the toolbar menu, then select "Export Audio";
10. Export your notched audio file into a file folder on your computer;
11. Import the notched audio file into your playback device.

If you have a music or soundscape audio file that you want to use instead of a noise file, follow steps 1 through 3. At step 4, open Audacity, click "File," then select "Import." Navigate to the file on your computer and select it for import. Once you have imported the file, follow steps 6 through 11. Keep in mind that if the audio file you import doesn't contain a sufficient range of frequencies, the notched audio file will not be effective.

The next chapter discusses the different color noise files and suggestions for choosing the best one based on your tinnitus.

44
THE COLORS OF NOISE

Why are colors assigned to noise signals? The simple explanation is because noise has a frequency which correlates with the color spectrum.

Let's start with white noise, the most popular masking noise. White noise includes all frequencies and is analogous to white light, which is a combination of all light wave frequencies, thus the name "white noise." White noise combines high and low frequencies into one even spectrum, with equal energy in each frequency. Therefore, white noise has the same intensity for every frequency within it, which gives it a somewhat flat sound. You hear white noise in the sound of a rotating fan, in a car radio when it tunes in to static, or an air conditioning unit running on a hot summer night. It cuts through and overrides environmental and background sounds. That makes it a great sleeping aid when someone is trying to cover other sounds in their environment. Babies respond well to white noise, and one 1990s study suggested that babies fall asleep quicker when listening to white noise. Because it encompasses all the human-audible frequencies from 20 to 20,000 Hz, white noise is often incorporated into the sound of emergency sirens on ambulances and police vehicles. This helps anyone within hearing distance to easily locate the source of the siren and to take appropriate action.

You'll recall from Chapter 12, "Why Me," that backup emergency beepers have become so commonplace that people have a tendency to ignore them. Experiments have now proven that there's another problem with beeping noise: people cannot tell where the sound is coming from. Researchers have discovered, however, that people can easily locate the source of white noise. In the future, those annoying beepers may be replaced by white noise emitters, a nicer and more useful sound. They will also be a lot easier on the ears for people who suffer from hyperacusis and/or reactive tinnitus.

Pink noise is similar to white noise, but every octave carries the same power. This gives pink noise a balanced consistent frequency, and it's the reason why many people prefer it to white noise. It has a more gentle overall sound. Who doesn't love the sound of falling rain, a waterfall, or wind in the trees? That's pink noise. In fact, research is beginning to show that pink noise can contribute to a higher quality of sleep. Pink noise slows and regulates your brain waves, leading to deep and restful sleep. Slower brain wave activity is also correlated with calming of tinnitus. Pink noise is an ideal choice for creating a notched audio file to help your brain work on repairing neural connections while you sleep.

Brown noise is white noise with emphasis on the lower frequencies. It sounds less like static and more like running water, similar to a fast-running stream or heavy winds. If white noise is too harsh for you, try brown noise. Incidentally, brown noise is recommended if your tinnitus is in the lower frequencies.

Blue noise, or azure noise, is a form of high frequency white noise. As the frequency increases, the power and energy of the signal will increase as well. Blue noise has more of a hissing sound due to its emphasis on the higher frequencies. It's called blue noise because the color blue is located at the higher end of the spectrum for visible light. It's less harsh than white noise but not as relaxing as pink noise. Blue noise may be a good choice if you like a sound which mimics spraying water.

Violet noise is a sizzling sound, which is a wonderful masker if your tinnitus has a hissing and/or sizzling quality to it. There are many people who describe their tinnitus as the sound of something frying in hot grease. Violet noise is a more intense version of blue noise, with a concentration of energy in the highest frequencies. This may also be a good choice if your tinnitus has a screechy quality to it.

Grey noise has equal loudness for every frequency within it, but grey noise doesn't sound the same to everyone who hears it because everyone has a unique hearing curve. It's a noise which is generally well-tolerated and thus it's often used to treat hyperacusis, as well as tinnitus. The article "Gray Noise," on www.Techopedia.com, describes it as "designed for the psychoacoustics of the human ear."

www.myNoise.net has sound generators for different color noises. Every sound generator includes a description of the type of noise and the effect it's intended to simulate. There are also specially calibrated Presets you can select on the right side of the screen. Click on them to test which of the variations you prefer. You can adjust components of the sound generator by moving the individual sliders up and down. Four popular sound generators are:

- White noise, "White Rain"
- Brown noise, "Impulse Noise"
- Pink noise, "Waterfall Noise"
- Grey noise, "White Noise & Co." - choose the Grey-like Noise Preset link on the right side of the screen.

Sound generators on the myNoise website can be ordered as MP3 audio files. The option to purchase is located under the "Current Slider Settings" header. By the way, when you donate to myNoise, you will earn generous credits toward your purchase of MP3 files.

YouTube has many color noise videos, some of them as long as 12 hours. The three listed below are suitable for both masking and audio notch therapy. The combination noise video reminds me of an air conditioner and is more soothing than plain white noise. One comment by a YouTube user described it as "wind and rain."

- Blue noise, "Ten Hours of Ambient Sound - Blue Noise"
- Violet noise, "Ten Hours of Violet Noise - Ambient Sound"
- Combination "Grey Brown Violet and Pink Noise"

You can record noise files through streaming audio or purchase an MP3 if available. Import it into Audacity and create an audio notch file, following the instructions in the prior chapter. This will give you the benefit of both masking and sound therapy. Purchasing an MP3 not only helps to support those who create the sound generators and videos, it will give you much better sound quality than the compressed version obtained by directly recording streaming audio.

45
ACRN (ACOUSTIC CR NEUROMODULATION)

Acoustic Coordinated Reset® Neuromodulation (ACRN) is a promising treatment which uses sound frequencies to remap the brain. This unusual sound therapy was developed to improve tinnitus by taking advantage of brain plasticity as a way to correct the false signaling of hyperactive neurons.

You will recall that audio notch therapy involves creating a notch filter in music or colored noise that removes your tinnitus frequency from the audio. ACRN takes somewhat of an opposite approach. The treatment consists of listening to four brief tones, two of which are above your tinnitus frequency and two of which are below it. These tones are played repeatedly and are based on a sophisticated algorithm. The four tones in ACRN activate the frequencies which surround the misfiring neurons that match your tinnitus frequency. In time, this disrupts the abnormal neural synchronicity of the misfiring neurons in your auditory cortex. In between the tones are brief intervals of silence, strategically timed to allow your brain to adjust and reset as it processes what it has heard.

That is a very simplistic explanation of an extremely complicated neural process. If you would like more detailed information, please read "Acoustic Coordinated Reset Neuromodulation in a Real Life Patient Population with Chronic Tonal Tinnitus," published by BioMed Research International, on www.hindawi.com. It's an excellent scientific summary of a study involving 200 tinnitus patients, most of whom were followed over the course of 12 months in an ACRN trial. More than half of the participants experienced improvement within three months. Information was provided by Germany, the United Kingdom, and also participation by Stanford University in California, U.S. If you prefer a more informal approach, The Tinnitus Clinic in the UK has created a YouTube video, "Acoustic CR Neuromodulation Tinnitus Treatment," which explains how ACRN works in their treatment protocol.

ACRN is a time-intensive method that requires listening to the audio from four to six hours per day over the course of at least three months, with the recommendation that you stay with the program six to nine months, or longer if you continue to experience improvement in your tinnitus. You can play it in your environment as background sound, or you can listen to it directly by using a playback device such as a smartphone or MP3 player with high quality earbuds. Be sure to keep the volume low enough so that it's either at or slightly above your hearing threshold. It doesn't need to be any louder than that for your brain to process the ACRN tones. By keeping the volume just low enough to be able to hear it and no louder, it will be easier for you to ignore the tones as time goes on.

At the beginning of my do-it-yourself ACRN treatment, I limited my listening time to six hours each day, usually for six consecutive hours. After a month, feeling confident that there was some improvement, I simply played my ACRN audio all day long and didn't limit the listening time. At the end of two months, I was convinced there was definite improvement. At that point I decided that not only would I play the ACRN all day, I would keep my iPhone on the nightstand, turn the volume to where I could just barely hear it, and play the ACRN all night. It didn't keep me from falling asleep, and even though I would still wake up once or twice during the night, I attribute that to the tinnitus, not the tones.

Within six months the very loud intrusive tinnitus dropped from a fairly consistent level of 8 or 9 out of 10, to more days when it was 7 out of 10. Some days the volume and intensity still went up to an 8. However, I was encouraged by the fact that there were also more days of mild to moderate tinnitus. Before the ACRN treatment, I would have four loud intrusive tinnitus days in a row, followed by one and sometimes two mild or moderate days, and then the loud intrusive tinnitus would begin again. Within three months, there was no definite pattern, but the number of severe tinnitus days decreased. In fact, there were even a couple times I experienced three mild days in a row. For me, a mild level means I still hear it all day long but I'm able to concentrate on work, and it doesn't wear me down like it did when it was severe day after day.

For six months I listened to ACRN for most of the day and all night. Then I changed the routine and stopped listening during the day, and instead just let it play throughout the night. My tinnitus is remarkably better than it was at the beginning of the program. On most days, I still hear it all day but it doesn't interfere too much with my work. It tends to get more intrusive at night, but that may be partly due to less things going on to distract me. Every week or so, the tinnitus will drop to a barely noticeable level of 2 or 3 for a day or two, then ramp up in volume the next day. There are still days when it's annoying and difficult to ignore, but those days are far fewer than a year ago. In fact, it's been months since I used masking to help me cope.

One of the criteria for being a suitable candidate for ACRN is that you can hear all the tones at a reasonable volume. If you don't hear them, it means the nerve impulses for the necessary frequencies will not reach the auditory cortex. ACRN depends on the neurons of the surrounding frequencies being able to stabilize the abnormal misfiring neurons. I have been told by people familiar with this therapy that if you cannot hear the surrounding frequencies, then the remapping of your brain will not occur. Despite that, I would suggest giving it a try anyway. Everyone is different, and the brain is a complex organ with intricate neural pathways. There is perhaps a chance that ACRN may help, whether you can hear all the frequencies or not. If you are seeking ACRN treatment through a professional service, the issue of being unable to hear the different tones should be addressed during your initial appointment. If you are creating your own ACRN files, as outlined in the next chapter, it's up to you how to proceed with the tones you are able to hear. If you don't wear a hearing aid, now would be a good time to invest in one, as that would improve your ability to hear all the tones.

Another criteria established by The Tinnitus Clinic is that your tinnitus be tonal; that is, the sound of your tinnitus is a constant tone, often described as "eeeeeeeeeeee." Many people do not have tonal tinnitus. They have buzzing, hissing, sizzling, roaring, et cetera. According to The Tinnitus Clinic, these people would not be good candidates for ACRN. My tinnitus consists of a persistent whine that could be considered as tonal, but I've also had hissing, whistling, screeching, squealing, and other assorted sounds. Despite that, ACRN definitely helped me. Perhaps those with tonal tinnitus get the best results, but you might experience some improvement even if you have tinnitus that doesn't fall into that category.

If you have very high frequency tinnitus in the 14Hz to 15Hz range, it can be a bit more difficult to target your frequency. In particular, if it's tonal, listening to a constant tone while trying to zero in on your frequency might result in temporary residual inhibition, which could interfere with determining the correct frequency. Try having a friend help you by asking them to operate the frequency matcher while you listen with your eyes closed, until you feel like you've got a match. (Remember that hearing becomes more sensitive when sight is shut off.) If the frequencies begin to sound too much alike, give your ears some time to rest and try it again later. It's easy to get sensory overload. This is why people who shop for perfume are advised not to test more than three to five perfumes in one day, as their olfactory system simply becomes unable to differentiate one scent from another. Your auditory system can likewise become unable to discriminate between two similar frequencies.

Please note that ACRN has not been shown to be helpful for tinnitus caused by a somatic disorder or disease, such as temporomandibular joint problems or Ménière's disease. The reason for this is because the problem does not lie within the auditory cortex and misfiring neurons, but rather that the tinnitus is caused by dysfunction in other systems of the body. Pulsatile tinnitus falls into that category as well, since it is generally a symptom of a vascular disorder. Tinnitus can actually get worse if you have Ménière's disease and use the ACRN protocol. If you have tinnitus due to Ménière's, please consult with your healthcare practitioner if you're thinking of trying ACRN.

At this time, ACRN apparently is only available under professional supervision in Germany and the United Kingdom. It is also fairly expensive if you are on a limited or moderate budget. Fortunately, there is an alternative do-it-yourself ACRN treatment available that has been tried by members of Tinnitus Talk, with positive results. I am one of those members, and because my tinnitus has improved using the DIY ACRN, I want to share it with you. It was created by General Fuzz, a member of Tinnitus Talk. He describes it as a protocol designed to replicate the ACRN treatment offered by The Tinnitus Clinic. Obviously there is no professional consultation included with this type of do it yourself treatment, so if you have doubts please consult your healthcare practitioner.

General Fuzz first introduces himself and his website on page 6 of the "Acoustic CR Neuromodulation: Do It Yourself Guide" thread on Tinnitus Talk. If you want to know as much as possible about ACRN, and are comfortable with technical discussions by professional sound engineers, read the entire thread of the Do It Yourself Guide from the beginning. It includes anecdotal comments on the results of the DIY treatment, as well as messages posted by a few members who participated in clinical trials of ACRN.

There are several do-it-yourself ACRN websites, but my familiarity (and modest success) has been with the General Fuzz generator. Please feel free to research the Internet for alternative ACRN do-it-yourself or professional treatments. However, for the purposes of this book, and to keep it simple, the next chapter utilizes the General Fuzz ACRN generator. It's free, it's easy, and it just might work for you.

46
ACRN - DO IT YOURSELF GUIDE

In this chapter I'll show you how to create a free personalized Acoustic Coordinated Reset® Neuromodulation audio file. Screenshot images in this chapter were made on a Mac.

Step 1. Go to www.GeneralFuzz.net/acrn for the ACRN program. There is some explanatory text at the top of the page, and some settings that look like the image below. For this example the frequency is set at 8125.

Play Single Frequency	Play ACRN	Stop Audio

Frequency: 8125 hz

Volume:

Frequencies in current pattern: 6236 hz, 7315 hz, 8908 hz, 11360 hz

Note: My Internet Explorer browser doesn't work well with the General Fuzz website. If you have the same problem, try Chrome, Firefox, or Safari. I have tested the site on those browsers and it works fine.

Step 2. Press the "Play Single Frequency" button. Put your cursor on the Frequency bar marker. If you think your tinnitus frequency is higher than the tone you hear, slide the marker on the Frequency bar to the right. If you think your frequency is lower, slide it to the left. Keep moving the marker until the tone sounds the same as your tinnitus frequency. Each time you move the marker, you can then use the right-arrow or up-arrow key which increases the frequency by 1 hertz. The left-arrow and down-arrow keys will decrease the frequency by 1 hertz. If you experience residual inhibition while trying to match your frequency, give your ears a break for a few minutes and try again. The higher the frequency of your tinnitus, the more difficult it may be to match, because our perception of sound isn't as precise between 14 kilohertz and 15 kilohertz as it is, say, between 5 kilohertz and 6 kilohertz.

In this example, let's say the Frequency bar when it's set at 7345 seems like a fairly accurate match. It doesn't need to be a perfect match, but it's important to get it as close as possible. When you get the right frequency, press the "Stop Audio" button.

Play Single Frequency   **Play ACRN**   **Stop Audio**

Frequency: 7345 hz

Volume:

Frequencies in current pattern: 5633 hz, 6611 hz, 8058 hz, 10272 hz

The four frequencies generated which target the 7345 tinnitus frequency are 5633, 6611, 8058, and 10272. To hear what your own sound therapy program will sound like, find your tinnitus frequency, then press the "Play ACRN" button. As each frequency is played, it will light up in red. After you've listened for a moment, go ahead and press the "Stop Audio" button.

If you could hear all four frequency tones, you're a good candidate for ACRN sound therapy. If you could not hear all the tones, the general belief is that it will not work for you. At this point you'll need to decide if you want to pursue this, just in case it does reduce your tinnitus. Time is going by anyway, so you might as well spend that time by using a therapy that has been shown to help some tinnitus patients. As noted in the prior chapter, supposedly ACRN only works on tonal tinnitus. However, it has helped reduce the severity of my tinnitus, which for the most part is not tonal. As an interesting side note, one member of Tinnitus Talk support forum mentioned that when he gets a spike, he listens to his ACRN audio for five to 10 minutes and the spike settles down.

Step 3. You can create your personal ACRN file using Audacity software if you don't have recording software on your computer. Download and install Audacity for free at www.AudacityTeam.org. Here's a March 2017 screenshot from their Home page:

Audacity® is free, open source, cross-platform audio software for multi-track recording and editing.

Audacity is available for Windows®, Mac®, GNU/Linux® and other operating systems. Check our feature list, Wiki and Forum.

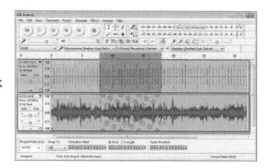

If you need help with installing Audacity, visit YouTube and type "install Audacity" into the Search bar. There are several good tutorials that will walk you through the procedure. Choose one for your operating system, whether Mac or a Windows version.

Step 4. Open Audacity. Return to the frequency matcher and make sure it has your frequency displayed. Press the "Start ACRN" button to begin playing the ACRN frequencies. Then press the round Record button in Audacity to start recording. When your file is the length you want, press the tan/yellow Stop button in Audacity, and then press the "Stop Audio" button on the frequency matcher.

Note: If you're going to play the audio file in a playback device that has a loop (repeating) option, then a 10-minute file is sufficient. If your device doesn't have a loop or repeat option, you should make the file 30 minutes to an hour long. ACRN sound therapy requires listening for four to six hours each day. It will be distracting if you have to restart the audio file more than once or twice every hour. Looping is the best way to listen to ACRN audio.

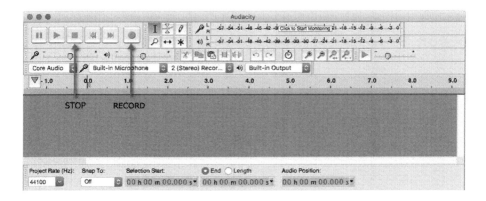

When it's recording, you'll see the graphical representation of the different frequencies in the Audacity window, as shown in the next screenshot. The height of the triangular shaped elements may be different than what's displayed here, depending on the frequency of your tinnitus, the volume at which you're recording, and the size of your monitor.

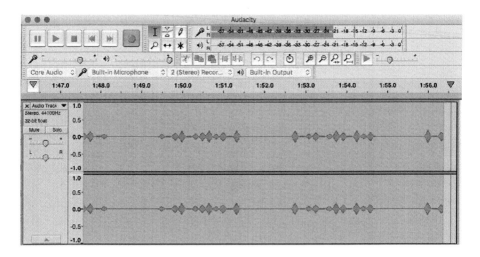

If you're in Record mode but all you see is a straight blue line going across, that means it's not recording. This sometimes happens the first time you use Audacity for recording, and there can be different reasons for it. For my Windows 7 system, I fixed it by right clicking on the volume icon in the task bar tray, then clicking on the Recording devices option, selecting "Stereo Mix Realtek High Definition Audio," then clicking "OK." This easy fix was from the "Fix Audacity not recording!" tutorial on YouTube. If this doesn't work for your system, try a different YouTube tutorial, using the search term "Audacity not recording." Also check to see that your computer sound volume is set at an audible level.

When the file is the right length, press the square button to stop recording.

Step 5. Click File on the toolbar menu, then click Export Audio in the dropdown menu.

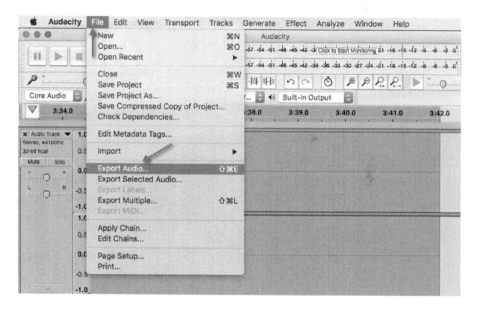

Step 6. At this point the steps are basically the same as Steps 8 and 9 in Chapter 43, "Audio Notch - Do It Yourself Guide." In the window that opens, choose a folder where you want to export the file. I created a folder in my Music Library and named it "ACRN." The file name reflects that it's an ACRN file customized for tinnitus frequency 7345, created on June 28, 2017. You should test your tinnitus frequency at least once a month to see if there are any changes. By naming the ACRN file in this manner, it will help you to keep track of those changes.

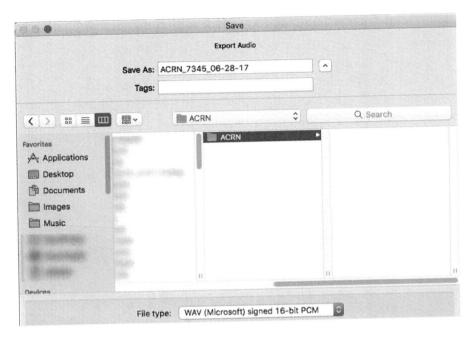

I've chosen to export as a WAV file because it has less data compression than an MP3 file. Data compression affects the quality and accuracy of frequency representation in audio. FLAC is an excellent choice for high quality encoding of frequencies if your device accepts FLAC files. Be aware that it will be a larger size file than if you export as WAV or MP3. For a highly detailed explanation of the lossy quality of various audio file formats, visit the www.SoundOnSound.com website and read their article, "What Data Compression Does to Your Music."

When you click "Save," you may get a popup message, "Your tracks will be mixed down to two stereo channels in the exported file." Just click "OK" to continue. Then a popup menu to insert metadata tags will appear. It isn't necessary to add metadata information for this type of audio file, so just click the "OK" button. Your ACRN file will be saved to the folder you assigned it.

Step 7. Now you can import the file into your playback device. It's no different than the procedure you use to import any music file from your computer to another device. If you don't have a playback device, you can play it directly from your computer. As long as you can hear it, your brain can utilize it. The obvious advantage of creating an audio file and loading it into a playback device is you can take it with you wherever you go. When you use earbuds to listen to it, be sure to keep the volume at a safe level to protect your hearing. Just above hearing threshold is sufficient for the therapy to work.

There is one thing you need to be aware of in the beginning stage: As the auditory cortex is adapting to these new sounds and trying to correct its misfiring frequencies, you may experience some unusual increased intensity and volume of your tinnitus. In my nonprofessional opinion, it's probably due to the brain experiencing more intense cortical reorganization than it's been used to. The tinnitus should go back to baseline soon. If the increase in volume or intensity persists for more than two or three days, take a break from the ACRN therapy for a couple of days. Re-check your frequency again to make sure you've got as close a match as possible, then try again. If you continue to experience negative results, this type of sound therapy is probably not suitable for you.

Keep in mind that this is a long-term therapy. It requires patience and discipline. You will need to listen to the audio four to six hours every day for a minimum of three to six months, and perhaps up to 12 months. There may be some improvement within the first month, but it might take longer than that to notice a difference, especially if you've had tinnitus for several years.

If you believe this ACRN is helping you, or you just want to show your appreciation, please consider donating some dollars to General Fuzz at http://generalfuzz.net/donate.php for his generous contribution of time, talent and effort in creating this great program for the tinnitus community.

47
BACK TO SILENCE METHOD

The Back to Silence method was developed by Terry, a member of Tinnitus Talk. He used it with great success to overcome loud, intrusive tinnitus that he had struggled with for four decades. Terry's tinnitus was brought on by excessive noise exposure and migraine medication. As early as high school, he began to experience the distressing symptoms of tinnitus that tormented him until he found a remarkably simple solution. The solution was to acknowledge his tinnitus when he heard it, to state his emotional response to hearing the tinnitus, make a mark on a piece of paper to show that he had responded to it, and then to go about his business. Terry admits that he can still clearly hear his loud tinnitus when he actively listens for it, but that otherwise he is completely unaware of it in his day-to-day life. As an example, he mentioned one day that he hadn't even noticed it while sitting in the relative quiet of a dentist's office.

How can this be, that someone with a decades long history of loud intrusive tinnitus no longer hears it, even though it's still there? If you read Chapter 23, "The Amygdala and Limbic System," you'll recall that the key to reducing emotional distress is to alter the pathway of the tinnitus signal from the limbic system to the frontal lobe. The limbic system is a reactive and emotional creature, whereas the frontal lobe is cool and logical. If you watched the original Star Trek series, you can see that Doc would be the limbic system and Mr. Spock the frontal lobe. Doc would become almost hysterical whenever the survival of the Enterprise crew was at stake, whereas Mr. Spock would assess the situation objectively and figure out a logical approach to the danger at hand.

The dynamics of the Star Trek characters is very similar to what Terry is doing. In other words, the intrusive sound of tinnitus is the danger signal. Doc wants to go into high alert about it, but Mr. Spock listens to it and says, "There is no danger here. Ignore this." In time, Doc realizes that the best way to handle the tinnitus signal is to simply transfer it to Mr. Spock, who in turn pays no attention to it because it isn't important to the survival of the Enterprise. In fact, no one on the

Enterprise even hears it anymore until someone says, "Hey, what happened to that sound?" That's when it reappears. Mr. Spock calmly takes control once again, and soon the signal fades away.

There's scientific research to support this method. Back in 2007, psychologists conducted brain imaging studies which showed that naming what we're feeling lessens the emotional impact. Subjects were asked to look at photographs of faces depicting anger or fear. In response to those images, the amygdala showed heightened activity. However, when the subjects were asked to name the emotion, that activity decreased. At the same time, heightened activity occurred in another region of the brain, the right ventrolateral prefrontal cortex. This is the part of the brain which we use when assigning words to emotional responses. The prefrontal cortex plays an important role in managing tinnitus, and is covered in more detail in Chapter 64, "Train the Brain - Basics."

If you want to know more about how naming an emotion can lessen its power, read "Putting Feelings Into Words Produces Therapeutic Effects In The Brain," published on www.ScienceDaily.com. The article explains how naming emotions utilizes some of the same principles as mindfulness meditation, which is another proven method for increasing activity in the prefrontal cortex and tamping down the amygdala.

What to do when you hear your tinnitus:

1. Tell yourself, "I hear it and I feel _____," (whatever emotion you're feeling);
2. Make a mark on a piece of paper to indicate you've had a response;
3. Look at the marks you've made at the end of each day, and see if they're becoming less as time goes on.

Step number 1 can be tough if you're not used to acknowledging your emotions, and even tougher if you have no idea how to describe them. It may help you to understand that common emotional reactions when experiencing tinnitus distress are anger, frustration, annoyance, irritation, agitation, resentment, depression, sadness, hopelessness, fear, anxiety, and panic. So for step 1, you might say, "I hear it and I feel depressed," or, "I hear it and I feel annoyed," or, "I hear it and I feel anxious," or, "I hear it and I feel angry," and so on. Some people are very uncomfortable with acknowledging so-called negative emotions. It isn't because they believe it's unhealthy to have a negative emotion. Instead, they feel that putting emphasis on a negative emotion over and over, which is what happens when you first begin this method, may cause that emotion to gain a stronger hold in the psyche. That isn't the case with this method.

If you are fortunate enough to have mild tinnitus, or if you have cycling tinnitus that brings you mild days from time to time, then write down your emotion whenever you become aware of your tinnitus. If you happen to be feeling good, your response might be, "I hear it and I feel all right." If you have no emotional reaction at all, you could say, "I hear it and I feel calm," or, "I hear it and I don't care." Make your mark on the paper with each acknowledgment, and return to whatever it is you were doing when the tinnitus surfaced. When the louder or more intrusive tinnitus strikes again, carry on with the method like you did before. For example, "I hear it and I feel angry," or, "I hear it and I feel despondent."

It's a natural tendency to start something and look for improvement right away. I would recommend waiting at least a week or two before checking to see whether you're making less marks per day. If the number of marks have decreased, that's fantastic. It means Mr. Spock is taking control. If not, don't worry about it. We all know how incredibly stubborn and bullheaded Doc could be. Keep in mind that you only want to measure the number of reactions you're having, not the volume or nature of your tinnitus. The main objective of the Back to Silence method is to **focus on your reaction, not on the tinnitus.** Terry says that the more he described his feelings about the tinnitus instead of describing the volume of his tinnitus, the less it bothered him.

What you must avoid doing if you want to make progress:

- Monitoring your tinnitus to check its volume, even if you're only looking for improvement;
- Describing your tinnitus;
- Telling yourself you're going to beat your tinnitus.

When you monitor your tinnitus for changes in volume or other characteristics, that's the same as telling your brain that the tinnitus is important. You don't want that. You want your brain to respond to your tinnitus the same way it responds to the sound of your refrigerator humming in the background, or the sound of your keyboard as you type. You might notice your refrigerator's motor starting up, but then you ignore its ongoing sound because you're so used to it. If you're like most people, you've probably never paid attention to the tapping sound of your keyboard. However, the next time you're typing, you might remember this comment and notice the sounds of clicking keys for a few moments. When you're out walking, listen to your footsteps. This is another sound that most people never notice because they're simply used to it and have learned to tune it out.

"Wait a minute," some of you might say. "I wish my tinnitus were as mild as a refrigerator hum. It sounds like a swarm of cicadas in my head!" It can be a struggle to set aside the issue of volume, but the frontal lobe doesn't care how loud your tinnitus is. It really doesn't care about the existence of the tinnitus at all. Have you ever been driving down the road, thinking of things you've got to get done, when all of a sudden you realize there's an ambulance right behind you, its siren blaring at full force? The intense volume of that siren was audible long before you noticed it, but your brain was engaged in decision-making activity and didn't register the warning, despite how incredibly loud it was. It was only when the ambulance was perceived as a genuine danger by your limbic system that it took over and snapped your attention to the siren. This allowed you to take evasive action by pulling over and letting the ambulance pass.

Now you might say, "But a swarm of cicadas buzzing in my head all day isn't the same thing as a siren that sneaks up on me while driving and then goes away." As far as your brain is concerned, if enough time passes, it's very much the same thing. The key is to not deliberately listen for it. **Diminish its importance by making a decision that you will not listen for it.** In fact, promise yourself you won't listen for it. A promise carries enormous weight with most people and is usually emotionally significant. Let the limbic system handle the promise, and let your frontal lobe handle the tinnitus.

Describing your tinnitus is another way of giving it power. When you describe it, you're assigning importance to it. Think about it. Let's say you drive to work on the same old route. When you get to the office, you don't talk about what you saw, because there was nothing along the way that was interesting enough to talk about. But if you saw a white dog wearing a clown suit and riding a unicycle, with an orange cat wearing a purple bow tie balanced on the dog's head, you would get to the office and begin describing what you saw with great detail. Why? Because it stirred your emotions and so you paid attention. If you see that same dog and cat every day for the next three months, you'll stop paying attention. You don't react to them anymore because they've become part of your everyday scenery. You may not even notice them at all. We only describe things in detail when we have a vested interest in them. The limbic system creates an emotional attachment to that description. The frontal lobe does not. Stop describing your tinnitus, no matter how obsessed you currently are with its characteristics. **Diminish its importance by making a decision that you will not describe your tinnitus to yourself or others.**

Obviously if your healthcare practitioner asks you about your tinnitus, you need to provide an accurate description because it will affect the prescribed treatment. Also, if there's a sudden and extreme negative development in your tinnitus that's outside the norm of a spike, set aside the Back to Silence method and seek medical attention. Something serious may be going on.

Feeling angry, resentful, and frustrated are common strong reactions to intrusive tinnitus. Any of those three emotions can easily provoke a fight-or-flight response. When angry, you want to strike back at the attacker. If something of high value, like silence, is taken away, it can cause extreme resentment. If something constantly makes you miserable, you'll likely do anything you can to get rid of it. The problem is, you can't fight tinnitus and make it go away. Your brain isn't wired that way. It simply won't work. It does you no good to put up your dukes and tell yourself you're going to beat the tinnitus. Remember that tinnitus is a mindless beast under the influence of your amygdala. When you think about this beast with the attitude that you're going to beat it, that triggers the fight-or-flight mechanism of your limbic system and keeps it activated. You cannot "fight" tinnitus. You cannot "beat" it. As I mentioned earlier in Chapter 15, "Don't Panic (and Other Advice)," the best way to deal with tinnitus is to outsmart it.

RaZaH, a member of Tinnitus Talk, asked Terry, "What is the Back to Silence technique?" Terry answered, "It's a nickname for attention switching applied to tinnitus." In his words, this is how Terry described the technique in four basic steps:

- "You simply QUIT listening for the tinnitus, or describing it, or measuring it, or comparing it."
- "You START describing (to yourself) and measuring your emotional response to tinnitus as often as you'd like."
- "Hopefully in time, the responses become fewer; and for some reason, unknown to me, the tinnitus all but disappears."
- "A little harder than it sounds actually. I had a bad habit of 'checking in' on my tinnitus. Not anymore."

By the way, if you have cycling tinnitus and you happen to have a severe episode, you need to resist the temptation of comparing it to a milder day. Remember that comparing it is another form of describing it, which will get in the way of letting the method work.

When I first read about the Back to Silence method, I tried it for a few weeks and didn't seem to gain any benefit. I was stuck in a rut of measuring, monitoring, describing and comparing my tinnitus, and eventually abandoned the method altogether. A couple years later, I switched to another technique based on the guidelines of the method. Whenever the tinnitus intrusiveness became overwhelming, I would tell myself, "Don't measure it, don't monitor it, don't describe it, don't compare it." Sometimes I had to repeat that a lot in a day. Maybe it was just a coincidence, but there did seem to be a slight improvement in my tinnitus by consistently repeating the guidelines to myself.

I'm trying Back to Silence again, making sure I follow the four guidelines, and getting better results this time. However, I added something new to Terry's method. When I state how I feel about the tinnitus, I include the reason why and then say, "I prefer quiet." For example, "I hear my tinnitus and I feel annoyed because I want to concentrate on my work. I prefer quiet." Or, "I hear it and I feel frustrated because I want to sleep. I prefer quiet." I don't know why it works, but it definitely has made a difference. Maybe stating the reason why I'm feeling what I'm feeling, and then stating what I want, activates the decision-making or rational part of my brain. When you make your statement about how you're feeling, just add the reason why you feel what you feel, and then say in a calm voice, "I prefer quiet." Try it for a while, and see if it helps.

Terry has created a "Back to Silence" video which is available on the Tinnitus Talk Support Forum channel on YouTube. He tells the story of how he developed tinnitus, the years of struggling with it, and how it's no longer an issue for him. The video begins with a short version explaining the method, followed by a more in-depth version beginning at timeline 2:20. For the hearing impaired, the video has closed captioning.

The next chapter is a summary Q&A about the Back to Silence method. If you feel comfortable with the information already provided, you can skip the Q&A and start using the method right away. Follow the program faithfully for at least six weeks. Everyone is different, so it doesn't work for everybody, and it may take much longer to work for some people than others. When it does work, the suppression of tinnitus can be significant.

48
BACK TO SILENCE Q&A

The Back to Silence thread on Tinnitus Talk is filled with useful information about the method, as well as feedback from those who have tried it. I have chosen what I believe are the most often asked types of questions about the method. Answers were given by Terry and other members. This chapter is a summary of those questions and answers.

Q. It's hard not to listen to my tinnitus. My attention keeps going back to it because it's loud and intrusive.
A. Listening to your tinnitus is a habit that's hard to break. Like any bad habit, it takes time to establish a new and healthier habit. Turn your focus away from the tinnitus and immerse yourself in something that requires concentration. That will help.

Q. Do you say this to yourself or do you speak it out loud? For example, "I hear the tinnitus and it's making me angry."
A. Either way is good. If you say things out loud, you're getting it off your chest, so to speak. If you're around people and you don't want to speak out loud, or you just want to think of what you're feeling and note it mentally, that's fine. The important thing is to describe your emotion.

Q. Doesn't acknowledging a negative emotional reaction just highlight the irritation you feel and make the tinnitus stronger?
A. The opposite happens. It decreases the tinnitus.

Q. If I get annoyed at myself for checking on my tinnitus, will that make it worse or does it matter?
A. You only want to describe your reaction when you hear the tinnitus, not to something you're doing, so don't describe your response to what you're doing.

Q. Does this work with hyperacusis?
A. Unfortunately, hyperacusis can still flare up.

Q. Sometimes I say to myself, "There it is again! I'm so worried it will never go away." Is that okay?

A. That's a good response because you're talking about how you feel, not how loud or obnoxious the tinnitus is. Just make a note that your emotional reaction is worry.

Q. I can't help but compare how my tinnitus sounds from one day to the next. It affects my emotional reaction.

A. If you listen to your tinnitus in an attempt to measure it and compare it to the last time you heard it, the method won't work. In other words, do not measure the tinnitus. Measure your reaction to the tinnitus.

Q. Can I say something like, "It's hissing instead of screeching and I feel better"?

A. That won't be helpful. You don't want to describe your tinnitus. Maybe the change from screeching to hissing gives you hope. You can say something like, "I hear it and I feel hopeful," the key word being *hopeful*.

Q. I sometimes get spikes. Will this keep spikes from happening? What do I do if I get a bad spike?

A. It doesn't prevent spikes, which can be unpredictable. A spike can certainly shake you up, no matter when it happens. Take a deep breath, have confidence that the method has worked before and it can work again. Respond by describing your emotional reaction, and not by describing the intensity of the spike. "I hear it and I'm really scared," or, "I hear it and I'm hopeful that I'll feel better soon." Don't monitor or measure the tinnitus during a spike.

Q. I hear my tinnitus all the time, from the moment I wake up until I go to sleep, and sometimes it wakes me up. Am I supposed to constantly note that I hear it and how I feel?

A. As often as you react emotionally to it, that's how often you note it, even if it's 500 times a day. Every time you describe your emotion, you're telling the frontal lobe to deal with it. The interesting thing is that you may find yourself getting tired of noting your reaction, which means you're getting bored with noticing the tinnitus. This is another way of diminishing its importance.

Q. How long is it going to take before my tinnitus improves?
A. The question to ask is, "How long will it take until I feel better?" To say "My tinnitus is improving" is a measurement of your tinnitus. Usually within a few weeks of dedication to the Back to Silence method, you will probably begin to have less responses to your tinnitus throughout the day, and your emotions will be more on the positive side. "I hear it, and I feel okay," or, "I hear it and I'm looking forward to feeling better," that sort of thing.

Q. What if I'm not hearing the tinnitus? Do I still measure my response?
A. The idea is to measure your response when you hear the tinnitus, because that's when the signal is traveling along pathways in your brain. If you don't hear it and you realize you're not hearing it and that makes you feel good, you can just say, "I feel good," without mentioning the tinnitus at all.

Q. When my tinnitus is loud, I feel bad. When my tinnitus is low, I feel good. The volume directly affects my emotions. How can Back to Silence work for me?
A. It works because you're addressing your emotions, not the tinnitus. You may make more responses when your tinnitus is loud or intrusive, but remember to note your emotional reaction itself, without indicating the tinnitus volume. Instead of saying, "It's so loud, it's driving me crazy," say, "I hear it and I feel like I'm going crazy."

Q. My tinnitus level changes during the day. How do I deal with this?
A. You can say, for example, "I hear it and it's not bothering me as much as it was this morning." If you feel the opposite of that, you would say, "I hear it and I am really bothered by it," or whatever your emotion is. If you feel like it's getting worse, you would say, "I hear it and I'm afraid." Don't say, "I hear it and I'm afraid it's getting worse," because "getting worse" is a description of your tinnitus.

Q. When the method begins to get good results, does that mean you don't hear your tinnitus in a quiet room?

A. The tinnitus stays unnoticed in the background no matter where you are. However, if you deliberately think about it, and if you make a conscious effort to listen for it, it will likely reappear. If it does, tell yourself, "I hear it and I'm okay." Then go about your business of whatever you were doing, and it should recede again.

Q. Do you use masking?

A. I don't use anything except the Back to Silence method. No pills, no counseling, no masking. This lets me know that it's the method that's working to improve the tinnitus, and not some combination of treatments.

Q. My tinnitus is constant, and it's so loud and high pitched it could shatter glass. I'm desperate for this to work, but what am I supposed to do when tinnitus is like this?

A. Respond to it when it bothers you the most. Try to stay focused on something to distract yourself, even a little bit, from the tinnitus. When the tinnitus begins to overwhelm you, that's when you respond. "I hear it and I feel overwhelmed," or, "I hear it and I feel frustrated," if that's what you're feeling. Keep doing this, because this is how you alter the pathway of the tinnitus signal.

Q. I tell my tinnitus all day long to p*ss off, that I'm too busy to deal with it, but it's not working. I'm scared, and I cry all the time.

A. That's not how the method works. Back to Silence is not a pep talk, and it's not a fight-or-flight talk ("p*ss off"). Instead you would say, "I hear it and I'm scared," or, "I hear it and I'm sad." Do this as many times a day as you need to, all day long. Your responses will become fewer as time goes on.

Q. My honest feeling is that it's driving me insane, not just today, but every day.

A. Take it one day at a time. Don't think about how your tinnitus will be tomorrow, or next week, or next month, or next year. Stay in the present moment. "I hear it and I feel anxious," is a good response. We may feel like we're going insane when we believe we can no longer tolerate it. "I hear it and I feel hopeless," or, "I hear it and I feel so discouraged," or, "I hear it and I feel defeated," are all different ways to describe an emotional response in that sort of situation.

Q. Instead of naming an emotion, can I say something like, "I hear it and it's p*ssing me off"?
A. That will work. You could say, "I hear it and I feel very angry," but your brain gets the message either way.

Q. How precise do I have to be about naming my emotion? I need to know if that's important in getting this to work.
A. Giving your emotion a general description is all it takes. You don't need to say, "I hear it and I'm feeling apprehensive." If you say, "I hear it and I'm worried," that will work just as well. Your brain is involved in your emotions, so it understands what you're trying to convey.

Q. I don't understand how this works. It seems too simple.
A. Fortunately, you don't need to understand how it works in order for it to work. Even though the method seems simple, it actually involves a very complex change taking place in your brain and how it handles the tinnitus signal.

Q. I hear different sounds in each ear. Will this work for me?
A. Yes, as long as you focus on describing your emotion, and not on the sounds you hear.

If you still have questions, I encourage you to read the entire "Back to Silence" thread at https://www.tinnitustalk.com/threads/back-to-silence.7172/.

49
COGNITIVE BEHAVIORAL THERAPY

Cognitive behavioral therapy (CBT) is sometimes recommended to help people cope with tinnitus. This is such a baffling condition with unique challenges to everyone who has it, so you'll improve your chances of success if you see a CBT professional with experience in treating patients with tinnitus. That being said, if you cannot afford a therapist, you can try a do it yourself approach.

First let's understand what the phrase "cognitive behavioral therapy" means. The word "cognitive" relates to the process of knowing or perceiving. You use your cognitive skills when you assess a situation and decide how you're going to react to it. "Behavioral" is of course related to how you actually react to your environment and your individual circumstances. Behavior can include thought patterns as well as physical actions. "Therapy" simply means treatment, with the aim of either curing or improving a condition, or learning how to cope with it when a cure or improvement is an unrealistic goal. With CBT, people learn that even though they cannot change what has already happened or control everything in their environment, they can learn to control how they interpret what is going on in their environment and respond in an emotionally healthy manner.

For example, many people who experience their first heartache from a breakup tend to have self-defeating thoughts like, "I'll never love again," or they may criticize themselves to a severe degree, blaming themselves for the loss of the relationship. They withdraw from social interaction and can't imagine living a happy life without that other person. As time goes on, those negative thoughts tend to fade away and are replaced with healthier, more positive thoughts. Think of how emotionally unhealthy we would all be if we were never able to move on from that first heartache! Someone who cannot accept the end of a relationship, and remains obsessively attached emotionally to the other person, is an example of not being able to replace negative thoughts with neutral or positive thoughts. It's a bleak outlook and can seriously affect their overall well-being if something isn't done to change their thought patterns.

Very few people, if anyone, live their entire life free of pain, disease, vindictive people, or just plain bad luck. Why is it that some people seem to naturally bounce back from terrible events that would send other people into the depths of depression? For one thing, we all have a natural set point in our personalities, a basic way of responding to people and our environment. This set point is created both by our DNA and our upbringing. If your natural set point is doom and gloom, you've got a lot more work ahead of you to cope with tinnitus than someone who faces adversity with an attitude of taking it in stride. However, if you make a sincere effort to overcome that set point, you can change your pattern of thinking and in turn make living with tinnitus a lot easier.

Think about how you behave when you get stressed out, when things go wrong, when you fail despite trying your best to succeed at something. Write down some examples of how you've reacted to negative or painful events in your past. Be honest with yourself as you record what your thoughts were at the time and how you reacted emotionally and physically. Write down everything you can think of, and then look for patterns in your thoughts and behavior. This will help you to understand your basic psychological makeup for dealing with adversity.

Once you understand how you tend to think and react to misfortune, take the time to write down some thoughts you have about your current tinnitus situation. How does it make you feel? What do you think of your present life with tinnitus? How do you envision your life in the future if the tinnitus remains? That last question is very important. It reveals your underlying attitude about how much influence you believe tinnitus will have in your life and how much power it will have over you personally. The purpose of cognitive behavioral therapy is to take any thoughts that life is meaningless, or that you can't be happy if you have tinnitus, and reshape those thoughts into a more realistic and positive framework. This doesn't mean trying to transform yourself into a Pollyanna. But you do want to step outside of yourself, so to speak, and be as objective as possible in assessing your situation. In time, as hard as it may be to believe, you literally can change how much tinnitus affects you by making a deliberate effort to change your thoughts about tinnitus.

The first months are the worst months, and the thought of living with tinnitus for the rest of your life can be devastating. This is true whether you're young, middle-aged, or in your senior years. We all have plans, goals and dreams. Tinnitus can knock everything sideways for a while. The danger zone occurs in the initial weeks and months. This is when people are most likely to engage in what's called catastrophic thinking, the belief that the torment of tinnitus is permanent and that life will never be good again. The first months are usually when all-or-nothing thoughts tend to invade the mind.

Let's start with the most common catastrophic thought that plagues people when they first develop tinnitus: "I just can't live like this." This is an absolutely normal reaction. After all, tinnitus disrupts your sleep, it keeps you from enjoying peace and quiet, it interferes with reading a good book, listening to music, it affects your work and personal life, and is a constant presence no matter what you do. It seems like you can only escape it in your sleep or maybe when you shower. That's how it feels in the beginning, and that's why it's so hard to imagine a productive, happy life with tinnitus. But the truth is, you can live with tinnitus. Millions and millions of people do it every day. There are people in your social circle and possibly even in your family who have tinnitus but never mention it because they've learned to adjust to it and don't feel like it merits attention. They may deliberately avoid bringing it up in conversation, if only because they don't want to be reminded of it. When you find yourself obsessively thinking, "I can't live like this," stop a moment and consider a new way of thinking about it. For example, you might say to yourself, "Right now I feel miserable because of tinnitus, but I know as time goes on that I'll be able to deal with it much better." You're not lying to yourself when you say something like that. It's true because at the moment you do feel miserable (or whatever emotion you're experiencing). It's also true that as time goes by, the odds are definitely in your favor that you will in fact be better able to deal with it.

When you're discouraged or depressed because tinnitus is affecting your concentration and productivity, you might have a thought like, "I can't get anything done, this tinnitus interferes too much with my ability to think." That certainly is an honest reflection of how you *feel*, but you need to understand that it really isn't *true*. When that kind of thought hits you, try saying something to yourself like, "Beethoven was deaf and he had tinnitus, but still he wrote beautiful timeless music." Look at the list of celebrities and other famous people in Chapter 12, "Why Me?," and think about their lives as examples of how the obstacle of tinnitus can eventually be overcome.

You can also look back on your own life and remember times when you felt defeated, but you kept going because the goal you were aiming for mattered more than the disappointments in your path. Your goal now may be to return to as normal a life as possible. At the end of the day, even if your productivity is barely half of what it used to be, at least you have learned a solid truth, that you can in fact get something done. So instead of saying, "I can't get anything done," replace that with, "I can get some things done, and as time goes by it will get easier to concentrate and work." You can substitute the words "concentrate and work" with whatever applies to your life. For example, "As time goes by, it will become easier to keep up the house and yard." The important thing is to remove the false thought and replace it with the truth. Again, look around your social circle, look at people you encounter at the grocery store, at the ballgame, at the theater. One in 10 people experiences tinnitus to some degree or another, yet there they are, living life and getting things done. That's all the proof you need that you can be like them, that tinnitus can't keep you from working, from playing, or doing anything you did before. The exception, of course, is that you absolutely must not risk exposing yourself to loud noise or music. It doesn't matter whether your tinnitus stems from noise exposure or for some other reason. You will need to protect your auditory system from now on, even if you become habituated to your tinnitus to the point where you seldom notice it anymore. Now, there's a goal worth thinking about!

Most of us are familiar with the pro/con approach to making big decisions. This is when you take a sheet of paper and draw a vertical line down the middle of the page. On the left side you write the good things you envision about the decision, and on the right side you list the possible negative outcomes of that decision. When you review the pros and cons, usually one side is weighted more heavily than the other. You can now make your decision, knowing that you've viewed it objectively and considered all possible outcomes. You can use the same technique when considering your thoughts about tinnitus. However, instead of writing your false/true statements on a piece of paper, use index cards.

On one side write down a false thought, something like, "I'll never get used to this." Flip the card over and write something true that counteracts the false thought; for example, "I have learned to adapt to many things in my life, and I'll learn to adapt to tinnitus in time." Do this with every negative self-limiting thought you presently have about tinnitus. Write it on the front of a card, and write down a more positive approach on the back side of the card. Once in a while, take the cards out and read them. In time, you'll notice yourself agreeing more and more with the positive outlook. This not only helps your emotional health, it also helps to reduce the importance your brain assigns to tinnitus.

Cognitive behavioral therapy is not a form of lying to yourself. You're not engaging in wishful thinking. What you're doing is deliberately replacing negative false thoughts with positive truthful thoughts when you consider your life with tinnitus. If you're the kind of person who typically engages in catastrophic, all-or-none types of thoughts, using the substitution technique will require more time and effort than someone who adapts to adversity more easily. If you need to take baby steps, don't worry about the person who's already walking or running. Take your time, and be patient with yourself. Remember, tinnitus is a very complex disorder involving the auditory system and the brain, with the limbic system playing a large part. Your thoughts and emotions play a major role in how your limbic system reacts to tinnitus signals. Dwelling on negative thoughts reinforces the amygdala's tendency to overreact to tinnitus signals in the brain. Do your best to push aside doom-and-gloom scenarios. Even if you can't adopt a rosy attitude, at least try to keep your thoughts rational and objective. Somewhere down the road, you'll look back and wonder why you spent so much time and energy worrying how you would ever live with tinnitus.

Mental illness, of course, is a separate issue. For example, someone with severe depression or extreme anxiety cannot simply "think away" the depression with positive thoughts. In such cases, professional intervention is usually required for that person to gain more control over their emotions.

I have given just the basics of cognitive behavioral therapy and some examples of applying it to tinnitus. If you're interested in pursuing CBT on your own, I recommend that you do more research to understand the science of why it works. A good layman's explanation of the process of CBT is on the Very Well website, "What is Cognitive Behavioral Therapy." A more detailed article is on the Psych Central website, "In Depth: Cognitive Behavioral Therapy," by Ben Martin, a doctor of psychiatry. With regard to tinnitus, I urge you to read "Dr. Hubbard's Tinnitus Story." Dr. Bruce Hubbard has had severe tinnitus since 2005, but his life is productive and fulfilled. It's an excellent article from the perspective of someone who both specializes in cognitive behavioral therapy and has severe unrelenting tinnitus.

You will likely get better results if you are treated by a professional trained in CBT, such as a clinical psychologist. Be sure to ask what experience they have in treating patients with tinnitus. In your sessions, be honest about how you feel and what your thoughts are about living with tinnitus. This is not the time to put on a brave front. You can rest assured that no matter how bleak your current outlook may be, your therapist has heard similar expressions of frustration and despair from other patients.

If you prefer a do-it-yourself approach, Amazon offers many books about CBT, including workbooks with step-by-step programs. Read the reviews, and check out the "Look inside" feature of any books which interest you. Most of them are reasonably priced, and some are available in an ebook version for Kindle. They seem to be primarily focused on CBT to address anxiety and depression, but more than likely there will be enough information and useful techniques that can be applied to tinnitus as well. You can also look for books about CBT through other online booksellers, or at your local bookstore and library.

50
HYPNOTHERAPY

It's unfortunate that most people have only a limited familiarity with hypnosis. They think of hypnosis as a form of entertainment, with an onstage hypnotist getting laughs at the expense of those who volunteer to be hypnotized. The truth is, in comparison to its broad range of therapeutic uses, hypnosis as entertainment is a very narrow field. Aside from perhaps convincing some people that hypnotism does work, using hypnosis as entertainment is a disservice to professional hypnotherapists whose main goal is to relieve suffering or change unhealthy behavior of their clients/patients.

Our choices today to treat physical disorders are far more expansive than they were only a couple decades ago. One reason is because enough people were willing to set aside their preconceived notions about treatment and seek an alternative method. Patients didn't stop going to allopathic doctors such as M.D.'s, but they began exploring holistic methods of treating both physical and mental disorders. This is due in large part to the increasing acceptance within the general population that the mind and body are intertwined. What affects one will affect the other. It wasn't that long ago that the majority of people were dismissive of chiropractors, acupuncturists, osteopaths, and naturopaths. As time went on, more and more patients sought help from those professionals because they were either not pleased with conventional treatment, or they wanted a more holistic approach to health care and turned to a combination of allopathic and alternative remedies. Nowadays no one bats an eye if a friend or family member mentions that they're getting treatment from a professional other than a medical doctor. In fact, it's almost as likely that someone will recommend a chiropractor or acupuncturist as they are to recommend traditional conservative treatment, depending of course on the type and severity of the illness or disorder. Many cancer patients, rather than placing all their trust in conventional treatment, will choose to see a naturopath in addition to their medical doctor. This was certainly not a typical decision as recently as the end of the twentieth century. Hypnotherapy, too, has gained wider acceptance, although not to the same degree as naturopathy or acupuncture. People still like the idea of something tangible being done to or within their body. Treating disorders by working solely with the mind requires a greater willingness to set aside long-held beliefs.

As medical science continues to progress, our increasingly sophisticated technology will allow us to gain a greater understanding and appreciation of the mind/body connection. A lie detector test, although not infallible, is one example. You tell a lie, you consciously know you're telling a lie, and your body's parasympathetic system reacts. The results are printed out in graph form that a trained examiner can easily interpret. Likewise, neuroimaging through the use of machines such as MRIs can detect neural activity in the brain that directly correlates with pain sensation and tinnitus perception. An MRI technologist can read the results and notice anything unusual in the reading that should not be happening in a healthy brain. As noted in Chapter 26, "Brain Waves and Tinnitus," one example of how the brain reveals abnormal activity is that tinnitus has been linked to lower alpha waves and higher delta waves.

Science hasn't yet reached the point where neuroimaging can definitively measure the volume of tinnitus, but it isn't out of the realm of future possibility. For now, the generally accepted measure of volume is related to the distress it causes. Just like a machine can record the signs of lying, distress can also be measured by physiological responses. The level of distress usually correlates with perceived volume, but not always. If someone has little to no emotional reaction to their tinnitus, regardless whether it's loud or barely audible, then they usually don't suffer from their tinnitus. That person can function normally in their everyday activities, including sleep. They tune out the tinnitus and go about their lives, and are often completely unaware of their tinnitus until someone mentions it to them. Then they'll say, "Oh, yeah, there it is. I hear it." If you hook them up to electrodes and ask them to focus on their tinnitus, they simply will not have a negative emotional response, and their calm physiological response proves it. This lucky person has no need for hypnosis or any other type of treatment for their tinnitus. They have habituated to their tinnitus and it no longer causes them discomfort or misery.

On the opposite end of the spectrum are people who are greatly disturbed by the presence of tinnitus; again, regardless of volume. They obsess about it, their ability to function begins to break down, they often become depressed and truly suffer. They need help, something that will ease their torment and break the hold that tinnitus has on their limbic system. They need to close the open gate that's allowing the phantom sounds to intrude and be heard by the brain.

In many cases, underlying anxiety is keeping that gate open, particularly when tinnitus is idiopathic (no known physical cause). Anxiety is often the result of fear. Hypnosis is a great tool for getting to the source of fear and reducing or eliminating it. When the fear is gone, the anxiety lessens. Less anxiety means the body calms down. A calm body produces less harmful chemicals, which in turn helps to calm the hyperactive neurons in the brain. The result? You stop the vicious cycle where hearing the tinnitus increases frustration, which in turn increases anxiety, which causes the brain to ramp up the volume because your amygdala thinks you're in danger and initiates the fight-or-flight mode. Instead, with a calm mind, the opposite occurs. In a relaxed state when you're free of fear, the tinnitus is more easily shrugged off. The more it's shrugged off, the less attention the brain gives to it. The less attention the brain gives to tinnitus, the less you hear it. And of course the less you hear it, the less distress it causes. Eventually tinnitus becomes a fairly insignificant factor in your life, or at least its ability to negatively affect your life is greatly diminished.

People often seek the services of a hypnotherapist to treat psychological issues; for example, fear of public speaking, anxiety, negative self-esteem, et cetera. But hypnosis has also proven to be a valid tool for treating physical conditions as well. For example, a dentist trained in hypnotherapy can treat patients who either cannot tolerate or refuse to use medication. Under hypnosis, such patients can have a tooth filled and not experience pain, as shown in the YouTube video, "Hypnosis in Dentistry." This is an authentic demonstration of the mind overriding the body's response to painful stimuli. Smokers have been known to cut down or completely eliminate their dependence on cigarettes, even though it's an established medical fact that tobacco addiction is notoriously difficult to overcome. (Incidentally, chronic pain, addiction, and tinnitus share similar properties and pathways in the brain.) It's possible that under hypnosis, a person can be convinced that they will no longer be aware of the phantom sounds of their tinnitus. This is because tinnitus is not the sounds per se; it is the *perception* of those sounds by the conscious mind. It's similar to being asleep. While you sleep, the brain and auditory system are still manufacturing the sound, but your conscious mind is paying no attention to it. Most people do not hear tinnitus in their dreams. Dreaming is an example of a state of consciousness where tinnitus is being created by the brain, yet the dreamer is unaware of it.

If you find it easy to get lost in a daydream, then there's a good chance that hypnotherapy will work for you. Hypnotherapy can change your underlying thoughts so that even if you are still aware of your tinnitus, your emotional reaction to it may change to where it no longer disturbs you or interferes with your life. YouTube has some interesting videos to test whether you can be hypnotized or not. One of them, on the Morpheus Hypnosis channel, is called "Can You be Hypnotized? The Lemon Test." I expected the test to reveal how I would respond to an imaginary sour taste of lemon in my mouth. To my surprise, that is not what the test is about. It's a short video, and the hypnotherapist has a nice soothing voice. Try it, and see what happens. If you're like most people, you will discover that the power of suggestion, combined with your imagination, has a strong influence on how your body reacts.

If you're interested in hypnotherapy as treatment for tinnitus, I recommend first learning about hypnotherapy in general by either going to your local library or bookstore to get a book on the subject, or finding one online. Once you understand the scientific foundation of hypnosis, it will be easier to accept hypnotherapy as a potential treatment. If working with a hypnotherapist helps you, then you will be on your way to relieve the psychological distress of tinnitus. This will in turn either reduce the perceived volume or reduce your perception of its intrusiveness. From that point, it will be easier to habituate to the presence of tinnitus in your life.

Like many other skills, hypnosis can be self-taught through either video or books. If you think about it, we all practice self-hypnosis to a certain degree. We say both positive and negative things to ourselves. In time, we begin to believe them if we say those things often enough. When you say something negative about yourself over and over, it can take root in your subconscious mind, whether it's criticizing yourself for how you do something or the way you look or how you handle your emotions. The same is true for people who pump themselves up with positive self-talk. In time, they gain confidence and feel better about themselves. In a sense, your mind trains itself to accept repetitive thoughts and statements as fact, whether they are actually true or not. You can think of hypnotherapy as a more intense and short-term version of retraining the mind. It cuts through the barriers of the conscious mind and goes directly to the foundation of your beliefs.

Self-hypnosis through repetition is a form of cognitive behavioral therapy. One thing you can try is to tell yourself, "The tinnitus is not a real sound, I only pay attention to sounds that are real." You can say, "I'm too busy to listen to you, tinnitus." Or you can practice saying, "Go away, tinnitus, I can't be bothered with you." You may have to tell yourself those things over and over and over again in the first few months, maybe longer in more severe cases, but eventually your mind will come to accept what you're saying as truth. The more often someone is exposed to either a positive or negative statement, as long as they're receptive to that statement, the more likely they are to believe it. The repetitive statement becomes part of who they are. If you find yourself in despair and constantly saying things like, "I'll never get used to this, my life is ruined," you need to tell yourself the opposite: "I can deal with this tinnitus. Millions of others have learned to cope with their tinnitus and are living happy, productive lives. I can do the same thing." In other words, **replace the hopeless negative statements with comforting and positive statements, even if right now you don't believe they're true.** The point is, it's possible for them to become true. In time, the mind will accept the statements as true. When that happens, you will discover that you are paying less and less attention to your tinnitus, to the point where it becomes a non-issue in your life.

Most of us have heard the expression, "Fake it 'til you make it." That's basically what's happening when you constantly reinforce positive messages to yourself, when you deliberately act as if everything is going to be all right. The important thing is that you simply do not allow yourself to dwell on negative thoughts about your tinnitus. When they rise up, turn your attention to something else. Whenever possible, let your mind wander to a pleasant daydream. This helps to put you in a light trance of visualization and imagination. Alpha brain waves increase when you use your imagination to visualize positive scenarios. You not only get the benefit of focusing on something other than your tinnitus, the elevation in alpha brain waves will help you feel more calm and relaxed.

I mentioned earlier the role of the imagination in hypnosis. It isn't unusual for people to have imaginary conversations with friends and others, or maybe we're just kind of talking to ourselves in our minds. With tinnitus, it's easy to fall into the trap of creating mental conversations where we relate how hard it is to have tinnitus, or we describe it in great detail, justifying the misery it causes. This of course makes it more important to our limbic system, because there is a strong emotional component to that kind of imaginary conversation. Try something different the next time you start doing that. For example, imagine instead that you're talking to someone and telling them how much better you feel, that you used to hear your tinnitus all the time and it really bothered you, but now you hardly notice it. Embellish it with details, and make the conversation as vivid as you can. When you change negative thought patterns to a more optimistic or carefree outlook, you lessen the importance of tinnitus to your limbic system.

You can find a qualified hypnotherapist by searching online or looking for someone local. Some hypnotherapists offer sessions over the phone or via Skype, a free visual/audio telecommunication service. I cannot recommend anyone specifically, as hypnotherapy is an intensely personal decision. Many hypnotherapists offer a free initial consultation. You can then decide whether you want to pursue treatment with that individual or go to someone else. If you cannot find a hypnotherapist who specializes in tinnitus, look for one who has successfully treated chronic pain or addiction. As mentioned before, tinnitus shares the same neural pathways as those two conditions.

51
SELF-HYPNOSIS FOR SLEEP

If you've never practiced self-hypnosis before, it may take you a while to relax enough to trust the process. Eventually you should reach the point where you can induce a trance-like state within 10 minutes and fall asleep within another five or 10 minutes.

The technique described here is simple but effective. If you find it works for you, you can change the words you tell yourself as you breathe in and breathe out. Concentrate on your breathing. Do not monitor your tinnitus to see if its volume is changing as you begin to slip into a trance-like state. Otherwise you might return to full alertness and will need to start over.

---

1. Lie down and make yourself comfortable, with your arms at your sides. Self-hypnosis generally works best when you lie on your back because it's less likely that you'll shift around in that position. If you simply can't lie on your back due to pain or discomfort, choose the position in which you're most comfortable. A dark room is preferable because it has less sensory stimulation. It's okay to have masking sounds on, especially if they are soothing nature-type sounds that tend to fade into the background. Wear loose-fitting clothing.

2. Close your eyes, inhale deeply and then exhale slowly. As you inhale, either think the words to yourself or speak in a soft voice and say, "Breathe in calm" before each inhalation. As you exhale, either think the words or speak softly and say, "Release stress." Do this 10 times. If you prefer, you can use another word instead of "stress"; for example, "Release anxiety" or "Release fear" or even "Release tinnitus." The important thing is that the words you speak have personal meaning to you. The words you tell yourself are called auto-suggestion, and can be very powerful when combined with trust and belief.

3. A relaxed state usually happens naturally when you close your eyes and breathe slowly and steadily, but now you'll want to deepen the sense of relaxation. Keep your eyes closed, and focus your attention on your toes. As you do that, either think to yourself or say to yourself, "Toes tingle." Many people will be surprised to discover that with this simple

command, their toes will indeed start to tingle, even if only for a little bit. If it doesn't happen right away, don't worry about it. Give it a little time, another 10 or 15 seconds. You want to *allow* your toes to tingle, not *make* them tingle. If it still isn't happening, move on to the next step.

4. Now turn your attention to your feet and think or say to yourself, "Feet tingle." Once again, it may seem hard to believe, but it's very likely that you will feel a tingling sensation in your feet. If it doesn't happen, just continue to breathe deeply, and go on to the next step.

5. Slowly work your way up from your feet, turning your attention next to your calves, then your knees, your thighs, your hips, your stomach, your chest, your shoulders, your arms, your hands, then to your neck, your scalp, and your face. As you're reading this, it may seem like it would take a long time to go through this self-hypnosis exercise, but with practice it only takes a few minutes. Focus on each body area and give a gentle command for it to tingle. Each time the tingling sensation happens, move up to the next body area. Some people can easily induce tingling in one body part but not another, so if this happens to you, don't worry about it. Simply turn your attention to the next part of your body.

6. When you reach the final point and are able to feel your face tingle, return your focus to deep breathing and auto-suggestion. By this time, you are probably in a trance-like state and receptive to suggestion. Any suggestions you wish to tell yourself are up to you, but now you will want to use more direct commands to your subconscious. For example, you can use words like, "I ignore the tinnitus and go about my life." Maybe you prefer to say something like, "The tinnitus is becoming softer and quieter every day." Or from the prior chapter, "Tinnitus is a phantom and my brain ignores it." Repeat the auto-suggestion approximately 10 times. It doesn't need to be a precise number of repetitions. When you finish the auto-suggestions, continue deep breathing and you should fall asleep soon.

There is some controversy about whether the subconscious mind accepts a suggestion which contains a negative word such as "no" or "not." In other words, rather than saying, "My tinnitus doesn't bother me," you would instead say something like, "When I hear my tinnitus, I stay calm and relaxed." I personally believe that the subconscious mind responds to suggestions whether they contain negative words or not, but it's up to you as to which approach resonates more.

If you fall asleep before you can give yourself any auto-suggestions, don't worry about it. By that point you will already have thoughts in your mind about releasing the tinnitus and remaining calm. This is what your subconscious mind will be working on while you sleep. You can also create your own self-hypnosis audio. Record the first 10 or 15 minutes with a gentle soundscape. Something like ocean waves or rainfall is ideal. Then record your auto-suggestions, speaking in a calm, steady voice. When you begin a self-hypnosis session, start by playing your self-hypnosis audio at a level where you can hear it but it isn't distracting. As you listen to the relaxing soundscape, follow steps 2 through 5 at the beginning of this chapter. By the time you slip into a trance-like state, the auto-suggestion part of the audio will begin to play. If you fall asleep, your subconscious mind will continue to listen to your words.

Here's a hint: When you use soft and soothing words in your suggestions, your subconscious mind will be more receptive to what you're saying. A study conducted at Édouard Herriot Hospital in Lyons, France, found that patients who had anesthesiologists who spoke to them in calm, positive words experienced an even greater degree of relaxation than patients who were given hydroxyzine, a common medication for reducing anxiety. The American Association of Anesthesiologists website has published an online press release about this technique, "Soothing words do more than pills to calm anxious patients, study shows."

Some relaxing words you might want to try are: tranquil, soft, gentle, serenity, peaceful, harmony, ease, warmth, safe, silken, float, freely, and light. You can make your own personal list of words to use in your auto-suggestions, words that promote feelings of acceptance and trust.

If you want to try self-hypnosis during the day, begin in a seated position. It's okay to lie down if you prefer, but be mindful that you're more likely to fall asleep. When practiced regularly, with a consistent approach, daytime self-hypnosis can reduce some of the anxiety and tension that often accompanies living with moderate to severe tinnitus. If your intention is to awaken after the self-hypnosis session, you'll want to give yourself instructions at the end of the session. That can be as simple as telling yourself, "I am now returning to full alertness, feeling calm, awake and refreshed." Use words that feel natural to you. Whatever you choose to say, be sure to end the session on a positive note.

The sleep-inducing technique in this chapter is just one of many methods that can be used, and I encourage you to research other techniques. For example, a popular method is to close your eyes and imagine yourself slowly walking down 10 steps on a winding staircase. Breathe in and out with each step, counting backwards from 10 to 1. With each step, you tell yourself that you are going deeper and deeper into a trance. When you reach the count of 1, continue breathing slowly and steadily, and begin your auto-suggestions. Another method is to imagine that you're lying on a soft cloud. As you count downward from 10 to 1, you sink deeper and deeper into the softness and comfort of the cloud.

If self-hypnosis simply doesn't work for you, try yoga or mindfulness meditation. Whichever method you choose, as you guide yourself to become more relaxed and less captive to your anxiety, your body will begin to naturally balance its neurotransmitters. When you increase the inhibitory neurotransmitter GABA while also decreasing the excitatory neurotransmitter glutamate, it helps to calm the hyperactive neurons which contribute to tinnitus. Studies have shown that GABA levels are higher in the brain of someone who regularly practices yoga or mindfulness meditation. Self-hypnosis, which is a heightened state of focused relaxation, also increases GABA levels.

myNoise.net features an ASMR sound generator, "Healing Trees" created with professional hypnotist Isabelle Knight. ASMR stands for "autonomous sensory meridian response," which is usually described as a tingling sensation across the scalp and back of the neck. "Healing Trees" is intended to induce relaxation or even a trance-like state. A more detailed explanation of how it works is given on the website. Depending on your response to gentle whispering, it can be a relaxing and enjoyable way to deflect your focus away from tinnitus. You can listen to the different presets to see how they affect you, or experiment by adjusting the sliders.

52
LOW-LEVEL LASER THERAPY

Low-level laser therapy (LLLT) is a controversial treatment which aims to lessen tinnitus by addressing hearing loss caused by acoustic trauma. The theory behind LLLT is that laser light can help to heal or repair damaged hair cells. This in turn restores hearing to a certain degree and thereby reduces the nerve cell hyperactivity that contributes to the tinnitus. A specially designed handheld device is calibrated to emit laser light at specific therapeutic doses, and the light must be precisely aimed at a target point in the ear in order for the treatment to be effective.

The average cosmetics consumer is aware that laser light therapy has made its way into various skin improvement devices on the market. Dermatologists routinely use professional grade laser light devices to treat patients for everything from skin rejuvenation and age spot removal to leg vein treatment. The long-pulsed alexandrite laser is used for hair removal, but occasionally has the opposite effect of causing unwanted hair to grow, a condition called paradoxical hypertrichosis. Obviously something is going on at a molecular level which is causing the changes, whether positive or negative. Therefore, it doesn't seem like too much of a stretch to believe that laser light therapy might, in the right circumstances, promote the repair of damaged hair cells in certain individuals. Of course, hair cells are not actually hair. They are nerve cells that under a microscope appear to have a bundle of hair protruding from them, called stereocilia. What hair cells and body hair have in common is that both tend to be weakened by the natural aging process. That is, hair begins to thin out and lose its color, and hair cells become damaged beyond recovery. Years ago it was thought impossible to grow new hair on the head once the aging process took hold, but laser light therapy has shown that hair growth can in fact be stimulated. Even though hair cells in the cochlea cannot be salvaged once they have died, LLLT theorizes that damaged hair cells can be healed enough to function again.

When laser light therapy is applied, the body produces chemicals known as reactive oxygen species (ROS), which cause tissue to switch on a growth-stimulating molecule called TGF-beta. You may recall from Chapter 7, "Tinnitus Has Many Origins," that ROS are associated with pathogenic processes. Therefore, it's a delicate balance in how much light to administer, and at what intensity, to effectively stimulate the TGF-beta versus introducing too many ROS into the tissue. In one encouraging laboratory study, a Harvard-led team used laser light to stimulate stem cells located in the dental pulp of mice. After 12 weeks, the mice showed increased production of dentin, a primary component of teeth.

Laser light therapy is not science fiction. It definitely has real world applications, but at this point much of it is highly experimental. Any perceived success with LLLT restoring hearing and reducing tinnitus is limited to anecdotal evidence. There is no verifiable clinical evidence to support low-level laser therapy as a reliable or even recommended treatment for tinnitus. I would not dismiss LLLT entirely, on the off chance that it might help someone who is responsive to laser light that is properly applied. Overall, however, this is a treatment that promises much but apparently delivers very little benefit, and then only to random subjects. The typical benefit mentioned seems to be a reduction in the sensation of fullness in the ears, rather than improvement in the tinnitus itself. There are so many potential causes of ear fullness, however, that it would be difficult to determine exactly what the LLLT is doing to help that condition.

If you still want to consider low-level laser therapy despite lack of sufficient evidence that it works, visit www.Konftec.com. This is a rather unsophisticated website but they offer a decent explanation of their products and why they believe LLLT is a viable treatment. For more information, including actual user experiences, read the thread about this subject on the Tinnitus Talk forum, "Low-Level Laser Therapy (LLLT) for Tinnitus." It's a long thread covering pros and cons, as well as do-it-yourself devices and clinic locations for professional treatment. A similar thread, "Is LLLT for Tinnitus by Dr. Wilden a Scam?," discusses Dr. Lutz Wilden, a well-known promoter of LLLT. For the most part, it is sharply critical of Dr. Wilden and dismissive of low-level laser therapy as helpful for tinnitus. I recommend reading both threads before you spend your money and time on this questionable treatment.

53
MOZART THERAPY and
THE TOMATIS EFFECT

Mozart therapy is a curious phenomenon which seems to reduce tinnitus in some people. Obviously it doesn't work for the vast majority, or it would be a widely recommended treatment. Most people have never heard of it. The Mozart effect was discussed in a book by Dr. Alfred A. Tomatis in 1991 and promoted as a therapy to treat hearing and attention disorders. In 1993, researchers Rauscher, Shaw, and Ky discovered that students who listened to Mozart's Sonata k448 for 10 minutes demonstrated temporary improvement in spatial-reasoning skills lasting approximately 10 to 15 minutes. Their research was published in *Nature* magazine and resulted in a great deal of media attention, including the misguided and subsequently debunked belief that listening to Mozart regularly can actually make you smarter.

Four studies were conducted to test whether listening to Mozart's k448 could help people with epilepsy. In every study, there was a statistically significant improvement in most of the subjects.

- A 1998 study showed less epileptic activity in the brain for 23 of 29 subjects.
- A 2011 study in Taiwan showed improvement in 47 of 58 children.
- Another 2011 Taiwanese study, lasting six months, demonstrated improvement in eight of 11 children with refractory epilepsy, which is the form that is the most difficult to control with medication.
- A U.S. year-long study was conducted to determine whether the Mozart effect would work if the subjects listened to k448 while sleeping. Although 36 percent in the control group who did not listen to music showed improvement, 80 percent of the 73 adults and children in the study who did listen to Mozart's k448 showed a reduction in seizures, and 24 percent became seizure-free.

Please note that none of these studies indicate whether any follow-up was done regarding whether the improvement was short-term or long-term. The studies cited are from the article "The Mozart Effect and Epilepsy," which was previously published on the British Epilepsy Foundation website but at this time is no longer available.

Epilepsy and tinnitus share similar neurological characteristics, so it's logical to consider that a therapy for epilepsy may also prove beneficial for tinnitus. In a study out of Italy, "The Mozart effect in patients suffering from tinnitus," a group of patients between 22 and 78 years of age were instructed to listen to Mozart's Sonata k448 for one hour daily for one month. Following that, they listened to Beethoven's Für Elise sonata for one hour daily for a month. The patients attended a cognitive behavioral therapy session before beginning the study, as well as filling out questionnaires designed to measure their tinnitus distress level. One of these was the Tinnitus Handicap Inventory. In general, there was an overall significant improvement at the end of the one-month period. The study even noted significant improvement regarding perception of tinnitus intensity which was demonstrated *after a single listening exposure* to Mozart's sonata. The article did not address whether this was a form of residual inhibition, or how long the perception of reduced intensity lasted. Perhaps the brain remained temporarily preoccupied with the complexity of the music and was less focused on the tinnitus signal.

The YouTube channel Healing4Happiness has a three-hour Mozart k448 video, "Mozart Classical Piano Study Music & Alpha Waves: Ultimate Concentration, Mozart K.448 Study Music." The video embeds binaural beats, which are intended to enhance alpha wave activity. As you'll recall, people with tinnitus have alpha brain wave levels below normal. You must wear headphones for the binaural beats to be effective. There is another version approximately 24 minutes long, with a more leisurely pace, "Mozart - Sonata for Two Pianos in D, K.448," on YouTube channel Am4d3MOz4rt. The 24-minute version does not have binaural beats. You can play the music in the background as you go about your day, or take the time to sit and listen to the intricate notes, which will help your brain to focus on it more intently.

I could find no information online whether classical sound therapy for tinnitus is helpful if one listens only to Beethoven's Für Elise and does not listen to Mozart k448. Für Elise is a more soothing composition. If you enjoy Beethoven, listen for an hour every day for a month to see if you notice any improvement in your tinnitus. The Ludwig van Beethoven channel on YouTube has a 60-minute version of "Beethoven's Für Elise," accompanied by a symphony orchestra.

Beethoven began to experience hearing loss in his thirties. The condition was irreversible and eventually led to profound deafness. He was also plagued with severe tinnitus. He once wrote, "My ears whistle and buzz all day and night. I can say I am leading a wretched life." Perhaps his musical compositions were an attempt to soothe his ragged nerves by concentrating on the composition of the music instead of the torment of his tinnitus. There's no way to know for sure what inspired him, but Beethoven composed some of the most relaxing and yet uplifting music of all time, a blessing for anyone needing a break from tinnitus or other stressors.

In 2001, the Journal of the Royal Society of Medicine published a study noting that "Acroyali/Standing In Motion," by the Greek composer Yanni, also produces the Mozart effect. This is due to its similarity "in tempo, structure, melodic and harmonic consonance and predictability" to Mozart's k448. Yanni's music is copyrighted and cannot be shared by a link, but you can find it on YouTube. It's available for download through Amazon, and can be streamed free if you have a Prime membership.

If you enjoy listening to classical music and it eases the distress of your tinnitus, try to make it part of your everyday routine as much as possible. When you have time, either sit back or lie down and close your eyes as you listen. Imagine that you are in a concert hall, with a symphony orchestra and either Mozart or Beethoven are there at the piano, playing before the audience. Focus your mind on the music, and let your thoughts be swept into its beauty. When you're away from the music, you can replay it in your mind. As you recall the musical notes and instruments, it may help to distract from the tinnitus signal.

There are some who claim that sound therapy based on the Tomatis Effect can be helpful for improving tinnitus under certain conditions. In short, the idea is that we are normally able to exclude sounds from our environment and focus only on what we want to hear. One example of this might be listening to the strings section of an orchestra while being only slightly aware of the other instruments being played. This is what's known as selective listening. Proponents of the Tomatis Effect theorize that the middle ear can become worn out or damaged due to acoustic trauma or age, and at that point it becomes difficult to shut out unwanted sounds, including the natural anatomical sounds of one's own body, such as blood circulating, breathing, et cetera.

The method was initially developed 50 years ago by Dr. Tomatis, an otolaryngologist. He believed that many problems with hearing and listening were caused by an inability to hear the full spectrum of sounds, particularly in the higher frequencies. Sound therapy based on the Tomatis Effect uses Mozart compositions which are specially modified to emphasize certain harmonics. The end goal depends upon the condition being treated, whether it's attention deficit disorder, learning difficulties, communication difficulties, and other conditions related to hearing and/ or listening. However, one benefit they stress is that it improves concentration. If your tinnitus is seriously interfering with your ability to concentrate, this type of treatment may prove useful. An ability to concentrate on something other than your tinnitus can be helpful in the habituation process. It's also helpful if you can train your ear, so to speak, to listen only to sounds that you want to hear while ignoring sounds which aren't useful. You can read more detailed information at www.Tomatis.com, and www.ListeningCentre.co.uk in their article, "The Listening Therapy successfully treats: Tinnitus."

There isn't much information online to confirm that this sort of sound therapy has proven helpful for tinnitus. Eric Jordan, cited in www.SoundTherapyPerth.com, claims a 90% success rate for improving tinnitus. His theory seems to be based more on the idea that brain cells are revitalized with sound therapy, which calms the hyperactive neurons contributing to tinnitus. He does not claim that the tinnitus is eliminated, only that the therapy decreases the intensity or perception to the point where people suffering from severe tinnitus are once again able to enjoy life. Rafaele Joudry, who has authored three books on the subject, believes that sound therapy works by addressing the fundamental causes of tinnitus. In the YouTube video, "Rafaele Joudry Interview," she explains her interpretation of sound therapy and how it's used in the treatment of tinnitus.

Ms. Joudry makes an interesting point in comparing the persistence of tinnitus to the persistence of chronic pain, a theory that has support amongst many tinnitus researchers. It's possible for a condition which begins with negative physical stimuli, such as pain, to eventually be embedded in emotional circuits. Chronification occurs when the brain perceives pain via an emotional circuit rather than the normal response of pain receptors. A similar process occurs with chronic tinnitus. This is why it's important to avoid responding to tinnitus with strong emotional reactions, and to instead view it as objectively as possible. The Back to Silence method covered in Chapter 47 is one way of doing that, where you step back from what you're feeling and name your emotion, instead of obsessing about the tinnitus itself.

myNoise.net has a soundscape called Aural Scan which incorporates the theory of the Tomatis Effect. It's an interesting arrangement of tones and tends to have a stimulating effect when the sliders are set for the higher frequencies. Although it's popular for concentrating, one site visitor praised Aural Scan for helping him cope with misophonia, another auditory disorder. Misophonia is an intolerance, even hatred, of certain sounds that most people can either tune out or are not bothered by. The intensity to which someone with this affliction dislikes a particular sound can actually lead to uncontrollable feelings of rage or panic. Learn more at www.Misophonia.com.

If you enjoy the Aural Scan soundscape, try listening to it at a low volume for half an hour to an hour every day for a month to see if your brain begins to naturally tune in to more pleasant ambient sounds instead of your tinnitus. Even though you might not achieve that desired result, it may still be helpful when you need to concentrate.

According to Dr. Pigeon, "This generator covers the entire audible spectrum." That makes Aural Scan suitable for a notched audio file. If you enjoy listening to it, purchase the MP3 version and import it into Audacity, using the instructions in Chapter 43, "Audio Notch - Do It Yourself Guide." Adjust the sliders on the myNoise Aural Scan generator to your preference before placing the order.

54
NEUROFEEDBACK

Biofeedback and neurofeedback are based on the principle that it's possible to consciously and deliberately control or alter your body's physiological responses to stimuli, with the goal of improving a physical or mental condition. Neurofeedback is more narrowly focused and designed to affect brain functions relating to attention, mood, and cognition. For people with tinnitus, it may be useful in correcting abnormal brain wave activity, with the goal of reducing or eliminating symptoms of tinnitus. Neurofeedback is the offspring of biofeedback therapy, which has been in use since the 1970s.

Biofeedback, an abbreviated term for "biological feedback," is a medically accepted method of helping people to deal with physical ailments such as pain or high blood pressure. The treatment usually consists of attaching sensors to the skin which can read nervous system responses. These sensors transmit signals into a computer where they are then output as either lights or tones. When someone recognizes from the light or tone that their respiration rate is too fast or their blood pressure is too high, they practice relaxation exercises with the intent of bringing those responses back to a normal level. Over time, with practice, a person can learn to control these bodily functions without the use of a monitoring system. Biofeedback is best taught with a qualified therapist, with the eventual goal of being able to stabilize responses on your own. No one really knows why biofeedback works, but, for some reason, the simple fact of being able to deliberately affect the signal of a light or a tone seems to give people a needed sense of control over how their body responds. Biofeedback is proof positive that the conscious mind and physical body are intricately and mysteriously connected.

Neurofeedback uses basically the same technique as biofeedback, except that electrodes are attached to the scalp and a person's brain waves are being monitored instead of their physiological responses. These electrodes read and record the electrical activity of your brain as reflected by your brain waves. This reading is known as an electroencephalogram, or EEG for short. The brain waves of a normal adult in her waking state will show mostly alpha and beta waves. Both the right and left hemispheres will generate the same amount of electrical activity, and there will be no spikes of electrical activity or slow waves on the EEG reading. Neurofeedback, when properly done, is an excellent tool to normalize abnormal brain wave activity and induce calm in stressful situations. Remember that brain wave measurements of adults with tinnitus reflect lower alpha brain wave activity and abnormally elevated delta and gamma brain wave activity.

Neurofeedback has been successfully used to treat a range of neurological problems such as ADHD, anxiety disorder, depression, drug addiction, and epilepsy. Is it possible for someone to lessen or eliminate their tinnitus by learning to actively control their brain waves? There isn't a lot of information online which addresses this question, but I did find a few reliable studies. In one instance, a 38-year-old woman who had sudden hearing loss followed by bilateral (in both ears) tinnitus was discovered to have lower brain waves than normal, and it was most pronounced in the alpha bands. She underwent nine neurofeedback sessions of 90 minutes each, twice a day. At the end of the treatment regimen, she only noticed her tinnitus occasionally. This was published in *International Tinnitus Journal*, Volume 8, No. 2, 2002. Another study, "Neurofeedback for treating tinnitus," published in *Progress in Brain Research*, showed that normalizing the oscillatory brain wave activity between the alpha waves and delta waves led to elimination of the tinnitus. This result was achieved by those patients who were able to successfully modify the oscillatory patterns.

Researchers analyzed EEG biofeedback (neurofeedback) studies of people whose epilepsy was not controlled effectively through medication. They discovered that seizure activity was in fact significantly reduced in the patient group that participated in the EEG studies. The subjects in this patient group were unable to control their condition with medication, which makes the finding all the more important. Because epilepsy and tinnitus share similar neurological characteristics, and because there have been encouraging results reported regarding epilepsy, then neurofeedback would seem to be a beneficial treatment for tinnitus. Details of the study are in the article, "Meta-Analysis of EEG Biofeedback in Treating Epilepsy," published on www.eeginfo.com.

There are many practitioners of therapeutic neurofeedback. I recommend finding someone who has experience with tinnitus patients or at least is knowledgeable about the abnormal brain wave activity associated with tinnitus. Also, you might be willing to try neurofeedback on your own with one of the many products that are now available for brain wave training. One such device is BRAINtellect. They advertise their product as guiding the brain to "self-adjust to more balanced rhythms." Another device is NeurOptimal, described as helping to "Reduce stress and anxiety" and "Improve and deepen sleep," among other benefits. These are relatively inexpensive devices, but I do not have any experience with them and cannot offer an opinion as to whether they are helpful for tinnitus. Neither company provides any information with regard to whether their devices are suitable for treatment of tinnitus, but, again, reducing anxiety and normalizing brain waves is usually helpful in reducing the perception of volume or intrusiveness.

Information about neurofeedback from a clinical perspective can be found at BrainMaster Technologies at www.brainmaster.com. Their Products page features research grade neurofeedback devices. This will give you a good idea of what to expect if you decide to undergo neurofeedback therapy at a clinic.

If you attempt to change your brain waves via neurofeedback but the results are disappointing, or if you have no access to a neurofeedback practitioner, you still have the option of treatment with biofeedback. Studies have shown that being able to influence your body's automatic responses can improve symptoms of depression, anxiety, and sleep disorder, which in turn makes it easier to cope with tinnitus. It's generally easier to achieve habituation when a person believes they have some control over what is happening in their brain and body. Biofeedback has been proven to be useful on a psychological level, with most subjects reporting anywhere from modest to significant gains in their ability to cope with the stress that accompanies chronic tinnitus.

Although there are many devices sold for do-it-yourself biofeedback therapy, there is only one that I'm aware of which is FDA approved. RESPeRATE is a sister product to 2breathe which was mentioned in Chapter 35, "Methods for Better Sleep." RESPeRATE is specifically designed to reduce blood pressure and promote relaxation. It measures your respiration and uses gentle tones to guide your breathing. If tinnitus

55
NEUROGENESIS

There's an old saying, "You can't teach an old dog new tricks." That was back in the time when most people believed that we couldn't change our ways after a certain age. Part of that belief was based on the prevailing idea that every person has a finite number of brain cells critical to the learning process, and that once those brain cells died, they were gone forever and could not be replaced. Therefore, without new brain cells to replace those that had died, it was supposedly too difficult for seniors to meet and overcome new life challenges. Fortunately, everyone knows by now (or should know) that there's plenty of evidence to show that seniors certainly do learn and master new things. It might take a little bit longer than their younger counterparts due to the complex biological changes that occur with age, but getting older doesn't mean that your body stops producing brain cells.

So what does this new evidence have to do with tinnitus? In one word, neurogenesis. Basically, neurogenesis is the growth of new nerve cells. Neurogenesis essentially occurs in two locations in the brain. One area is the subventricular zone (SVZ) of the lateral ventricles. The ventricles contain cerebrospinal fluid (CSF). This fluid cushions the brain and helps to circulate nutrients as well as removing waste. Scientists are researching the phenomenon of neurogenesis in the SVZ as a possible means of neuroregenerative therapy.

The other location where neurogenesis occurs is the hippocampus. That's the organ in the limbic system which is associated with mood and memory, as well as spatial navigation, which is the ability to know where we are and how to reach our destination. You may recall from Chapter 24, "The Brain Creates Tinnitus," that the hippocampus is considered to be the GPS of the brain.

Neuroimaging studies have shown that people with tinnitus have decreased grey matter in the hippocampus. Grey matter is basically a mass of neuronal cells. The question is, does a person develop decreased grey matter in the hippocampus which then predisposes them to tinnitus, or does the tinnitus cause the decreased grey matter, perhaps due to stress or other factors that accompany the tinnitus condition? Studies have verified that stress inhibits neurogenesis within the adult hippocampus, as noted in the Science Daily article, "Neurogenesis In Adult Brain: Association With Stress and Depression." It is not unusual for people with tinnitus to blame it on stress, either chronic stress in their lives or a major emotional upheaval just before the onset of tinnitus. It's well-known in the tinnitus community that perception of volume, severity and intrusiveness, as well as a person's ability to cope, are often made worse during stressful periods. In contrast, stress-relieving practices like meditation and exercise or going for a walk on a sunny day, as well as anti-anxiety medications such as Xanax, can reduce the symptoms of tinnitus. In addition to relieving stress, exercise has been shown to increase grey matter in the hippocampus. This is explained more thoroughly in the Scientific Reports article, "Physical Exercise Habits Correlate with Gray Matter Volume of the Hippocampus in Healthy Adult Humans." If you have tinnitus, you will most likely benefit by engaging in activities with the specific goal of increasing the amount of grey matter in your hippocampus.

When you lose your hearing, and in particular when it's noise-induced hearing loss, your entire brain is affected, not just your auditory system. Some studies suggest that hearing loss in and of itself is a factor in decreased hippocampal neurogenesis. Research has definitively shown that hearing loss in the elderly is linked to cognitive decline. Acquired sensorineural hearing loss from excessive noise exposure is associated with impaired learning and decreased cognitive functioning in both animal and human subjects. These deficits continue beyond the initial exposure to noise. The interesting thing about hearing loss and its relationship to neurogenesis is that the degree of hearing loss correlates with its negative effect on neurogenesis. In other words, severe hearing loss equals greater impairment of neurogenesis. One theory for why this occurs is that changes in auditory input affect the cognitive brain, as well as neural connections and interactivity with the limbic system. Because the hippocampus is part of the limbic system, it's not surprising that dysfunctional auditory input could result in declining neurogenesis.

Neurogenesis is a complex process. One of the most important factors in neurogenesis is a protein called brain-derived neurotrophic factor (BDNF). "Neurotrophic" is the medical term for substances that nourish nerve cells; therefore, BDNF is a protein derived from the brain that nourishes nerve cells. Think of it as a type of Miracle-Gro that your brain produces in order to sustain new nerve cells. When BDNF levels are low, neurogenesis is weak and grey matter decreases. When BDNF levels are normal or high (but not too elevated), this promotes sustaining neurogenesis at a healthy level. This helps to prevent grey matter from diminishing to the point of causing correlating neurological problems. The connection between BDNF and tinnitus has been proven through the testing of plasma BDNF, as demonstrated in the study, "Various levels of plasma brain-derived neurotrophic factor in tinnitus patients." Patients who complained of severe tinnitus had demonstrably lower levels of plasma BDNF than patients who reported having only mild tinnitus. Insufficient neurogenesis and decreased grey matter in the hippocampus have been linked to other neurological-based conditions, not just tinnitus. Evidence points to a connection with dementia and Alzheimer's as well. You can read more about this connection on www.BioMedCentral.com, "Adult hippocampal neurogenesis and its role in Alzheimer's disease."

Researchers who study traumatic brain injury (TBI) have learned that the presence of a TBI and prognosis for recovery are related to blood serum levels of BDNF. The blood must be drawn within 24 hours of injury in order to be a reliable predictor of outcome. Higher levels correlate with greater severity and longer recovery time. Physicians can now use this information to tailor treatment regimens, whereas in years past, the severity of someone's TBI may not have been evident from their symptoms alone. PsychCentral's article, "New Blood Test May Detect Traumatic Brain Injury," covers the details of this medical development. Since lower blood serum levels of BDNF are linked to tinnitus severity as well, the next time you have a complete blood panel test done, ask your physician to include measuring BDNF. A healthy person will have approximately 60 nanograms per milliliter (ml) of BDNF in their blood. If your level is abnormally low, there's a chance you can improve your tinnitus by working towards naturally increasing BDNF.

In summary, it appears to be a predictable cycle: less BDNF equals

56
TIPS TO INCREASE BDNF

There are some things you can do on your own to increase bone-derived neurotrophic factor (BDNF), with the goal of promoting neurogenesis. Some are fairly easy, such as getting enough sunshine. Others are more of a challenge in terms of time and effort. It's up to you to decide how motivated you are. Remember that none of these are guaranteed to reduce your tinnitus, but they all have the benefit of making you healthier and reducing stress, which can make it easier for you to cope with your tinnitus.

---

1. Exercise. Walk every day for as long as you can. Even if it's only a few blocks or maybe half a mile to begin with, that's fine. Stick with a schedule and gradually increase the distance until you're walking two to four miles every day, rain or shine. If there's no place safe to walk, put on some lively music and dance in your living room for 30 minutes a day. Buy a mini-stairstepper, or a treadmill if you have the room and budget, and build up to 30 minutes every day. If you can't exercise for 30 minutes, begin with five or 10 minutes and gradually increase the time as your endurance improves. Lifting weights is also good exercise, but aerobic exercise such as walking or running is more beneficial. Brain plasticity, which is the ability of the brain to change and remap itself, is strongly influenced by BDNF when it's induced by exercise. When you're exercising, give your brain remapping an extra boost by combining it with learning something new. For example, you can set a goal of learning a new language with audio-based lessons.

2. Stimulate your brain. Most of us have heard the expression, "Use it or lose it." When it comes to neurogenesis, you might say, "Use it to improve it." Chapter 65, "Train the Brain - Exercises," lists ways to improve the function of the frontal lobe. These exercises apply to promoting neurogenesis as well.

3. Practice calorie restriction. More evidence is emerging that fasting, when done properly, is healthy both for the body and the mind. As cited in "Don't Feed Your Head," published in *Johns Hopkins Magazine* online, studies have shown that intermittent fasting promotes the growth of new

brain neurons. The good news is, fasting for neurogenesis doesn't mean zero food intake. The same benefits can be achieved with severe calorie restriction for as little as two days a week, while still eating normally the other five days of the week. The 5:2 diet described by Dr. Michael Mosley on www.fastdiet.co.uk is enormously popular, with pros and cons being voiced about its benefits and drawbacks. I decided that a 5:2 plan wouldn't work for me, so I chose a 1:1 schedule instead, alternating fasting and non-fasting days. I definitely lost weight, but that was not the goal; it was strictly for the neurogenesis benefit. In case you're wondering, my tinnitus is improving, but that may also be attributed to following the ACRN protocol as outlined in Chapter 45, "ACRN (Acoustic CR Neuromodulation)." Perhaps it's the combination of both which is making a difference.

For more information about Dr. Michael Mosley and his path to creating the 5:2 diet, watch the BBC documentary, "Eat, Fast, and Live Longer," on YouTube. I recommend watching the entire video so you'll understand the foundations of different fasting regimens. However, if you want to get right to the basics, the discussion of the 5:2 diet begins at timeline 37:07. Its effect on neurogenesis is explained at timeline 43:02 in the video, and more specifically at 46:28. If you think this diet sounds like a good match for you, be sure to check with your healthcare provider first. You may have medical issues that would make you a poor candidate for severe calorie restriction. Additionally, according to neuroscientist Dr. Mark Mattson, fasting offers limited benefits for people over 70.

If the 5:2 diet is too extreme for you, you can still gain some benefit if you fast for 12 hours a day, for as many days of the week as possible. This can be done by simply not eating for 12 hours between your dinner meal and the next day's breakfast. If you finish dinner at 6:30 p.m., wait until at least 6:30 a.m. the following morning before eating anything. This fulfills the 12-hour fasting requirement, plus it's likely to improve your sleep because your digestive system will have already done its work by bedtime.

4. Say good-bye to high fat, refined sugar, and processed foods. There's no doubt that sugar has become the villain of the century in our food supply, with good reason. It's been positively linked to obesity, diabetes, and even depression, among other ailments. What most people

don't know is that sugar suppresses BDNF. In short, eating sugar means your brain is producing fewer new brain cells. Sugar consumption has been linked to shrinkage of the hippocampus, a clear hallmark of Alzheimer's disease. To make matters worse, sugar causes a cascade of chemical reactions in your body which lead to chronic inflammation. If your tinnitus is caused or made worse by any sort of inflammation, eliminating refined sugar as much as possible from your diet might help to ease your symptoms. It's not uncommon for people with tinnitus to complain of a spike after eating sweets. Is that chocolate chip cookie or slice of pie really worth the ringing, buzzing, or hissing? Maybe it's more than "you are what you eat." Maybe for some of us, it's a matter of "you hear what you eat."

Like sugar, a high fat diet also has negative effects on the brain, particularly the hippocampus. Too much fat in the diet increases the level of the enzyme histone deacetylase (HDAC). When this enzyme level raises, it signals the presence of neuronal death. This effect can be observed in the dorsal hippocampus and ventral hippocampus. Medical science is investigating the use of HDAC inhibitors to improve adult memory and promote hippocampal neurogenesis. It's clear from all the research that the hippocampus is the critical site for neurogenesis. It would be wise to avoid foods that could harm its functions, the most important of which is the formation of memories and the connection of emotions and the five senses to those memories. When someone with Alzheimer's no longer recognizes you, when they seem to be actively reliving events from many years ago, what you're witnessing are some effects of a severely damaged hippocampus.

5. There are good foods that help with neurogenesis, such as foods that are rich in omega-3's. By studying patients who had suffered traumatic brain injury (TBI), scientists discovered that omega-3's helped to normalize the BDNF level, thereby assisting in the survival of neuronal cells. Your first thought might be to simply take an omega-3 fish oil capsule, but be mindful that fish oil can go rancid. Be sure to choose wisely amongst the many supplements available over the counter. Your best bet is to obtain omega-3 from natural food sources whenever possible. A comprehensive list of these foods is on the Self Nutrition Data website, "Foods highest in Total Omega-3 fatty acids."

6. The foods you eat and the beverages you drink can have a positive effect on your BDNF level. You can start by eating more foods which contain flavonoids. It has been proven that cognitive decline is slowed down by the regular consumption of flavonoid-rich foods. In particular, BDNF in the hippocampus is enhanced by anthocyanin, the flavonoid typically distinguished by a red, blue, or purple color. Blueberries, strawberries, and blackberries are very rich in anthocyanin content, but there are many fruits and even legumes and vegetables with high levels of anthocyanin; for example, kidney beans and black beans, eggplant, purple asparagus, red onions, and red cabbage. Although there is controversy about the findings, some research has shown that bananas are also abundant in anthocyanin. The article "Anthocyanin-rich foods you should be eating," from www.NaturalNews.com, focuses on delicious foods to add to your BDNF-enhancing diet.

Add some curcumin to your diet. You can do this by using curry to add some flavor to your foods. If you aren't fond of the taste, you can take a turmeric supplement with a high concentration of curcumin. Curcumin helps to reverse the negative effects of chronic stress on BDNF levels. Another useful addition is resveratrol, which is found in red wine and, of course, red grapes.

Have a cup of green tea every day. Green tea contains the compound epigallocatechin gallate (EGCG), which is able to cross the blood-brain barrier and stimulate the BDNF signaling pathway. Green tea has about 70% less caffeine than coffee, but if you prefer caffeine-free, choose a green tea that has had the caffeine removed using a process called effervescence. Look for organic green tea, and if you have any questions about their decaffeination process, contact the company. Some products that claim to be naturally decaffeinated use the chemical solvent ethyl acetate, which can leave an aftertaste and isn't a healthy choice.

7. Get your recommended dose of sunshine. That's 15 minutes, three times a week. Sit outside in the morning sun when the sun's rays are safer, and drink your cup of coffee or tea. Your morning work break is another opportunity. Leave the office environment and step outside. Exposure to sunlight boosts serum levels of BDNF. However, you need to protect your skin from the damaging effects of the sun by avoiding going outside when the sun's rays are strongest. The American Cancer

Society's online article, "What Is Ultraviolet (UV) Radiation," discusses sun exposure and how best to protect yourself from harmful UV rays.

You have probably heard of seasonal affective disorder, also known as SAD. The amount of serum level of BDNF corresponds with exposure to sunlight. Low BDNF is linked to depression, so it's no wonder that when people are deprived of sufficient sunlight, it can result in depression, particularly in individuals who are more sensitive to lack of sunlight. If your work or personal life circumstances prevent you from getting adequate sunlight, or if you'd rather not expose yourself to the sun, take a vitamin D supplement to help maintain a healthy level of BDNF. Take only the recommended amount of vitamin D supplement, as too much vitamin D in your system can lead to serious side effects.

8. Create and nourish personal relationships. Spend time in joyful activities with people you care about. Share hugs and laughter, and be open to adventurous activities. Social and personal intimacy raise both serotonin and endorphin levels. Serotonin is involved in the regulation of BDNF signaling, so a healthy level of serotonin also helps to maintain a healthy level of BDNF. It goes without saying that whenever possible, you should avoid or limit toxic relationships that leave you feeling drained of emotional, mental, or physical energy.

9. Sleep for at least seven hours every night, and more if your body requires it. Sleep deprivation is an epidemic in modern society, taking its toll in numerous ways. Continuously burning the candle at both ends places great stress on your mental and physical health. Scientists have conclusively determined that sleep deprivation leads to significantly decreased serum BDNF levels. For people with tinnitus, it is critical that they get an adequate amount of sleep. You might be doing everything else right by making lifestyle changes to raise your BDNF levels, but you're undoing a lot of the good you've done if you shortchange yourself in the sleep department. Chapter 34, "Sleeping," covers the issue of sleep as it relates to tinnitus, including some helpful tips for going to sleep. If natural methods don't work, if you've tried everything you can and yet you still can't go to sleep easily or stay asleep long enough to feel rested, it's time for you to consider sleep aids. There are many effective over-the-counter sleep aids, such as those containing either the ingredient diphenhydramine, or doxylamine succinate. Read online reviews by users

to determine which one you think is best for you. If you have any medical condition, be sure to discuss it with your healthcare practitioner before taking a drug strong enough to induce sleep.

10. Pamper yourself with aromatherapy massage. Chapter 41, "Aromatherapy," discusses why it's helpful for tinnitus in general, and includes a review of the essential oils that are most conducive for relaxation. A study was conducted on women receiving aromatherapy massage for 40 minutes twice a week. At the end of that four-week period, their plasma BDNF levels had significantly increased. One surprising result is that after only one treatment, saliva tests indicated that their cortisol levels were reduced. Excessive cortisol acts as a suppressor of BDNF. If you can reduce cortisol, your BDNF levels are more likely to stay at a healthy level. Not only is this good for neurogenesis, but it also helps to combat depression. The other benefit is a change in brain waves. I've noted several times that people with tinnitus tend to have lower than normal alpha brain waves and higher than normal delta brain waves. Aromatherapy massage helps to reverse this abnormality; it increases the alpha and decreases the delta.

Massage always feels better when performed by a professional masseuse, but you can do it yourself and still reap the benefit. There are videos available online for self-massage, depending on which area of your body is showing signs of holding in stress; for example, tight muscles in the back, shoulders, or neck. One video for neck massage which has positive feedback from YouTube viewers is "Neck Massage: Do It While You View It." The video doesn't say anything about using massage oil, as it is only about technique and not enhancements to massage. Because of its therapeutic properties, you might try placing a few drops of lavender-scented massage oil on the palm of one hand, then rub your hands together to evenly distribute the oil before beginning the massage. Don't wear valuable clothing that can come in contact with the oil, as it can be extremely difficult to remove from fabric and may leave a permanent stain.

11. Look for ways to reduce stress. Some amount of stress is good. It keeps us on our toes. Too much stress can make us feel overwhelmed and defeated. In addition to some of the natural stress relievers outlined in these tips, there are other ways to reduce stress that are simple and easy

to do at almost any time of the day. Among these are doodling, taking a brief time-out to close your eyes and imagine something peaceful, writing a heartfelt letter of gratitude (for your eyes only) about something positive in your life, stretching out your arms and taking deep breaths, doing a couple yoga moves, listening to your favorite song, or playing a CD of gentle classical music. Soft, soothing music has been shown to provide benefits such as slowing the heart rate, lowering blood pressure, and even decreasing stress hormone levels such as cortisol. You can buy stress-reducing toys like fidget spinners or squish balls to channel negative emotions or pent-up energy without needing to leave your desk. At break time, a cup of tea is a better stress-buster than coffee or soda, and there are many varieties to choose from. Celestial Seasonings makes some delicious flavored teas, including Peach Passion and Raspberry Zinger. Another popular tea is Tension Tamer, which contains eleuthero, mint and lemongrass. Eleuthero is an herb which promotes better mental performance at times of stress-induced fatigue, so it's a great pick-me-up when the afternoon doldrums set in.

A major reason for stress is unrealistic expectations and demands that we place on ourselves or allow others to place on us. This is often caused by not taking the time to establish priorities. Get in the habit of spending five minutes every evening to make a list of what you need to do the next day, as well as the things you want to do. In time you will learn what you can reasonably expect to accomplish versus how much is simply too much to ask of yourself. Knowing your strengths and limitations will help to break the self-defeating habit of setting unrealistic goals. It will also increase your self-confidence when you experience the satisfaction of finishing the tasks you set out to do, with enough time left over to relax and pursue pleasurable activities.

Promoting neurogenesis to build more grey matter is not an overnight process. It takes time to repair damage and establish new nerve cells. Don't push yourself by trying to do too much at once; that just adds to stress. Ease the changes in gradually, until they feel like a natural part of your everyday routine.

57
OVER-THE-COUNTER SUPPLEMENTS

Supplements can help, but unfortunately they won't cure your tinnitus. Some of them may soften the sound a bit for some people, which in itself can be a great comfort. If your tinnitus is caused or worsened by an underlying inflammation in your ear canal, there are supplements that are helpful in treating the inflammatory process. Keep in mind that the FDA does not regulate the manufacture or distribution of supplements, so it's very important that you buy products manufactured by reliable companies. Look for testimonials on their websites to learn how others are using the supplement you're interested in. Amazon is an excellent source for customer reviews. You can read what other customers are saying about a particular product, and, as an extra benefit, you can post questions about whether the product is helpful for tinnitus even if it isn't advertised as such by the manufacturer.

Can you guess how many ingredients in over-the-counter vitamins and supplements are promoted as helping tinnitus? Would you believe more than 50? Among them are ginkgo biloba, bioflavonoids, vinpocetine, magnesium, NAC, pycnogenol, melatonin, zinc, vitamin B12 (methylcobalamin), taurine, citicoline, piracetam, alpha lipoic acid, CoQ10/ubiquinol/idebenone, fenugreek, cat's claw, l-tyrosine, l-theanine, GABA, niacin, astaxanthin, grape seed extract, apple cider vinegar, fenugreek, sesame seeds, black cohosh, goldenseal (do not use if pregnant!), passionflower, horsetail, 5-HTP, fish oil, moringa oleifera, and valerian.

You don't need a prescription to buy most supplements, but they still create chemical changes in your body and should be used with care. Whether you use the services of a practitioner or you're a do-it-yourself kind of person, be sure to research any supplement before buying it. And of course, if you have any sort of adverse reaction, stop using it and report the reaction to the company from whom you purchased the product. A reputable company keeps track of bad reactions through Adverse Event Reports. Feedback about negative effects is important to them. They also like to hear from consumers who benefit from their product. Contact the company to let them know their product works for you, or write a positive comment in the consumer review section of the website where you bought it.

Practitioners of homeopathy also offer a few remedies for treating tinnitus and its associated discomforts. These include, but are not limited to: Kali Sulphuricum, Salicylicum Acidum, Silicea, Calcarea Sulphurica, and Thiosinaminum. The homeopathic remedy is chosen depending on whether you hear crackling, hissing, ringing, chirping, buzzing, or humming. There is a lot of controversy regarding homeopathy for treatment of physical ailments, and its use has been strongly discouraged by most medical practitioners and often mocked in the general community. However, if you have a favorable attitude towards this form of alternative treatment, please consult with a naturopath or other expert. Even if homeopathy is just a placebo effect, you're more likely to experience that effect if you're being treated by someone you trust. The same recommendation applies if you want to use traditional Chinese medicine, usually referred to as simply "TCM." Find someone who is qualified and has experience in treating patients with tinnitus.

In the next chapter, I'll review 12 popular supplements that have shown some benefit for people with tinnitus. Although many supplements are studied in objective clinical trials, the reports of improvement published on public forums tend to be subjective and anecdotal. It's important not only to read reviews, but also to do a bit of extra research before making up your mind which supplements you think are most likely to help you.

58
POPULAR SUPPLEMENTS FOR TINNITUS

Let's take a look at some popular supplements that are generally accepted as safe and worth trying if you suffer from tinnitus. I'll include my own experience with a few of the supplements that are recommended by a significant number of people. The inclusion of any particular supplement doesn't mean it will necessarily help your individual case of tinnitus; it's just a suggestion based on a high number of positive reviews and online reports of improvement.

Ginkgo biloba is probably the first supplement your healthcare professional or others will recommend that you try. However, even though this medicinal herb has a long-standing reputation of helping to ease the symptoms, the truth is that it rarely does unless the tinnitus is directly related to poor circulation in the inner ear. Studies have shown that ginkgo biloba can be useful for treating health issues related to poor circulation. Among these are memory loss, headache, and vertigo. If the sounds in your head or ears are low frequency roaring or rumbling sounds, this herb is a good choice, because tinnitus that manifests in the lower frequencies is said to be related to blood pressure. Unfortunately, the consensus is that ginkgo biloba does not help with annoying high frequency sounds such as high-pitched buzzing, hissing, chirping, and squealing. Some users report that this herb actually increases the volume or intensity of their tinnitus. If you experience that, stop using it and your tinnitus should return to baseline within a few days.

In a small sampling survey on the Tinnitus Talk forum, members who had used ginkgo biloba were asked to rate their results. Of 126 who responded, nine noticed an improvement, nine indicated their tinnitus became worse, 30 weren't sure about its effect because they were taking other supplements in their regimen, and 78 reported no difference at all. In other words, approximately 7% reported improvement. The survey did not indicate a relationship to the severity of their tinnitus, its origin, or the type of sound.

As noted, ginkgo biloba affects the circulatory system. Be cautious about using it, and be sure to check with your healthcare provider about possible interactions if you are using other medications or supplements. If you are on a blood thinner medication, it's likely that you will be advised against taking ginkgo biloba or any similar supplement. Be mindful that a daily aspirin is considered to be a blood thinner. For more information about this type of herb-drug interaction, please read the article "Ginkgo and blood thinners" on the Medical Herbalism website.

Bioflavonoids are another popular remedy for treating tinnitus symptoms. Again, this is a suggested treatment that works for some people, while others receive no benefit at all. Bioflavonoids are anti-oxidants, sometimes called super anti-oxidants, found in everyday foods. Taking a supplement simply makes up for what may be lacking in your diet. Nature's Life also adds hesperidin complex and rutin complex in their product. I did a lot of research on those two compounds before buying the supplement and felt confident that they would create a synergistic effect with the bioflavonoids. I began taking the supplement about six months after developing tinnitus. It softened the tinnitus somewhat and lessened its intrusiveness. I took two 1,000 mg tablets daily for several months, and then dropped the dosage down to 1,000 mg per day. You can read customer reviews for Nature's Life Bioflavonoids on Amazon. (The first Q&A relates to tinnitus.) Various bioflavonoid products are generally available wherever supplements are sold.

If you prefer to get your bioflavonoids from food rather than a pill, you'll need to add or increase the following foods in your diet: red bell peppers, strawberries, citrus fruits, tropical fruits, spinach, broccoli, Brussels sprouts, garlic, and green tea. If your tinnitus worsens with caffeine, buy the decaffeinated version of the tea. You'll still reap the benefits of its other ingredients.

Vinpocetine is the synthetic version of the beautiful lesser periwinkle flower, also known as Vinca minor. It requires considerable laboratory time and work to create vinpocetine, so it straddles the border between being classified as an actual prescription drug versus a supplement. In Japan and Germany it is available only by prescription, whereas in the United States and Canada it is available over the counter. It is considered to be neuroprotective and to increase cerebral blood flow. Neuroimaging studies of tinnitus patients have shown that blood perfusion in the brain may be abnormal and therefore a cause or contributor to tinnitus or its severity. (Perfusion is the flow of blood through the vessels of an organ.) If vinpocetine helps to normalize cerebral blood flow, that may in turn decrease the severity of the tinnitus, hopefully to the point where it becomes a slight annoyance in one's life instead of a major disruption.

Fish oil, an excellent source of omega-3 fatty acids, is a popular supplement for many reasons. Clinical trials have repeatedly demonstrated that omega-3 fatty acids provide benefits to the heart, the blood system, and the skin, as well as reducing pain and swelling. Once again we have a supplement for tinnitus that supports the circulatory system, a recurring theme in treating tinnitus. Fish oil is also considered to be an excellent anti-inflammatory. If there is some sort of inflammation within the auditory system, it's possible that regular intake of omega-3 fatty acids will reduce or eliminate the inflammation and in turn ease the symptoms of tinnitus. Whether or not fish oil actually helps you with tinnitus, you will at least reap the other health benefits. Look for fish oil capsules with no aftertaste, and be sure to check the source to verify that the oil is derived from fish that have not been exposed to mercury.

Keep in mind that although fish oil can decrease triglyceride levels, it can also increase your cholesterol levels. Check with your healthcare provider before adding supplemental fish oil to your diet if you have high cholesterol levels.

Magnesium is an extremely popular and inexpensive supplement for treating tinnitus. Like fish oil, it has wonderful health benefits and is an excellent supplement for adults, since almost 70% of American adults have a magnesium deficiency. It helps your body absorb and process calcium more efficiently, it's good for your skin, and, like the other supplements, helps to keep your circulatory system in proper working order. Poor blood flow creates stress on the hair cells of the inner ear. If the hair cells are already weakened, that's all the more reason to protect them from further damage.

Magnesium is an essential mineral for maintaining healthy muscle and nerve function. When the nerves of your auditory system are stressed or damaged, magnesium may not be able to reverse the damage that exists, but it can help to prevent further damage as long as you take precautions to protect your hearing and general health. Magnesium is also great for helping you to sleep better. In fact, its nickname is the "relaxation mineral." Getting a good night's sleep is one of the most important things you can do to ease the symptoms of tinnitus. If you suffer from nighttime leg cramps or restless leg syndrome, magnesium has been shown to improve those ailments as well. Take it before bedtime for best results.

When you go to the store or search online for your magnesium supplement, choose chelated magnesium. It has the highest absorption rate and your body utilizes it more efficiently than magnesium citrate. Look for "magnesium glycinate" on the list of ingredients. It is the easiest chelated magnesium for your body to absorb. Magnesium supplements are not recommended if you have kidney disease, heart disease, or take certain medications. As always, discuss it with your healthcare provider first.

There are so many great-tasting foods which contain enough magnesium to meet your minimum RDA, you might just prefer to fill up your grocery basket with them rather than buy a bottle of pills. Among these are salmon (also great for omega-3), spinach and other dark leafy greens, avocados, bananas, pumpkin seeds, beans and lentils, brown rice, low-fat plain yogurt, artichokes and dates, to name a few. Excess magnesium intake can adversely affect a heart condition or kidney disease. If you have either of those health issues, be sure to check the magnesium content of your servings and be careful not to exceed the recommended daily allowance guideline set by your physician.

NAC, short for N-acetyl-L-cysteine, is a precursor of glutathione. A precursor is a chemical that is transformed into another compound. Glutathione is produced by the liver, as well as being present in meats, fruits, and vegetables. It has the important role of tissue building and repair. It makes chemicals and proteins that the body needs, and is helpful to the immune system. Although there is no conclusive proof of its effectiveness for improving tinnitus, NAC is generally recommended to prevent further harm to the auditory system. In other words, it won't help to repair what damage has already been done, but it serves to help protect against additional damage.

The U.S. military conducted a clinical trial to determine if NAC would be helpful in protecting ears at risk of damage from loud noises. Their conclusion was that taking NAC proved to be more helpful than earplugs alone for Marines who were exposed to gunfire. The recommendation is 1,200 milligrams taken 12 hours before exposure to loud events, for example a drag race. If you're exposed to an unexpected loud noise, take 1,200 milligrams as soon as possible, followed by 900 to 1,200 milligrams three times a day, with meals, for the next three days. Keep in mind that NAC is not a substitute for earplugs. If the acoustic trauma is severe enough, such as gunfire at close range without hearing protection, then taking NAC before and/or after exposure will not be adequate. That type of damage requires an immediate trip to the emergency room for prednisone treatment. (The use of prednisone for treating acute severe auditory trauma is discussed in the next chapter, "Prescription Drugs.")

Because NAC is believed to have antioxidant properties, and because free radicals damage the hair cells of the inner ear, it doesn't hurt to add NAC to your daily regimen. At the very least it will give you a sense of comfort to know that if you're walking down the street and someone suddenly revs a motorcycle nearby, or honks a horn, your ears have an extra level of protection with daily supplementation of NAC.

Quality NAC is not cheap. One popular brand is Jarrow Formula N-A-C Sustain, 600 milligrams, taken with a small glass of juice first thing in the morning, 30 minutes before breakfast. This recommendation is based on the research I did when I first experienced tinnitus. I was looking everywhere for something that would help reduce the volume of my tinnitus. I can't say for certain that NAC did reduce the volume, but it did help a bit to ease my anxiety about encountering unexpected loud noises in my everyday life.

Melatonin is a must-have supplement in your tinnitus arsenal if you are experiencing insomnia or disrupted sleep, especially for older adults, as melatonin production decreases with age. Melatonin is a hormone secreted by the pineal gland, an endocrine gland which is no bigger than a pea and situated deep in the center of the brain between the right and left hemispheres. Clinical studies are absolutely conclusive that melatonin is helpful for promoting sleep. It appears to be most effective at a dose of 3 milligrams, and is recommended to be taken 30 minutes before bedtime. Taking melatonin creates no negative feedback in the body; that is, the body does not begin secreting less melatonin while you are taking the supplement or after you stop taking it. Some people report vivid dreams when taking melatonin, but these are anecdotal reports and not verified in clinical studies. Because it is a hormone, melatonin supplements are not recommended for children, or women who are pregnant or nursing.

In addition to being a sleep aid, studies have shown that melatonin reduces the perceived severity of tinnitus. Subjects who took 3 milligrams of tinnitus daily over a 30-day period reported subjective improvement in their tinnitus. It's generally accepted that as one's sleep quality of sleep improves, their tinnitus will improve as well. Whether it's caused by the melatonin itself or simply better sleep, a perception of reduced severity is helpful in coping with tinnitus.

Some European countries, including the United Kingdom, do not allow melatonin to be sold except through prescription, but in the United States melatonin is readily available and very inexpensive. Many people prefer the timed-release version which more closely simulates the body's natural production. A reputable brand for melatonin is Source Naturals. Their product includes 31 milligrams of calcium with the 3 milligrams of melatonin. Calcium is a nutrient which is helpful for inducing sleep, which is why a warm glass of milk before bedtime is a well-known sleep remedy.

Melatonin is especially beneficial for older adults whose level of melatonin has begun to naturally decrease. It's a great supplement, and is generally considered safe for adults at 3 milligrams or less each night. However, keep in mind that melatonin is a hormone and should not be taken without considering its powerful properties. If you are taking any prescription medications or other supplements, check with your healthcare provider to ensure that it's safe for you to take melatonin.

B12 is a water soluble vitamin which is important in the formation of red blood cells. It also plays a role in the metabolism of sugars, fats and proteins. Like other supplements recommended for tinnitus and noise-induced hearing loss, B12 helps to maintain a healthy nervous system. It is essential for formation of the myelin sheath that surrounds and protects nerve fibers. A deficiency can make nerves more susceptible to inflammatory damage. Food sources for B12 include liver, red meat, soy products, whole grain fortified cereals, cheese, eggs and dairy products, and fish such as shellfish, tuna, salmon and sardines. Most people get enough B12 from eating those foods, so it isn't likely that you would have a B12 deficiency with that type of diet. However, it's not unusual to find B12 deficiency in vegetarians, and even more so in vegans, who eat no animal-derived products. If you suspect you have a B12 deficiency, you can get a blood test to measure the level in your system. Request a blood test for active B12 rather than serum B12, as the latter only measures your stores of B12.

If you decide to take a B12 supplement, choose the methylcobalamin version, which provides better absorption. Jarrow manufactures a high quality Methyl B-12. Their recommended dose is 5,000 micrograms per day. You may want to take less or more than that, based on your body weight and other factors. Because it's a water soluble vitamin, your body will excrete what it doesn't need. Risk of overdose is very small, but it's still best to stay within recommended limits. If you are severely deficient in B12 because your body simply cannot maintain proper levels, your healthcare professional may recommend B12 injections. This is actually the most effective method of administering B12.

Taurine is an essential amino acid that people generally associate with the diets of cats and dogs. In the 1970s, thousands of cats and dogs began mysteriously dying of cardiomyopathy, a disease of the heart where the ability of the myocardium to contract begins to deteriorate. In addition, thousands of cats were going blind. The mystery was traced to the gradual substitution of grains and meat byproducts in pet food instead of the more expensive muscle meat which contains the necessary taurine. Taurine is now added to pet food to make up for the deficiency.

Humans are also susceptible to disorders arising from insufficient taurine intake. Taurine helps control the flow of calcium into and out of the hair cells within the ear. Taurine has been shown in clinical studies to protect against progressive hearing loss, and is potentially helpful for tinnitus. This may be because taurine also improves blood flow. If compromised blood flow is contributing to someone's tinnitus, taking a taurine supplement may help. In addition, taurine has been proven to reduce oxidative stress on the light sensory cells in the retina. Taking taurine gives older individuals an extra bit of protection not only for their ears, but for their eyes as well.

Candida, an all-too-common infection, interferes with the body's taurine production, as do other bacterial and fungal infections. MSG (monosodium glutamate) is a synthetic flavor enhancer added to many common grocery foods. MSG degrades taurine and thereby decreases the amount of taurine that the body has to work with. It's worth noting here that MSG is implicated as a factor contributing to tinnitus due to its adverse effects on the nervous system. Check your food labels. If MSG is listed on them, which is highly likely, it's a good idea to add taurine to your daily supplement regimen. As with B12, vegetarians and vegans are at risk for taurine deficiency because taurine is found in food sources like red meat, fish, and eggs. People whose diets either do not include those foods, or when those foods are not part of their regular diet, would benefit from taurine supplementation.

A quality taurine supplement is somewhat pricey, but it's worth adding to your tinnitus regimen. It's even more important if you are over 40, have hearing loss in addition to tinnitus, and want to be proactive about protecting your eyes against age-related damage. Because of its reputation for high quality supplements, I bought Solgar brand taurine, 500 milligrams. They suggest one capsule up to four times a day, between meals. Their product is suitable for vegetarians because they use a vegetable-based capsule instead of a gelatin-based capsule. Gelatin is an animal byproduct derived from collagen.

CoQ10 (coenzyme Q10), is recommended by healthcare providers for many reasons. If you're over 40 and regularly take supplements, it's possible that CoQ10 or ubiquinol is already part of your daily regimen. In the years following CoQ10's splash on the supplement scene, research indicated that ubiquinol is a more potent and effective form of CoQ10 for adults over 40. Since then, an even more powerful synthetic analogue of CoQ10 has been shown in clinical studies to be helpful in neural transmissions. That relatively new product is idebenone, a supplement which falls under the nootropic category. A nootropic, commonly referred to as a "smart drug," is a supplement that has been shown to improve mental functioning. Idebenone stands out amongst these smart drugs because it is considered to have properties which directly affect the brain, specifically in the areas of mental cognition and neural health. Nootropics can be harder to find than better-known supplements. I purchased mine through www.SmartDrugsForThought.com, and was pleased with the customer service and quality of their products.

Research also indicates that idebenone is neuroprotective against excitotoxicity, particularly regarding suppression of excess glutamate. You can read more detailed information about this benefit on www.Examine.com/supplements/idebenone.

Theanine, also referred to as l-theanine, is an amino acid derived from green tea. Studies have demonstrated that theanine crosses the blood brain barrier. It promotes relaxation, as evidenced by increased alpha brain wave activity and decreased beta brain wave activity, but it does not have a sedating effect. It has been shown to reduce the perception of stress while improving attention and focus. Because people with tinnitus have lower than average levels of alpha brain wave activity, theanine may help to bring the brain waves back into balance, at least temporarily. Typical dosage of theanine is between 200 and 250 milligrams per day, taken away from food. Doctor's Best is a reputable manufacturer of supplements. They offer a high quality l-theanine product.

Theanine can reduce blood pressure, so it is not recommended for people who have hypotension or are already taking medications to lower their blood pressure. Theanine can also interact with sedatives, stimulants, and drugs for treating cancer and high cholesterol. Be sure to consult your healthcare professional before adding theanine to your supplement regimen.

Magnolia bark, or *Magnolia officinalis*, is a species of the magnolia plant native to China, and has been used in traditional Chinese medicine since 100 AD. Magnolia plants are considered to be protective against cancer, and much of the research about *Magnolia officinalis* concerns that aspect. The active properties of magnolia bark are magnolol and honokiol. Magnolol has been shown to have potential anti-epileptic benefits. Honokiol is a potent anxiolytic (anxiety reducer), similar to anti-anxiety medications such as Xanax and Valium. Similar to the actions of benzodiazepines, honokiol works by increasing levels of GABA. The difference is that honokiol targets specific GABA receptors in the brain, whereas benzos target GABA receptors throughout the entire body. Since tinnitus is now considered to be a brain disorder, it makes sense to limit the target area to the brain rather than the entire body. Benzodiazepines such as Xanax have the reputation of decreasing volume of tinnitus, but I could find no studies confirming that either magnolol or honokiol can reduce tinnitus volume or severity. However, magnolia bark is a very potent antioxidant, thereby helping to protect the delicate hair cells of the inner ear from further damage and hearing loss. This is important when considering the role that hearing loss plays in the development of tinnitus. Recent scientific studies are pointing to the formation of free radicals in the inner ear from noise exposure. These free radicals contribute to the hair cells being damaged. This is why supplements such as NAC and magnolia bark are being studied as a means of protecting the sensory cells of the inner ear.

Anecdotal reports indicate that magnolol and honokiol may reduce evening levels of cortisol, but I could find no clinical trials on this. If you have difficulty sleeping or other problems associated with high levels of cortisol in the evening, consider taking honokiol to see if it helps you to get a good night's rest. Signs of a high cortisol level include difficulty sleeping, persistent fatigue, increased sensitivity to pain, a thickening midsection (cortisol tends to deposit fat in the abdomen), craving sweets, and anxiety. If you suspect your cortisol level is too high, consider having your blood cortisol level tested. Remember that stress not only increases cortisol, it tends to make perception of tinnitus worse. If your cortisol levels are consistently too high, you will need to resolve the issues that are causing excess stress in your life.

For in-depth information about any of the above-listed supplements, visit www.Examine.com. Enter the supplement name in the Search field. On the results page, click on the link that most closely matches what you're looking for. Examine publishes extensive information on supplements, including how to take them, scientific research conducted, potential side effects, and more. I encourage you to visit this website and thoroughly research the supplements you're considering taking for tinnitus or any other condition.

59
PRESCRIPTION DRUGS

We are so used to taking a pill for whatever ails us, that it's a natural tendency when tinnitus strikes to look for a medication-based cure, or at least something that will reduce the volume or intensity. Unfortunately, there simply is no cure. Furthermore, treating tinnitus with prescription drugs can be a tricky trial-and-error process, with the potential of some unpleasant side effects. If you can avoid taking prescribed medications, give it your best shot to cope without them. Taking over-the-counter supplements is the best option if your tinnitus is mild or moderate. However, if you have severe tinnitus, particularly in the first few months when tinnitus is new and likely to cause greater distress, over-the-counter supplements may not be enough.

There are books on tinnitus wherein the authors totally shun the idea of using prescription drugs. I disagree with that approach. In my opinion, it is not a character weakness for you to rely on prescription drugs for tinnitus if you need them, just as you would use antibiotics to prevent infection if you sustain a severe wound or have a tooth pulled. Think of the harm that's being done to your body by a prolonged, relentless toll of insurmountable stress and/or lack of sleep. Don't try to be super human. Be willing to admit that everyone needs help when faced with something traumatic for which they are totally unprepared.

Talk with your healthcare provider to weigh risks and benefits. Here are some warning signals indicating you need professional assistance:

- Your tinnitus is constantly interfering with your ability to get more than a few hours sleep each night;
- Your moods have become erratic;
- Your tolerance level has dropped to the point where you've started snapping at co-workers, friends, family members, or pets;
- You're reacting with extreme anger or hostility to even the slightest provocation;
- You're so depressed that you've shut yourself off from everyday life;
- You're seriously considering suicide.

Any of those warning signals, **and especially if you're contemplating suicide**, is a clear indicator that you may benefit from something powerful to adjust the chemicals in your brain and help you to gain a more balanced outlook. If depression is part of the burden, it would be a good idea to find a counselor who is knowledgeable about tinnitus and can help guide you through all the conflicting emotions you might be experiencing. The same is true if your anxiety is spiraling out of control; you need professional guidance.

The observations about medications for tinnitus that I'm including here are based on what I've learned by reading about the experiences of others. I have also included information from reputable websites such as Drugs.com, MedicineNet.com, WebMD.com, and RxList.com that publish information about pharmaceuticals, diseases, and disorders. Please keep in mind that I am not a physician or any other type of professional healthcare provider. I have done my best as a non-medical person to present accurate information based on extensive research, but your healthcare provider and your own proactive research should be the deciding factor on what course you take regarding prescription drugs. With those qualifiers out of the way, let's review the most commonly prescribed drugs for tinnitus.

Prednisone is a corticosteroid with a bad reputation for side effects like weight gain and irritability, as well as more serious side effects such as blurred vision and pancreatitis, but there have been reports of its usefulness in treating tinnitus when administered early. If you review online articles about prednisone as a treatment for tinnitus, you will find that recommendations of how soon you need to take it will vary from 24 to 48 hours to as long as three months. The general consensus is, the sooner the better. It also seems to be more helpful when tinnitus is the result of acoustic trauma or sudden sensorineural hearing loss. Furthermore, prednisone has been shown to be helpful in some instances to stop or reverse sudden hearing loss. Because this is not a common treatment for tinnitus, many doctors are unaware of its possible usefulness. The success rate for improving or eliminating tinnitus through the use of prednisone is not encouraging, but if you are in that early window of time, especially 24 to 48 hours, it might be worth trying.

You never know if you'll be one of the lucky ones for whom it works. For more information on the use of prednisone to treat tinnitus, Medscape has published an article comparing oral therapy and intratympanic therapy (via injection into the middle ear). You can find the article online, "Steroid Injection an Option for Sensorineural Hearing Loss." This is information you can take to the emergency room or your personal physician.

Many reports indicate that after initial relief and silence, the tinnitus returned when the prednisone regimen ended. Again, the sooner you get this treatment, the more likely it is to provide benefit. The chance of having a better prognosis is noted in the PubMed article, "The efficacy of medication on tinnitus due to acute acoustic trauma."

Keep in mind that even though prednisone can be an effective treatment in the acute stage of tinnitus, it is still considered an ototoxic drug and is not to be taken lightly. It is also very important that you taper off a course of prednisone according to your doctor's recommendations. This will help you to avoid withdrawal symptoms of fatigue, weakness, body aches, and joint pain. When you take prednisone, your adrenal glands decrease their production of cortisol. Tapering off gives the adrenals time to resume their normal function.

Benzodiazepines ("benzos") are useful for treating anxiety and depression, and are sometimes prescribed to help people cope with tinnitus in the early stages. They can be helpful for those who are unable to sleep, and are especially beneficial for treating panic attacks or extreme anxiety. The top four prescribed benzodiazepines for tinnitus patients are clonazepam (Klonopin), alprazolam (Xanax), temazepam (Restoral), and lorazepam (Ativan).

To understand how benzodiazepines work and why they're so powerful, you need to know a little bit about the neurotransmitter GABA. Remember that neurotransmitters are chemicals that either promote or inhibit neural activity. GABA is the most abundant inhibitory neurotransmitter in the brain. GABA's role is to keep the neurons from becoming overly excited and hyperactive. When GABA is either inefficient or insufficient, anxiety can occur. Benzodiazepines are effective at reducing anxiety because they enhance the natural effect of GABA. Unfortunately, benzos are so good at what they do, the ability of the body to produce its own natural GABA becomes compromised, which can lead to serious problems. One of these problems is addiction, which can occur within a short time period, even at recommended doses. Benzo addiction is notoriously difficult to treat because benzos target GABA receptors which may become impaired from the benzos, and these receptors need time to return to their prior level of functioning.

Clonazepam (Klonopin) is generally prescribed to treat and prevent seizures, anxiety disorders, and panic attacks. It is not unusual for anti-seizure drugs to also be prescribed for tinnitus. In one study where subjects were randomly assigned either a course of clonazepam or a course of ginkgo biloba, with none of the participants knowing what they were taking, the clonazepam group showed highly significant improvement in terms of tinnitus loudness, duration, and annoyance, as well as markedly better Tinnitus Handicap Inventory scores. Keep in mind that clonazepam can have serious side effects. It is habit-forming and should not be taken long term. Drugs.com has reliable information on its website at www.drugs.com/clonazepam. You will want to take some time to read about possible side effects before asking your healthcare provider about this or any other drug as a possible treatment for acute or severe tinnitus.

In researching medications prescribed for tinnitus patients, it soon became clear that the one mentioned most often in online tinnitus communities is alprazolam (Xanax). It was first approved by the U.S. Food and Drug Administration in 1981 and fairly rapidly replaced Valium as the anti-anxiety drug of choice. In the 1990s, the U.S. was sometimes referred to as "Prozac Nation," but in the 21st Century we have become "Xanax Nation." In fact, Xanax and its generic counterpart, alprazolam, are the number 1 prescribed psychiatric medications in the United States, with 50 million prescriptions written every year. Based on the number of prescriptions, it's obvious that many of us grapple with anxiety on a regular basis. If you ask people what problems their tinnitus causes, they will often mention difficulty handling their feelings of anxiety. This is not surprising, as tinnitus does tend to raise fears about what the future holds and how one will be able to cope with the chronic intrusive and often distressing sound.

Like clonazepam, alprazolam has been shown to reduce the volume of tinnitus. It is believed that even though alprazolam helps with anxiety, that the reduction in volume is actually due to it being a GABA agonist. In other words, it acts upon GABA receptors to stimulate a higher level of activity, essentially acting as a counterbalance to glutamate-induced hyperactivity. Remember that GABA is an inhibitory neurotransmitter, and glutamate is an excitatory neurotransmitter. User Reviews on the drugs.com website, written by people who take Xanax for tinnitus, will give you a general idea of the benefits and drawbacks of this benzodiazepine.

Temazepam (Restoril) is usually prescribed specifically for sleeping difficulties, another common complaint of people with tinnitus. Temazepam has a pronounced hypnotic effect and should not be taken during the day, even if you feel "normal" while on the drug. That feeling can be misleading. One of the major drawbacks of temazepam is that tolerance can build in your system very quickly. You may take it for two nights in a row, and if on the third night you don't take it, you may experience what's known as rebound insomnia. Temazepam is another benzodiazepine which temporarily calms tinnitus, so it can work wonders for quick relief if you absolutely need to get a good night's rest. However, keep in mind that it has the reputation of being quite addictive, with a likelihood of eventually disturbing normal sleep patterns.

Lorazepam, sold under the brand name Ativan, has been shown to be effective in decreasing the annoyance of intrusive tinnitus. Lorazepam is a high potency benzodiazepine and can cause dependence in as little as four weeks. Basically it creates a state of indifference to your tinnitus (and other life frustrations), which makes the tinnitus much easier to cope with. This can be a good thing if you are also undergoing counseling to deal with the negative emotional and mental aspects of tinnitus. Unfortunately, if those are not addressed, then you will not benefit in the long run by taking lorazepam. Once you are no longer taking it, you will be right back where you started from. With intrusive tinnitus, it is especially important to learn how to cope with the psychological challenges without relying on addictive drugs that disrupt the delicate balance of your neurotransmitters.

Some people with tinnitus will only take benzos when they feel like their anxiety level has gone beyond their ability to cope. Benzos act quickly in one's system, which is why they can be useful as a last resort when someone cannot handle either the tinnitus or the accompanying anxiety. Whether on a regular schedule or an intermittent as-needed regimen, the use of benzos must be carefully monitored by a healthcare professional. Take them only at the lowest effective dose and for the shortest period of time. In addition, you must be very careful about tapering off, as too sudden a withdrawal from a benzo can have severe withdrawal effects, including psychosis. Improper tapering off, whether it's an improperly administered dosage or an inaccurate tapering schedule, has been linked to an increase in tinnitus and is known to cause tinnitus in people who previously did not have it. Your physician should certainly be aware of all this and caution you about it, but it's better for you to understand ahead of time how powerful benzodiazepines can be and the different ways they can affect you, for better or worse.

The online forum BenzoBuddies, which you can access through www.BenzoBuddies.org, is an excellent resource for information if you have questions or concerns about taking benzos for your tinnitus. The members of this forum are very aware of both the benefits and risks of benzodiazepines, including their use as a treatment for tinnitus. They readily admit that benzos can decrease the volume of tinnitus due to artificially enhancing GABA levels and thereby tamping down the neural hyperactivity associated with tinnitus. If you want to benefit from the hard-earned knowledge of people who have been treated with benzos, I recommend perusing this forum in addition to consulting with your healthcare practitioner.

Another excellent source of information is the online article, "Benzodiazepines: How They Work and How to Withdraw," available on www.benzo.org.uk. It was originally published in 2002 by Professor C. Heather Ashton, DM, FRCP, following her 12 years of experience in treating benzo withdrawal patients. I cannot stress enough that if your anxiety level is motivating you to seek benzodiazepines as treatment, you really need to learn as much as you can about them, especially their addictive properties that can arise with even very short-term use.

Although it's usually prescribed specifically for depression, mirtazapine (Remeron) has been shown to provide the dual benefits of a reduction in tinnitus volume and restoration of deep sleep. Mirtazapine is not a benzodiazepine. It works by increasing the level of the neurotransmitter norepinephrine. It does this by blocking the receptors that inhibit norepinephrine. Norepinephrine is a hormone and a neurotransmitter, secreted by the adrenal glands into the bloodstream. As a neurotransmitter, it helps to conduct nerve impulses between neurons. Norepinephrine is important in regulating our blood pressure, energy levels, and even our moods. Mirtazapine also increases serotonin levels. Serotonin is a neurotransmitter which helps to regulate mood, body temperature, sleep, appetite, and metabolism. As with any drug that affects neurotransmitter and hormone levels, proceed with caution and aim for short-term treatment with mirtazapine.

Because tinnitus is a neurological disorder with some similarities to epilepsy, anti-seizure drugs are sometimes prescribed for severe tinnitus. One of the more commonly prescribed drugs is gabapentin (Neurontin). Other drugs that have been used successfully in some patients, but not all, include levetiracetam (Keppra), pregabaline (Lyrica), carbamazepine (Tegretol), and flupirtine (Katadolon). These are anti-epileptics and should only be taken under the supervision of a neurologist or a physician who has experience in treating tinnitus with these drugs.

Another drug which showed a bit of promise is ezogabine or retigabine (Potiga or Trobalt), an anti-seizure drug. According to anecdotal reports, it reduced severe tinnitus for some sufferers, but others experienced no improvement. Ezogabine has the potential for drastic side effects, including urinary retention, skin discoloration, and pigment changes in the retina. It was originally developed for the treatment of epilepsy. Somehow the word got around that it could also be helpful for some cases of tinnitus, but there have been no clinical trials in that regard. Because of safety issues and limited use, the manufacturer elected to stop production of the drug in June 2017. Perhaps in the future a medication with the same mechanism of action that made ezogabine effective can be formulated, one that will be safe for both epileptics and people with debilitating tinnitus.

In late September 2016, Brazilian researchers published their preliminary findings that oxytocin was shown to reduce tinnitus. Oxytocin is a hormone manufactured in the hypothalamus. It is then transported to and released into the bloodstream and certain regions of the brain by the pituitary gland. Oxytocin is a hormone and a neuropeptide. A peptide is a compound containing two or more amino acids. Neuropeptides influence the function or activity of nerve cells.

Oxytocin has been nicknamed "the love hormone" and "the cuddle chemical" for its well-known properties of promoting feelings of affection and closeness and enhancing the desire to bond between couples and friends. With sexual intimacy, oxytocin is released in greater amounts during orgasm and tends to strengthen relationships. For a nursing mother, the suckling infant stimulates the nipples, whereupon oxytocin is released into the mother's system. This also causes the milk to flow from her breast to feed her baby. Oxytocin intensifies the maternal bond that the mother feels toward her child. In this respect, oxytocin is considered vital for the preservation of the species.

The Brazilian study on the effects of oxytocin on tinnitus included only 17 participants, some of whom were administered oxytocin via nasal spray, and some of whom were given a placebo. Average age was 63, with no mention of tinnitus severity. Results were reported 30 minutes after administration of oxytocin or placebo, as well as 24 hours later. Those who were given oxytocin reported that either the tinnitus disappeared, was significantly reduced, or was lowered to what they described as a non-distress level. None of the participants who received a placebo reported any improvement. Obviously this is a very small study, but oxytocin is a hormone/neuropeptide which is known for its calming feel-good effects on the nervous system. In this regard it's somewhat like Xanax, promoting a sense of well-being and relaxation. Xanax tends to reduce the perception of tinnitus volume and/or intrusiveness. It makes sense that a hormone which naturally promotes relaxation and blissful feelings would have a similar effect on tinnitus. Oxytocin has the additional benefits of regulating blood sugar, lowering blood pressure, relieving stress, increasing immunity, regulating sleep patterns, and protecting against heart disease.

You can purchase oxytocin supplements over the counter in either nasal spray or capsule form. However, oxytocin is not an herb or vitamin. Despite its purported benefits, it is still a hormone and neuropeptide which can have significant effects on your system if not properly dosed and monitored. Among these side effects are abnormal heartbeat, high blood pressure, breathing difficulties, and vomiting. Please check with your healthcare provider before using an oxytocin supplement, especially if you are currently taking any prescription drug or other over-the-counter remedy. I have included the oxytocin study in this chapter as an example of just one of many clinical trials that have been conducted in the search for an effective treatment for tinnitus. However, I do not endorse the use of oxytocin supplements because of the potential for serious side effects.

If you are seeing a healthcare provider for your tinnitus, be a proactive patient in your treatment. Some physicians encourage their patients to stay informed through online research. Others prefer that their patients not do so, out of concern that they will be misled by false claims. Scientific research into the use of prescription drugs to treat tinnitus is an ongoing process, and there are several reputable online sites to keep up with the latest news on medications and therapies for tinnitus. It's in your best interest to stay informed and share what you've learned with your provider. The section "Resources," page 391 in the Appendix, includes links to online sites for professional organizations which report on recent developments in the treatment of hearing disorders and/or tinnitus.

60
rTMS AND tDCS

Because tinnitus is associated with hyper or abnormal electrical activity in the brain, researchers have come up with interesting ways to treat tinnitus by attempting to directly influence the electrical activity. The general term for this type of treatment is "neuromodulation," which means to alter neural pathways and thereby change the function of the part of the body controlled by those neurons. Neuromodulation can be accomplished by either chemical means, such as prescription drugs or supplements which affect neurotransmitters, or by stimulating neural pathways with electrical impulses. Laypersons sometimes refer to such treatments as "brain hacking," an informal term for influencing your brain neurons through electrical stimulation devices.

One controversial treatment for severe tinnitus is repetitive transcranial magnetic stimulation (rTMS), wherein neuromodulation is applied via electrical impulses. The word "transcranial" means to pass through the cranium, what we commonly call the skull. A coil of wire encased in plastic is held next to the skull, and a pulsed current is then passed into that coil of wire. This creates a magnetic field which penetrates the skull and focuses on the cortex, the surface of the brain. This magnetic field directly affects the underlying neurons wherever the magnetic field is focused. The current is intermittently pulsed, meaning applied at regular intervals rather than a steady flow; thus the term "repetitive."

Repetitive transcranial magnetic stimulation may sound similar to electroshock therapy, which has a notorious reputation due to its past history of abuse in the treatment of patients with severe mental illness and emotional pathologies. However, the procedures are quite different. Electroshock therapy, now called electroconvulsive therapy (ECT) is still being used, but with safeguards in place. These safeguards include the use of anesthetics and much lower electrical currents during treatment. ECT is used to treat extreme cases of mania, severe depression or anxiety, catatonia (profound nonresponsive stupor), and other conditions that fail to respond to conventional treatment. The current that is generated induces a brief seizure in the patient, which alters the brain chemistry.

The patient, who is unconscious during the session due to anesthesia, is completely unaware of the seizure. ECT generally requires a series of treatments given over time. In patients who do not respond to conventional treatment, or those with severe mental illness, ECT alters the brain chemistry and appears to reset the brain's electrical activity to a more normal state.

Instead of electroconvulsive therapy, the application of repetitive transcranial magnetic stimulation has been successfully used to treat milder cases of depression. The magnetic coil is usually placed over the area of the prefrontal cortex, the part of the brain which is involved in emotional responses. The prefrontal cortex is also connected to other parts of the brain that are important in the regulation of norepinephrine, serotonin and dopamine, three neurotransmitters that are critical for mood regulation. Magnetic stimulation of the neurons in the prefrontal cortex can help to stabilize the levels of those neurotransmitters and thereby alleviate depression.

Repetitive transcranial magnetic stimulation is administered while the patient is awake. It requires no anesthesia or medication. It is generally a painless procedure, although some people have reported that their teeth knock together when the magnetic stimulation is applied. Other side effects include post treatment headache or toothache, and sometimes there is muscle twitching during the session. One very rare side effect is seizures, which is why it is not recommended for epileptics. Because epilepsy and tinnitus both have abnormal brain wave patterns and hyperexcitable brain neurons, it raises the question why anyone thought it would be a good idea to treat someone who has tinnitus with repetitive transcranial magnetic stimulation. Studies conducted on tinnitus subjects have shown very limited success with the use of rTMS. Any perceived reduction in tinnitus volume appeared to be a temporary effect with no statistical difference noted at four months follow-up. In fact, even though Johns Hopkins Hospital uses rTMS for treatment of depression, they do not mention it as helpful for tinnitus.

At this time no one knows precisely which tinnitus-related neurons are being targeted during any application of rTMS. Not only that, there's no way to know how an individual's brain wave characteristics will be affected by any particular duration or strength of the magnetic field generated. Even though anecdotal accounts from Internet forums are not considered scientifically valid, the general opinion from those who have tried rTMS is that it either results in little to no improvement, or it makes the tinnitus significantly worse. In addition, this is a very expensive treatment and, because it's classified as experimental, it is not covered by many health insurance companies.

Transcranial direct-current stimulation (tDCS) is another experimental treatment for tinnitus. With tDCS, a constant low electrical stimulation is applied via two electrodes attached to the skull. The stimulation can be anodal, which excites the underlying neurons, or it can be cathodal, which reduces neural activity. Transcranial direct-current stimulation is relatively inexpensive and easy to administer. Kits are available online for those who want to try do-it-yourself brain hacking, but medical scientists advise strongly against it. Researchers at Oxford University experimented with using tDCS to relieve anxiety in performing math tasks. They discovered that tDCS did in fact decrease anxiety and subjects performed better with their anxiety lessened. Unfortunately, it had the unwanted side effect of decreasing performance in another brain-related task. It was like the brain was compensating for enhanced performance in one area by reducing performance in another area. Studies conducted at Oxford were not related to tinnitus, but one should proceed with caution regarding any treatment utilizing electrical stimulation of the brain.

There is no doubt that tDCS can affect the brain's neural activity. Since we know that tinnitus is the result of abnormal brain activity, how then does tDCS affect the perception of tinnitus? For tinnitus patients, the anodal and cathodal electrodes are placed on the skull so that the current is applied to the dorsolateral prefrontal cortex. That's a fancy way of saying the part of the brain near the forehead but slightly back from it, on each side of the brain. The important thing to remember here is that the prefrontal cortex is very much involved in our emotional responses. When an anodal electrode is placed on the right side and a cathodal electrode is placed on the left side, some patients have reported that tinnitus distress is reduced, as well as perception of loudness and discomfort. When the cathodal electrode is placed on the right side and the anodal electrode is placed on the left side, tinnitus annoyance is reduced even though perception of loudness doesn't change. This finding bolsters the claim of tinnitus retraining therapy practitioners that tinnitus annoyance is based more on an emotional reaction to the tinnitus itself and not the perceived loudness.

One interesting aspect of tDCS is that females seem to respond better than males. Generally speaking, women have more neural connections going from left to right in their brains, whereas men have more connections from front to back. Perhaps the electrical stimulation travels more efficiently in the prefrontal cortex of the female brain. Although men are more likely to have tinnitus, studies have shown that women tend to be more distressed by their tinnitus. It's possible that women experience a stronger sense of relief and therefore report a greater benefit.

I am neither a scientist nor a medical doctor and cannot make a recommendation for transcranial direct-current stimulation. My general impression from researching the information available is that it appears to be a milder and safer treatment than repetitive transcranial magnetic stimulation. If you're interested in pursuing this form of neuromodulation, please investigate as much as you can about the potential benefits and side effects of this treatment. Adjusting neural activity via electrical stimulation is a serious matter, and there is not a great deal of data to support its use as a treatment for tinnitus. However, if you believe your tinnitus is severe enough that you're willing to try this procedure, be sure to find a qualified and experienced professional, and ask them to provide solid evidence that tDCS has helped their tinnitus patients.

61
RESIDUAL INHIBITION

Residual inhibition refers to the phenomenon that after hearing certain sounds for a period of time, your tinnitus perception is temporarily suppressed. This may last for a few seconds, or as long as several hours. Listening to the different color noises can have this effect (white, pink, violet, etc.), as well as exposure to sounds that match the frequency or characteristics of your own tinnitus. For example, if your tinnitus sounds like cicadas and you listen to an audio of cicadas singing, it's possible that your tinnitus may seem to fade away for a brief time after the audio ends. Many people with tinnitus get residual inhibition from being in the shower. Their tinnitus can temporarily seem to disappear or at least become much less noticeable.

You may recall that audio notch therapy works by lateral inhibition to suppress dysfunctional neurons from firing spontaneously in a hyperactive manner. Residual inhibition, on the other hand, works by increasing the auditory output at your exact tinnitus frequency. The result is that your auditory system stops turning up the gain, so to speak, at the damaged frequencies. You might say that residual inhibition fills in the missing gap, fooling your brain into thinking that the missing frequency is not missing at all and that you can hear normally in that range. In other words, audio notch targets *functional neighboring neurons* and is a long-term treatment with the goal of long-term results, whereas residual inhibition targets the *dysfunctional misfiring neurons* and is a short-term treatment that usually produces only short-term results.

Residual inhibition has been studied as a treatment method for many years, using different variations to suppress tinnitus perception. Masking is one method of doing this. By listening to a sound that matches your tinnitus frequency for an extended period of time, the tinnitus is suppressed long enough to bring some relief. Another method involves listening to an audio loop which plays short segments of tinnitus-matching sounds, followed by periods of silence. (An audio loop is any audio file that is set to play over and over again until the listener stops the playback.) The theory behind all residual inhibition treatments is that the firing of the dysfunctional neurons becomes less and less until eventually the phantom sounds are reduced or eliminated for extended periods of time; i.e., days, weeks, or months.

HushTinnitus is one product which was developed to take advantage of the residual inhibition effect. It is marketed as being more effective and longer lasting than simply listening to flat white noise, shower sounds, or nature sounds. You can take a test on www.HushTinnitus.com to see if you're a candidate for residual inhibition therapy. When you visit the website, you are presented with an online preview to find your frequency. Then the website plays a sound specifically designed to match your frequency. (It doesn't matter if you have tonal or non-tonal tinnitus.) If you experience relief or a reduction in volume, you can then decide whether to purchase a downloadable set of custom audio files for the treatment program.

I tried the HushTinnitus system soon after acquiring tinnitus. Although I was impressed with the quality and number of the audio files, as well as the clear instructions, it was not suitable for me. The audio was not abrasive or irritating; it simply wasn't something I could listen to for more than a few minutes at a time. Your experience may be different. Therefore, I would not discourage you from giving it a try.

People with long-term chronic tinnitus are naturally wary of any treatments that don't have a long, established track record. Anyone with recent onset tinnitus should also be wary of companies that claim their products will reduce or eliminate tinnitus. HushTinnitus makes no claims that it will eliminate tinnitus. It relies on the natural phenomenon of residual inhibition as a way to obtain relief, but not a cure. The company's founder, Clyde Witchard, joined the Tinnitus Talk forum and answered questions about the product in great detail, in a friendly and nondefensive manner. The forum thread is "Hush Tinnitus Sound Therapy Experiences?"

Residual inhibition can occur from the strangest sounds. One example of this is available on YouTube, a video uploaded by user MedExamTools. The video is titled "Experimental Tinnitus Sound Treatment," but the explanation given by its developer is so technical that I can't convey it adequately. Basically it's white noise with random flat frequencies within a given range that play over and over in a continuous loop. The creator of the video makes no claim that it will reduce or suppress tinnitus, and that it was initially developed for an unrelated project. However, the Comments section indicates that it has definitely had a positive effect on more than a few people who have tried it.

The sound is not your typical static white noise, but instead has somewhat of a beeping tone sci-fi effect blended with a gurgling underwater effect which is hard to describe. Back when my tinnitus was severe, I listened to it for a while and experienced some residual inhibition. It wasn't long-lasting, although I will readily admit that it did provide some temporary relief. If you dislike the flat sound of white noise, this experimental treatment provides a much richer listening experience. Because the audio includes frequencies from 11 to 24,000 hertz, and because the frequencies are relatively flat across the spectrum, people with high-pitched tinnitus can benefit from it. For that reason, if the sound is acceptable to you, it's a good choice for creating a custom audio notch therapy file as described in Chapter 43, "Audio Notch - Do It Yourself Guide." Even if your tinnitus frequency is in the 20,000 range, you should still be able to create a notch filter to match and surround your frequency.

Residual inhibition doesn't work for everybody. Even though I've listed it in the Treatment section of this book, it could also have been included in the Coping section. The science behind the theory of residual inhibition is valid, which is why many clinical trials have attempted to replicate residual inhibition and make it work long-term. Like every other treatment for tinnitus, it depends on the individual as to how well it works for them. It's certainly worth trying. The benefit may only last a few minutes at a time, but that in itself can be a great blessing for those who need a bit of escape from their moderate or severe tinnitus.

62
TINNITUS RETRAINING THERAPY

Tinnitus retraining therapy (TRT) is a treatment with the goal of helping you to manage your tinnitus reaction and perception rather than aiming for a reduction or elimination of the tinnitus itself. If you visit a tinnitus therapy clinic, chances are TRT will be a primary or at least secondary part of their treatment program.

TRT is the brainchild of Dr. Pawel Jastreboff, a pioneer in the field of tinnitus studies. In 1990, he developed his Neurophysiological Model of Tinnitus. The premise of his model is that people who have clinically relevant tinnitus experience distress not because of the volume or intrusiveness of the tinnitus itself, but rather because their limbic system and autonomic nervous system are dominating their reactions. This belief is the foundation upon which tinnitus retraining therapy is built, to address the issue of the errant dominating systems that have been triggered in response to what is basically an auditory system dysfunction. Before going further, let's look at three scenarios that illustrate how people can react to sound in general, not just with the auditory system, but with emotions and provoking the survival instinct.

Scenario 1: Richard values privacy and appreciates classical music. To his horror, a new neighbor has moved in who plays country music outside on his deck. The neighbor rudely dismissed Richard when he politely asked him to turn down the music. The sound of the neighbor's music drifts into Richard's house, invading his space. Richard hates country music and responds to this intrusion with rising blood pressure and an increasing impulse to go next door and punch his neighbor. Richard fumes inwardly and fantasizes about packing up his belongings and moving elsewhere, but it isn't practical. He feels trapped and out of control of the situation. He misses the considerate neighbor who moved away. The two of them shared many of the same interests and attitudes, including the desire for a peaceful environment.

Scenario 2: Suzi loves Chihuahuas and thinks they're fantastic. They can be notorious barkers, but Suzi doesn't mind hearing them bark because it reminds her of the pet Chihuahua she had as a child. Her new neighbor moved in and he's got a Rottweiler. It doesn't bark much, but when it does, it's a big booming bark. Suzi hasn't had much experience with big dogs, and some of them terrify her. The neighbor's dog seems well-behaved, but Suzi is constantly on edge, knowing that a Rottweiler is next door.

Scenario 3: Jan thinks children are adorable. The more the merrier. Her new neighbors recently moved in, and they have three small children. The kids love to play outdoors. They're boisterous, with loud voices, laughing and sometimes shrieking with joy. Jan's kids have left the nest, and she's thrilled to have the presence of children in her life again.

In Scenario 1, you can see that the problem is not the intrusion of the music itself. The style of the music and his inability to control the situation is the source of Richard's rising blood pressure and his feeling that he wants to fight his neighbor. If the new neighbor were a classical music lover, it very likely wouldn't bother Richard to hear the music drifting into his home. He might even welcome it as a pleasant diversion.

With Scenario 2, although a Chihuahua's high-pitched bark is more irritating to most people than the bark of a big dog, Suzi connects the Rottweiler with her fear of big dogs. She could get to know the Rottie (as they're affectionately called), and discover that it has a good disposition. Shortly after moving in, her neighbor comes over and introduces himself. He assures her that his dog has been trained to be sociable with people and other dogs. In time, having this protective dog next door gives her a greater sense of security in her neighborhood. Suzi still doesn't like to hear it bark, but she begins taking notes of each time it barks and discovers that it really isn't that often during the day, and she never hears it at night because it stays indoors. After a while, when she hears the Rottie, Suzi simply shrugs it off as the dog warning someone to stay away or voicing its opinion about something going on in its territory.

In Scenario 3, loud children is a trigger stressor for many people. Children's voices tend to be high-pitched and after a while it can be an irritant to listen to them shriek and shout while they're playing. But this isn't always the case for folks who adore kids and miss having their own around the house. Their emotional reaction is a positive one. The sound of children is a reminder of happy memories.

With all three scenarios, the individual history and emotional makeup of each person drives their reaction, not the sound itself. No one is wrong to have the reaction they have. It takes many years of life to develop a strong like or dislike to something as fundamental as sounds in the environment. You might be saying, "Well, I am who I am. How am I supposed to change my reaction to a sound that I hate and it never stops? I don't want to hear this tinnitus and it's driving me mad!"

That's exactly the point where you need to begin. You have unconsciously trained your brain all your life through countless experiences to have a certain reaction to sounds you hear. You may be skeptical of any program that seeks to undo such a deeply ingrained reaction, but people with tinnitus have managed to do exactly that through tinnitus retraining therapy. It isn't easy, it takes time and it takes self-discipline, but it pays off when you finally realize that you can gain control of your reactions and emotions. Incidentally, emotions provoke the fight-or-flight response. Anger makes us want to fight; fear makes us want to flee. When your emotions are stable, your autonomic nervous system is stable as well, which in turn decreases your perception of tinnitus.

Sound is a *stimulus* that we react to. We smile when we hear a favorite song from our past come on the radio. We laugh when those around us are laughing, because it's so contagious. We startle when somebody drops something and it hits the floor with a bang. The hairs rise on the back of our neck when creepy music is played during a suspenseful scene in a scary movie. Most of us love the sound of a thunderstorm, but not everyone. Some of us value the gentleness of silence around us, and take to the woods for a tranquil space where we can hear only the sounds of nature and the thoughts in our head. Others flock to venues that are filled with rowdy noise, such as drag races, high stakes football games, and loud nightclubs. When we're driving, we usually don't notice the sound of the engine running unless something is amiss. We tune in to sounds we love to hear, and we tune out sounds every day that aren't important to us or that we have become accustomed to over time, just as we no longer notice our furniture arrangement unless somebody moves the couch and then it instantly gets our attention.

Think for a moment about all the stimuli you encounter every day and how you react to it. For instance, are you wearing shoes right now? How do they feel? A little bit tight maybe, now that I mention it. But before I brought your attention to it, your shoes and the comfort of your feet were probably the furthest thing from your mind. You're so used to wearing shoes that unless you happen to be wearing an extremely uncomfortable pair, you simply don't notice them throughout the day. Now think about someone who for whatever reason has always gone barefoot but now has to wear shoes. That person would likely feel the pressure of those shoes every day for a long, long time. The sensation of shoes for you is a neutral stimulus; you just don't pay attention to it. The sensation of shoes for the former barefooter is a negative stimulus; he dislikes it intensely and wants it to stop.

Consider all the stimuli in your environment that at one time held your attention. That stimuli may be positive or negative, but maybe now it doesn't even register on your conscious mind unless you reinforce its presence either through your words or your emotional reaction. For example, let's say there's a broken-down pickup in the city parking lot that you pass by every day on your way to work. You probably couldn't tell anyone whether it's still there five minutes after you drove by. However, the trashy vehicle parked in the driveway of a neighbor gets your attention every single day, because each time you see it you say to yourself, "That ugly thing is ruining the looks of the neighborhood." It's your reinforcement of negative perception which makes that particular vehicle hold your attention, versus the one in the city lot that evokes no emotional reaction. The pickup in the city lot is a neutral stimulus and has faded from your awareness. The vehicle in your neighbor's front yard is a negative stimulus and remains in your awareness because it stirs emotions of revulsion or hostility. If it makes you want to confront your neighbor in anger or move from the neighborhood because you can't stand it anymore, it's also engaging the fight-or-flight response, which increases the intensity of your reaction.

What does all this have to do with adapting to tinnitus? Tinnitus retraining therapy is about changing your perception of tinnitus from a *negative* stimulus to a *neutral* stimulus. Your brain prioritizes stimuli according to the importance you assign to it. The less importance you attach to a stimulus, the further in the background your brain places it. We would be unable to concentrate, wouldn't get much done, and would likely be in a persistent overwhelmed state if our brain didn't filter out the neutral stimuli we're constantly exposed to. If you're a nervous wreck because of your tinnitus, the sad truth is that it's because you steadfastly perceive it as a high level negative stimulus, so your brain classifies it as a high priority threat and makes sure you hear it as clearly as possible. I'm guilty of doing the same thing myself, with the rationale that I've always loved peace and quiet, and that's why the loud tinnitus distresses me so much. See how that works? Now think about the barefooter, and imagine if you had had tinnitus all your life, just as you've worn shoes all your life. Would you still have such an adverse reaction? Imagine if everyone had tinnitus from birth and it were just the natural human state. It would be nothing more than a neutral stimulus unworthy of our attention. Of course, that's not the way it is, but we can reprogram how we react to tinnitus and how we perceive it, thereby changing it from an important negative stimulus to an unimportant neutral stimulus.

Clinicians who use tinnitus retraining therapy in their practice report a success rate of approximately 80 to 85 percent. The success rate is defined as, number 1, the reaction to hearing tinnitus is significantly decreased; and, number 2, perception of the tinnitus is consequently decreased as well. Tinnitus can be a negative cycle, where you hear it and become agitated, which makes it seem louder, which agitates you more. It can also be a positive cycle, where you hear it, you have little to no reaction, which decreases your perception, which makes it seem less loud. If you were to have an actual decibel comparison test by a certified audiologist, the decibel level of your tinnitus would be the same in either case. It's only your *perception* of it that makes it seem louder or softer and therefore more, or less, distressing. The brain is a trickster when it comes to what we perceive, whether it be a magician performing sleight-of-hand tricks, or the tinnitus signal residing in your brain and performing in accord with your perception.

The next chapter covers what makes a good candidate for tinnitus retraining therapy, and what you can expect if you decide to try it. It may sound counterintuitive to say that volume doesn't matter, but TRT has helped countless people adjust to severe, debilitating tinnitus, regardless of the cause of their tinnitus and despite the perceived volume.

63
WHAT TO EXPECT WITH TRT

Any clinician can offer TRT services, which can make it difficult to find the right therapist. For best results, tinnitus retraining therapy should be performed by someone who is certified and has experience in successfully treating patients with moderate to severe tinnitus. There are some things you can look for and questions to ask that will narrow down the field.

First, you will want your case handled by an expert who is trained in diseases and disorders of the auditory system. That would include audiologists and otolaryngologists. Psychologists can be trained in TRT, but the full workup of hearing tests must be performed in a clinic or hospital outpatient facility specializing in audiology or otolaryngology. You can begin by visiting www.AmericanTinnitusPractitioners.com. It's a good starting point for finding clinicians who advertise expertise in treating tinnitus. A link to each practitioner's website is included by their name, so you can follow up to learn more about them. Please note that there are many qualified audiologists and otolaryngologists who treat tinnitus that may not be included in the American Tinnitus Practitioners database. Again, it's a starting point. An important qualification for TRT is that the practitioner is certified by the American Speech-Language-Hearing Association. Their mission and purpose are explained on www.asha.org/about.

When you arrive for your appointment with the clinician, be prepared for an intensive pre-treatment evaluation to determine your course of therapy. TRT is a comprehensive therapy and is not a one-size-fits-all program. At the beginning, though, you can expect the following things:

1. You will have a verbal interview and likely will be requested to write down the history of your tinnitus. You will need to provide any relevant personal information, such as your job, noise exposure history, diet, your smoking or drinking habits, and stressors in your life. You will be asked questions about where you hear the tinnitus (one ear, both ears, in your head); what sound(s) do you hear; is it high-pitched or low-pitched; do you know or can you estimate the frequency; is the volume loud or soft; is it worse at night or in the morning; do any particular

foods or drinks aggravate the tinnitus; does the tinnitus interfere with sleep and/or concentration; et cetera.

2. Your auditory system will be thoroughly examined to check for any abnormalities or conditions that could be causing or contributing to the tinnitus.

3. You will be given a pure-tone hearing test and should also be given an ultra high frequency audiometry test. A pure tone test will identify your hearing threshold to determine the degree, type, and configuration of your hearing loss, if any. An ultra high frequency test goes beyond the typical hearing test which measures up to 8 kHz, and tests your ability to hear high frequencies up to 14 kHz. Some audiologists test beyond that level. This is useful in finding which frequencies you can no longer hear, even though such frequency losses are usually not noticeable in everyday life except to people who work in audio engineering and similar jobs.

4. You will be given speech reception and/or word recognition tests. You can get an idea of what to expect in this type of test by taking the test at www.Starkey.com/online-hearing-test.

5. You will have an otoacoustic emissions test. This is to determine the health and status of the cochlea. A normal cochlea will not only receive sound, it will produce low-intensity sound on its own by the contraction and expansion of the outer hair cells. Simply put, this test provides information about the type of hearing loss and what components may be involved, as well as the degree of hearing loss within a limited range of frequencies.

6. Depending on the results of your tests and the assessment of the clinician, additional tests or evaluations may be required.

The main foundation of tinnitus retraining therapy is counseling. If you have moderate to severe tinnitus that is causing you great distress, much of that distress may be due to lack of understanding about the condition itself, as well as how you perceive and react to the sound of the tinnitus. You will learn how your reaction and attitude can influence the perceived volume and intrusiveness. This is probably the most difficult thing for people to accept, because it's absolutely counterintuitive to how we normally react to sounds in our environment. Because tinnitus is generally a persistent and constant sound, and because it's a sound we believe we can never get away from, we develop a deep negative reaction to it. TRT will help you to perceive tinnitus in much the same manner as you perceive any other constant sound in your environment, such as traffic sounds outside, the hum of your air conditioner, the refrigerator motor running, and the sounds of the dryer tumbling clothes. All these sounds are intrusive but we have adapted to them and, unless hyperacusis is present, we tune them out rather quickly after we first notice them.

TRT will also teach you about the importance of sound enrichment. Dr. Jastreboff believes it is critical in the treatment of tinnitus to avoid absolute quiet. Sound enrichment can be as simple as a table fountain in your work space, or playing some kind of nature sounds at low volume throughout the day. The natural inclination for some people with tinnitus, and to a much greater degree with hyperacusis, is to avoid any sounds. Unfortunately, this can contribute to a worsening of hyperacusis, and it can extend the time it takes to habituate to tinnitus.

Your clinician will review different methods of employing sound enrichment, and will also discuss options for sound therapy. The goal here is to select the most compatible therapy for your lifestyle and the type of tinnitus you have (tonal versus hissing, for example). Nature sounds such as streams, waterfalls, meadows, wind in the trees, crickets, and rainfall are popular sound enrichment choices. If your clinician thinks a sound therapy device will be helpful, she will explain what's available and how they work. Again, your lifestyle will play a big role in choosing which device is best for you. For example, someone who is active in sports or works in construction and moves around all day will be better off with one style of sound therapy device, whereas someone whose job is basically sedentary with a less active lifestyle would do well with a different device. If you have not already done so, please read Chapter 32, "Sound Enrichment." It discusses the theory behind sound enrichment and why it's used in tinnitus retraining therapy and habituation protocols.

Tinnitus retraining therapy is not a quick fix, and it can be rather expensive. It took a long time for your brain to become wired in its responses to stimuli, and it will take a long time to rewire your brain for a healthier response to tinnitus. The general consensus is that you can begin to see a level of noticeable improvement within six months. The entire course of TRT usually lasts 18 to 24 months. Beware of unreasonable expectations. TRT is not a cure. It is intended to help you reach the point where you are not bothered by your tinnitus. TRT breaks the cycle of hearing tinnitus, becoming distressed, tinnitus seems louder, distress rises again. The new cycle will be that you hear the tinnitus, you accept it as a neutral sound, the emotional center of your brain is not activated, and the tinnitus either fades from your awareness or it simply does not bother you when you notice it.

Some people dismiss the value of TRT in habituating to tinnitus, since statistics indicate that habituation for many people will occur within the first two years whether they undergo a program such as TRT or not. However, I believe that being proactive in coping with one's tinnitus is a much better option than simply waiting for time to go by, hoping that eventually you will no longer be disturbed or distracted by the sounds. Whether you choose TRT or any other treatment method, it usually feels better to do something about tinnitus if it's troubling you, rather than waiting for it to resolve on its own. As long as you're not obsessively engaged in monitoring or worrying about it, the simple action of taking positive steps to deal with it might lessen the time it takes for the tinnitus severity to decrease or for habituation to take place.

64
TRAIN THE BRAIN - BASICS

Chapter 23, "The Amygdala and Limbic System," briefly covered why training the brain can be helpful for tinnitus. The following paragraph contains excerpts to refresh your memory:

The amygdala is an emotional center and thus incapable of being swayed by the cerebral cortex, which is the seat of complex thought. Why is this important if you have tinnitus? Recent clinical studies are pointing to an intriguing connection between the role of the amygdala and the level of distress that people experience with their tinnitus, independent of perceived volume. The researchers discovered that those who experienced more distress from their tinnitus also engaged their amygdala more when processing emotional sounds. Those who claimed a lower level of distress from their tinnitus engaged the executive processing region of their brain, the cerebral cortex. They had somehow found a way to react to their tinnitus without engaging their emotions. Over time, their reaction to tinnitus became less dependent on using the amygdala pathway and instead used the pathway of the frontal lobe, located in the cerebral cortex. Researchers theorize that actively engaging the frontal lobe is helpful in controlling the processing and expression of emotions. In time, this could alter how one responds to tinnitus and thereby reduce the distress.

If you want to redirect the pathway of your reaction to tinnitus away from the amygdala's influence and instead reroute it to the frontal lobe, it will help to first understand the functions of the frontal lobe. When most people think of the brain, they envision the cerebrum, which is the main portion of the brain. Those with a good memory or medical training may also envision the cerebellum and the brain stem. The brain is an incredibly complex organ, with many fascinating aspects. For our purposes, though, let's review only the basics of the brain, just to get an overall idea of the roles assigned to its different regions.

We'll start with the brain stem, located between the spinal cord and the base of the brain. The brain stem is important for basic attention, arousal, and consciousness. Information received both to and from our body is transmitted through the brain stem to the brain itself. Because it's located in an area near bony protrusions, it is vulnerable to damage when trauma occurs to that area of the body.

The cerebellum, nicknamed "the little brain," is located on the back side of the brain around the brain stem. You can thank your cerebellum for your voluntary motor movements, your balance and equilibrium, and your muscle tone. The cerebellum helps in muscle memory, the ability to learn and remember muscle movements. For example, when someone throws a ball and you catch it automatically, that's your cerebellum at work. The cerebellum plays a role in most of our automatic, involuntary physical reactions, like instantly jumping away when we see a snake suddenly appear in our path while hiking. Think of the cerebellum as the gateway for the motor responses that pass to and from the brain.

The cerebrum includes the cerebral cortex, the basal ganglia, the limbic system, and the right and left hemispheres of the brain. The cerebral cortex is the wrinkly layer that surrounds the brain. The cerebral cortex is responsible for your ability to think. It's also where processing of the five senses takes place. The basal ganglia control eye movements and voluntary movements, and are important in learning routines or habits. The limbic system is considered to be responsible for our emotional life and the formation of memories.

The cerebrum essentially consists of two regions, the cerebral right hemisphere and the cerebral left hemisphere. They are connected by the corpus callosum, a large bundle of nerve fibers. The right hemisphere controls the left side of the body, and the left hemisphere controls the right side of the body. Each hemisphere has four distinct lobes: the parietal lobe, the temporal lobe, the occipital lobe, and the frontal lobe:

- The parietal lobe processes sensory information such as taste, temperature, touch, and pain. Damage to the parietal lobe could result in not being able to perceive touch. The parietal lobe is also responsible for spatial perception; that is, where you are in your space, the objects in your space, and your ability to navigate within that space. When you reach for a coffee cup and put your fingers on the handle, that's your parietal lobe telling you where your fingers are and where the handle is.
- The temporal lobe receives and processes auditory information

from the ears. It is able to discern different sounds as well as pitch. The temporal lobe is where meaning is assigned to sound. Without it, we wouldn't be able to comprehend speech.

- The occipital lobe processes visual information it receives from the eyes. If the occipital lobe is damaged, it results in visual confusion.

- The frontal lobe is the center of thinking, planning, problem-solving, being able to speak fluently and with meaning, and social interaction.

For now let's focus on the frontal lobe, because that's the part of the brain you want to train in order to suppress the negative emotional impact of tinnitus.

Imagine that you're planning a dinner for 10 people. You need to consider the time involved in preparation, the ingredients, perhaps the special diet needs of those you're inviting, the beverages you'll serve with the meal, the dinnerware, glassware, and silverware, the napkins, maybe a floral centerpiece and candles, what kind of music to play in the background and at what volume, the seating arrangement for the best conversation, and other factors unique to your situation that will contribute to a successful dinner party. You break that overwhelming task down into small sections and approach each of them one by one. Each small section probably is made up of its own individual pieces. When everything is in place, and your successful dinner party is underway, thank your frontal lobe for helping you coordinate all those moving parts with grace and skill.

The frontal lobe contains the prefrontal cortex, which is the executive part of your brain. It's the chief decision-maker. This is where a complex situation is analyzed and systematically broken down into its smaller elements so you can make sense of it and take care of whatever problem or challenge you might be facing at any given moment. When you think of the prefrontal cortex, think of reasoning, analysis, calculation, concentration, and planning. The frontal lobe is rational, as compared to the limbic system which is emotional. An interesting fact about the frontal lobe is that's where your personality is formed. Your higher mental processes and your personality are integrated in your frontal lobe. **Management of your emotions is located in the frontal lobe.** This is why it plays a significant role in how you deal with your tinnitus.

The next chapter contains exercises and recommendations on how you can train your brain, with the goal of rerouting your tinnitus reaction from the emotionally reactive limbic system to the analytical frontal lobe.

65
TRAIN THE BRAIN - EXERCISES

While researching who gets tinnitus and how they deal with it, I found some similarities between ADHD (attention deficit hyperactivity disorder) and tinnitus. Characteristics of ADHD are hyperactivity, impulsive behavior, and problems with maintaining attention. Researchers at McGill University, using magnetic resonance imaging (MRI), discovered that individuals with ADHD have decreased activation in their frontal lobes. Brain training is increasingly popular to treat and correct the hyperactivity and inability to focus that is common in children and adults with ADHD. The brain training exercises focus on activities that stimulate the frontal lobe. This creates an increasing reliance on the frontal lobe for daily decision-making, rather than relying on making impulsive decisions that tend to disregard consequences. As noted earlier, the prefrontal cortex in the frontal lobe is responsible for planning and carrying out complex tasks. People with ADHD have extreme difficulty with focusing. Their mind, specifically their frontal lobe, jumps from one thing to another to another. You might say their attention span is broad but shallow.

It's been proven that children and adults with ADHD benefit from brain training. They learn to focus, to concentrate, to carry out one task before beginning another. This is because the prefrontal cortex, the executive center of their brain, is now in control, instead of the limbic system which is impulsive and much more interested in instant gratification. When the task of doing laundry beckons, but instead you turn on YouTube to binge watch cute kitten videos, you're being controlled by your limbic system. When you start your laundry task first, delaying your desire for YouTube gratification, your prefrontal cortex is in charge.

What does this have to do with tinnitus? People with tinnitus have the same type of frontal lobe characteristics as people with ADHD. The brain training exercises that help people to overcome ADHD can also be helpful to people with tinnitus. In both cases, the goal is to increase reliance on the frontal lobe and away from the limbic system. By doing so, you slowly but surely change the pathway of your brain's response to the tinnitus signals. Not only will your distress level begin to subside, you may discover that the tinnitus begins to fade out of your conscious awareness. You'll discover the joy of realizing one day that you haven't heard your tinnitus for an hour, maybe two or three hours. Even if it's only for a few minutes, it's still an empowering feeling to realize that your tinnitus can completely fade away from your awareness.

At the beginning, it may be difficult to accomplish any of these brain-training tasks, and particularly if you have severe tinnitus. Even something as simple as getting out of bed can bring on an instant wave of fatigue, as you once again realize that your brain will be forcing tinnitus on you all day long. Start small. Read the list of brain training techniques, and choose one that inspires or motivates you. Give it a chance to work. It will take at least a month and in some cases much longer than that before the frontal lobe begins to gain control of your reaction to tinnitus. Don't monitor your tinnitus, "Is this technique working? Is my tinnitus getting quieter?" That just gets your amygdala agitated, the part of your brain responsible for anxiety. Instead, congratulate yourself every step along the way when you perform any part of an exercise. That soothes the limbic system, which loves the sense of reward for accomplishment. Be patient with yourself, allow yourself to make mistakes, but be committed to completing at least one of these exercises. If you want to start with something easy, that's fine. Do that, and then add something more challenging. Training your brain is similar to physical therapy to recover from an injury. It requires motivation, self-control, time, and a belief that you can do it.

As you continue to reinforce the frontal lobe as being in charge of your tinnitus reaction, the limbic system gradually loses its grip on the tinnitus signal. The frontal lobe, the chief decision-maker in the brain, says that there is no danger present and that the sounds of your tinnitus are not important. The limbic system plays an important role in protecting you from danger. However, if the executive function of your brain tells you that there is no danger, and if you keep reinforcing that message to and from the frontal lobe, then the tinnitus is no longer interpreted as a threat. The result? The tinnitus may continue to exist, the sound will still be there if you actively search for it, but your conscious mind simply has better things to do than to constantly ramp it up or pay attention to it.

These methods to strengthen the function of your frontal lobe aren't difficult, but they do require sincere effort on your part. The following tasks will help you achieve your goal. Some are simple, where you only need to make small changes in your everyday habits. Others are more complex and require long-term commitment.

---

1. **Concentration.** Stop multi-tasking and force yourself to do one thing at a time. While you're performing a task, pay attention to what you're doing. If you use a dishwasher to clean your dishes, wash them by hand instead as a concentration exercise. Don't watch television or listen to music or talk to someone while you're washing the dishes. Focus on the dishes, the glassware, the silverware. As you wash each item, notice the details of your dinnerware pattern, the silverware design, the shape of the glass or cup you're washing. Immerse yourself in the moment. If that sounds like a zen practice, it is. Monks are renowned for their ability to concentrate. Whenever you're online, stay focused on one website article. If you're reading something interesting and it triggers another interest in your mind, resist the temptation to open another window and search for that new topic you just thought of. If you're reading online, don't chatter with others, don't listen to music (unless it's sound therapy). Keep your mind on the task in front of you. Remember that the goal here is concentration, rather than scattering your attention across multiple interests or distractions.

2. **Make lists.** Every morning, as soon as you feel fresh and alert (as much as possible), make a list of five things you want to accomplish or need to get done during the day. Be sure to prioritize, and don't add too many little things you'd like to do, because that will only add to any sense of anxiety or frustration you already have if you don't get them done. As you go through your day, cross off each item as it's completed. When the day is over, review your list. Anything that didn't get done will be added to the next day's list. The frontal lobe is in charge of the thought processes required for making lists. This will keep it engaged on a daily basis.

3. **Plan menus.** If you've had tinnitus for some time, and/or if your tinnitus is severe, you've probably noticed that it's more difficult to make

a plan, whether it be organizing a birthday party or trying to set up a weekend getaway. Your brain simply does not seem to want to cooperate. The key is to start with something simple. Make a menu for this week's breakfast, lunch, and dinner. Start with tomorrow's meals, then move forward and create a menu for every day. Don't think about the menu for the entire week, because that falls under multi-tasking. Begin by keeping your focus on tomorrow's menu. When that's done, keep your focus on the next day's menu, and so on. It doesn't matter if you actually follow the menu, although that would be nice. The point is that you create the menu. As time goes on, you will prepare a menu and also include a list of ingredients you'll need to make each meal. However, don't get ahead of yourself. Keep it simple at this stage. Adding complexity will only lead to frustration, which activates the limbic system. Do only what you feel comfortable doing, knowing that in time you will move forward. Planning menus is a natural exercise for the frontal lobe. In the meantime, you may find that you want to add some creative cooking to your life. That's great, because it gives you another reason to take your mind off the tinnitus and direct your attention to something that inspires you.

4. **Enhanced reading.** Don't read everything that shows up on your attention horizon. Sandra Bond Chapman, Ph.D, is the director of the Center for Brain Health at the University of Texas at Dallas. She advises that it's much better to pick one or two articles and really think about them, than it is to read 10 or 20 articles and then dismiss them from your mind. The brain does not like to be overwhelmed with information and will not function at its best when subjected to information overload. Think of your brain as a complex container designed to hold information and absorb it a little at a time. Pour too much information into the container and it will spill over and be wasted. Pour in a little at a time, give the brain time to absorb the information, and then it's ready for more and can thrive.

Practicing reading comprehension is a useful exercise for information retention. Try it with one article every day. Read two or three paragraphs, turn away from what you're reading, and then recite your understanding of what was contained in those paragraphs. You might be surprised to discover how difficult it can be to do that. If you can't even begin to summarize the points of what you read, it's a sure sign that you were simply skimming the information rather than absorbing it. Your frontal lobe is a major player in reading comprehension. You can help to strengthen it by becoming actively engaged in what you're reading.

5. **Mind games.** Your frontal lobe is important in determining strategies and in problem-solving. Mind games were made for frontal lobe stimulation, such as games where you need to strategize, to think about potential consequences and outcomes before you make a move. These are games like chess, checkers, card games, bingo, Sudoku, and Scrabble. Assembling picture puzzles is another worthwhile mind game. When you assemble a puzzle, you first need to look at a missing area. Then you check the remaining puzzle pieces to see which one conforms to the missing area in shape and color. Assembling jigsaw puzzles involves both the right and left hemispheres, so it's a double benefit of being mentally and visually engaged. If the puzzle image is one that appeals to you emotionally, that keeps your limbic system satisfied. It helps to calm your tinnitus when you're immersed in a game that's both fun and mentally stimulating. Game apps are available through many online outlets, for all kinds of devices and fitting every budget.

Kristanix offers a fun app called Epic Puzzles, available on Amazon. It comes with several puzzle packages featuring different topics, and each day a new free puzzle appears on the app. You can purchase additional puzzle packages for a modest price. Amazon also has Scrabble game apps. A popular one is Classic Words by Lulo Apps, which includes an option to play solo against the Android device. You can think of these types of games as conditioning exercises for the brain. Because tinnitus is usually perceived as being more intrusive at night, it may help to add one or more of these games to your evening routine so your focus shifts away from listening to the tinnitus and onto something you enjoy. If your device has it, be sure to use the night-viewing option to reduce the blue light effect.

6. **Brain games.** These are games designed specifically to sharpen your mental skills. You can find them online by simply doing a search for "brain games." Some are free but have limited choices. Others are by subscription, but will offer a few free examples so you can try it out and see if it's something you'd be willing to pay for. One website with clever

thinking puzzles is www.sharpBrains.com, which devotes part of its content to free brain teasers to challenge and develop your frontal lobe. They also publish articles about neuroplasticity, brain fitness, and other brain-related content, as well as articles devoted to tinnitus research.

One subscription-based website is www.BrainHQ.com. It features different categories of brain training exercises, including attention, navigation, memory, brain speed, and others. There are some free exercises on the website, but I believe you need to sign up with an account in order to access them. BrainHQ advertises their online brain-training program as being based on neurological science and related medicine. Their team is led by Dr. Michael Merzenich, Ph.D., who won the prestigious 2016 Kavli Prize in Neuroscience. The Kavli Prize is awarded for outstanding achievement in scientific research and creativity. You can read more about Dr. Merzenich in the article, "Research Opened Door to Restoring Brain Damaged Function" on the University of California San Francisco website, www.ucsf.edu.

Chapter 55, "Neurogenesis," covered the important relationship between neurogenesis and the hippocampus. The MindSparke article, "Adult Neurogenesis in the Hippocampus," discusses the scientific basis for how brain exercises that emphasize focus, challenge and reward can lead to stimulation of hippocampal neurogenesis. Here's how it works:

- When you focus, the nucleus basalis region of the brain secretes acetylcholine, a vital neurotransmitter which helps signals to travel across nerve synapses.
- A challenging task requires us to use more of our brain in order to process and carry out the task. For example, solving an algebra problem such as $4(x-2) + 6x = 14$, uses more mental resources than simple addition like $4+4 = 8$.
- Reward is the sense of accomplishment and maybe even pride when we complete a challenging task. We know this feeling of reward when we successfully repair something ourselves rather than hiring someone to do it, or when we realize we've learned a new skill after months of practice. Whenever you feel satisfaction about something you've done, the brain releases dopamine, the feel-good neurotransmitter.

- The release of acetylcholine along with the release of dopamine creates a synergistic effect of stimulating neural growth and promoting neuroplasticity. This refers to the ability of the brain to form new connections and remove old connections that are no longer useful. Neuroplasticity is a lifelong process and relies on neurogenesis to strengthen and sustain healthy connections within the neural network of the brain.

7. **Exercise.** When you're moving, you're increasing blood flow to your brain, so more nutrients are being carried to your brain to keep it healthy. Exercise also increases the level of neurotransmitters in your brain. These are chemicals responsible for nerve impulses. More neurotransmitters means these nerve impulses operate more efficiently. One very important inhibitory neurotransmitter is GABA. This is a neurotransmitter that keeps your nerves from becoming overly excited and hyperactive. By calming the hyperactivity, perception of tinnitus can be reduced. Serotonin, another neurotransmitter, is increased with exercise. Serotonin helps to balance your moods and alleviate depression, a common side effect of tinnitus.

The best exercises to improve brain function include physical movement as well as hand-eye coordination, and require you to stay focused before making the next move. To help your brain, take time out at least twice a week for activities like bowling, golfing, tennis, ping-pong, or line dancing. These are activities that no matter how good you are, you can always aim toward improving your skill. One of the best ways to strengthen your frontal lobe is through ordinary cardio exercise, like walking. When you exercise, you take in more oxygen. Oxygen is fuel to your brain, and the frontal lobe thrives on extra oxygen. Maybe this is why so many people use their walking or jogging time to think about solutions to problems, or to work out the details of plans and schedules.

Yoga is an ideal activity for those who need or prefer a calmer form of exercise. It stimulates the brain because it requires concentration and focus, and you can practice yoga well into your nineties. Yoga instructional videos are available at your local store as well as online. There are also many websites with free illustrated yoga poses, as covered in Chapter 37, "Yoga."

8. **Meditation.** A Harvard Medical School study proved with MRI evidence that meditation, over time, increases the thickness of the cerebral cortex, including the prefrontal cortex, which as noted earlier is part of the frontal lobe. Among its other roles, this is the brain region associated with attention and sensory processing. There are many complex neural relationships in the brain amongst its different regions and functions. With regard to tinnitus, it's important to note that the frontal lobes are interconnected with the limbic system. Meditation produces an increase in positive feelings in the left frontal lobe, which in turn affects the limbic system. The limbic system begins to produce greater levels of melatonin, as well as serotonin, dopamine, and endorphins, the mood elevating neurotransmitters. When the limbic system is feeling good, it's much less interested in sending an alarm about tinnitus sounds. The result? Less distress in response to tinnitus.

9. **Learn a new language.** The frontal lobe is involved in both language and memory. Learning a new language is an excellent way to challenge the frontal lobe to put those capabilities to use. Maybe you've always wanted to go to France. In that case, now would be a good time to learn French. While you're learning the language, make plans to travel to Paris. Even if your finances tell you that you can't go, the act of making those plans is still beneficial to the frontal lobe. Do you have mixed heritage? If you're Italian, Russian, German, or no matter what your family background is, learning the language of your ancestors will create a connection to them. Did you take Spanish in high school and wish you had kept up with it? It's easier to relearn a language you've forgotten than to learn a new one, and there are many Spanish tutorials available on the Internet. One of the best is by Marcus Santamaria at www.spanish-is-easy.com. He teaches conversational Spanish in an easy and relaxed manner. Before you know it, you'll be packing your suitcase for a vacation in sunny Mexico, confident that you'll be able to mix and mingle with the natives, and maybe help a few non-Spanish-speaking tourists while you're there.

10. **Learn a new skill.** Many of us have a secret desire to do something special, but we never get around to it. If you've always wanted to paint with watercolors, go ahead and buy the supplies you'll need, plus a simple how-to book or instructional video. Set aside time and begin

practicing. You will be engaging a different part of your brain than you normally use, plus the concentration that's required to paint will help to strengthen the frontal lobe. Maybe you've always wanted to learn how to make fly fishing lures, or build a model train set with all the wonderful accessories that make them so much fun to watch. There's a good chance that you'll become so immersed in enjoying what you're doing that your tinnitus recedes into the background. Those kind of moments will give you the proof you need to accept and believe that your limbic system is not in control of your tinnitus.

11. **Volunteer.** When you volunteer in your community, you usually need to brush up on dormant skills or learn new skills. Even if it's only for an hour a week, turning your attention away from your tinnitus and toward helping someone else is a good way to let your limbic system know that you will not let your tinnitus stop you from getting out and trying something new. Volunteers report higher levels of satisfaction with themselves and their lives, and part of this is due to the increase of those "feel good" neurotransmitters when we do good deeds with no expectation of tangible reward. If you're not a people person, volunteer at your local humane society to walk dogs or provide other services based on your skills. Animal shelters are almost always in dire need of volunteers, and animals have a wonderful way of taking our minds off our troubles. If there are no shelters nearby, put an ad in your paper or post a notice on your community bulletin board and offer free dog walking for the elderly and disabled who love their pets but aren't able to take them out for proper exercise. Dogs are the perfect walking companions. Their happy-go-lucky nature will give you a positive emotional boost, plus you'll be getting the cardio exercise you need to circulate the nutrients that keep your brain healthy.

66
TRAIN THE BRAIN - SUMMARY

In meditation, when the limbic system is relaxed and stops sending out an alarm about tinnitus, it reduces the negative reactions associated with tinnitus perception. As those negative reactions decrease, tinnitus becomes less important for the brain to respond to. The less the brain responds, the more the tinnitus calms down, and that reduces the negative reaction even further. When both the limbic system as well as the conscious mind are less attuned to the tinnitus, this means tinnitus perception can now begin to move to the background where it belongs. Picture it being in a room all by itself where no one can hear it, not even you, unless you open the door to check on it.

You've probably noticed the emphasis throughout this book about keeping exercise in your daily routine as a means of improving tinnitus. If you don't like the word "exercise," think of it as maintenance for your body. You wouldn't expect your car, truck, motorcycle, or any vehicle to stay in good condition without proper maintenance. The same is true for your body. If you haven't exercised in a long time, start slow and make realistic goals. If you start off trying to walk two miles every day but you can only walk two blocks, you may become frustrated or angry, causing your stress level to rise. Your limbic system then goes into high alert, and before you know it, your tinnitus is raging, which only discourages you from exercising further because then you associate exercise with more intrusive tinnitus. Again, it's simply your limbic system making that connection in your mind. You don't want to form unpleasant memories. Take it easy when you begin any new routine, and congratulate yourself on every small step forward. Remember that the limbic system is happy whenever you receive a reward. It truly thrives on the positive.

The great thing about the Internet is that even though there's a lot of misinformation and outright deceptive information online, you can also find a tremendous wealth of online sites to help you with any brain training goal. Whether you want to increase your frontal lobe capabilities through physical exercise, mentally challenging games, learning a new language, discovering the benefits of yoga, or becoming an extraordinary cook as you plan menus for yourself or others, you can find a website where one person or a community has gathered all the information you need to work toward your goal. Take advantage of it, but remember to be patient with yourself. It may take weeks before you begin to notice the difference, but your dedication will be rewarded, in more ways than one.

You can probably think of some areas in your own life that can be changed or improved upon to help you train the brain. Look for things that involve exercise, meditation, single-task concentration, brain games, jigsaw puzzles, crossword puzzles, anything you can do that engages critical thinking skills. Basically you're looking to include more activities in your life that stimulate mental processes and keep the frontal lobe active and engaged. If it's something that ignites or sustains a passionate interest, so much the better. For example, dancing is a pleasurable activity for many people. It has been studied by neuroscientists for its benefits to the body's sensory and motor circuits while it stimulates the reward centers of the brain.

In summary, you can train your brain by improving the frontal lobe and by helping your limbic system feel better. You've now got two things going for you in coping with tinnitus. One, you're rerouting the tinnitus signal to the frontal lobe which will take care of it in a calm and rational manner; and, two, you're enhancing feel-good neurotransmitters in your limbic system so that it stops perceiving the tinnitus as a danger. Even if the volume of your tinnitus doesn't decrease as much as you would like, its negative impact on your life will decrease because you're generating so many positive feelings about your life otherwise.

67
OTHER TREATMENTS

There are a few more treatments for tinnitus that are worth mentioning. The costs for these treatments range from fairly affordable to prohibitively expensive. I'll briefly review three that have drawn attention on Internet tinnitus forums: stem cell treatment; high intensity focused ultrasound; and craniosacral therapy. The first two are generally classified as experimental, whereas craniosacral therapy falls within the realm of alternative medicine.

Stem cell treatment is not for the faint of heart, and the cost can be astronomical, from $15,000 to $25,000 and more. Stem cells are used from one of three sources: (1) donated cord blood stem cells; (2) adipose stem cells; or, (3) blood platelets and bone marrow stem cells. Cord blood stem cells are typically donated because it's rare that someone has stored their own cord blood since birth. Adipose stem cells are derived from abdominal fat. Blood platelets are isolated from blood taken from a vein, and mesenchymal stem cells are isolated from bone marrow.

Numerous tests must be conducted in order to qualify for stem cell treatment, as well as tests to monitor what progress, if any, is being made during the treatment regimen. This is an extremely complex procedure with no guarantee of good results. Stem cell treatment is still a fairly new frontier in treatment, not just for tinnitus but also for serious conditions like Parkinson's disease and multiple sclerosis. If you have the funds, and if your tinnitus is so debilitating that you're willing to risk stepping outside the boundaries of conventional medical treatment, please read the Tinnitus Talk thread, "My Trip to Bangkok: Stem Cell Treatment [Journal]," by member attheedgeofscience (At the Edge of Science). He gives an in-depth explanation of how stem cells are used to treat tinnitus, and relates his own experience with stem cell therapy. Many of your questions will be answered by reading both his journal entries and the comments from other members.

High intensity focused ultrasound (HIFU) is considered to be a radical surgical approach for treating tinnitus of neurogenic origin. This is tinnitus that arises from dysfunction or reduction of auditory input which in turn causes neural hyperactivity in the brain, the most common cause of tinnitus. It is not recommended for (1) tinnitus of idiopathic origin, (2) when there are no hearing deficits, and (3) if stress is suspected as a cause or contributing factor.

HIFU is another extremely expensive treatment, with no guarantee of results. According to what I've read, a high-intensity laser is used to ablate (surgically remove) a section of the thalamus. One member of Tinnitus Talk noted that the laser is used to "fry overactive cells on the hypothalamus." The hypothalamus is a structure within the thalamus. In Chapter 21, "Meet Your Neurotransmitters," I noted that the brain cells in the hypothalamus are particularly sensitive to excitotoxicity. It's also the part of the limbic system which receives signals from the amygdala and initiates the fight-or-flight response. It makes sense to target this area, but the procedure does carry risk because the hypothalamus is an extremely important region of the brain. To understand its crucial role, please read "Hypothalamus Activity and Hormone Production" on www.ThoughtCo.com.

The "HIFU (High Intensity Focused Ultrasound) Surgery" thread on Tinnitus Talk contains helpful information but is not up to date. Please visit www.SoniModul.ch to learn more. The page Our Therapeutic Offer, under the About link, indicates that they treat tinnitus from auditory nerve damage. SoniModul is located in Switzerland. The U.S. Food and Drug Administration has currently not approved HIFU as a treatment for tinnitus.

Craniosacral therapists use a light touch for what they say is gentle manipulation of the pelvis, as well as joints in the skull and spine. By doing so, they claim that changes occur to pressure and circulation in cerebrospinal fluid. These changes then lead to relief of pain and dysfunction. Craniosacral therapy (CST) is also promoted as helpful for dementia, back injury, fibromyalgia, learning disorders, and PTSD, to name just a few. People who undergo CST often speak of how relaxing it is, but I have been unable to find any scientific studies to indicate that tinnitus severity is reduced either during the session or after the relaxation wears off. Usually the treatment is given in pleasant surroundings, with soft music playing in the background. Combine that atmosphere with someone gently touching stress points around your neck to relieve tension, and it's no wonder that people tend to feel wonderful after a treatment session. I had CST many years ago for a problem unrelated to tinnitus, and felt positively euphoric for a couple hours afterwards. Unfortunately, it did not help the underlying problem. I eventually needed medical intervention for that. However, I wouldn't hesitate to recommend craniosacral therapy as a stress reliever.

Julian Cowan Hill is a fairly well-known name in the tinnitus community. He promotes CST along with psychotherapy as a potential cure for tinnitus. In fact, one of his YouTube videos is titled, "Stop telling people there is no cure for tinnitus!" My impression is that Mr. Hill sincerely believes tinnitus is caused by either unmanaged stress and/or the limbic system being out of control. I don't doubt his sincerity, but I disagree with telling people that tinnitus can be cured, as that leads to unreasonable expectations. It may well be possible that we'll have a cure in the future, but not in the current state of medical knowledge. I do agree with him that the limbic system has a lot of influence on perception of tinnitus severity.

Craniosacral therapy usually costs somewhere around $60 per hour, about the same as a professional massage. In Chapter 26, "Brain Waves and Tinnitus," I mentioned how aromatherapy massage has been proven to elevate alpha waves. In Chapter 56, "Tips to Increase BDNF," I discussed a study which proved that aromatherapy massage reduces cortisol and increases plasma BDNF levels. Whether CST can do the same thing or not is unknown, as those two benefits may simply be a natural effect of enhanced relaxation. If you have the funds, try both, and then decide which one either improves your tinnitus or helps you cope with it better.

68
SCAMS

No matter what your level of tinnitus is, you just want it to stop. Especially in the beginning, one can become quite obsessive about finding a way to get away from the relentless sound. For those with moderate or severe tinnitus, it can overwhelm you so much that you become desperate for a cure. And just like any other chronic disease or affliction, there are plenty of greedy and unethical people who are more than happy to take advantage of someone in a desperate situation. They are the scam artists who promise you amazing relief or a magical cure if you will only buy their product with its special combination of ingredients. If you search online for "tinnitus cure," you'll get millions of results. Many of the search results are nothing more than affiliate marketing sites promoting the same useless product.

Of all the millions of people with tinnitus, there might be somebody who will actually experience improvement by using one or another of these snake oil potions. Maybe it's the placebo effect, which is the mind-body interaction where a person takes a pill with no active ingredients and yet shows measurable improvement in their medical condition. This happens frequently in clinical trials when new drugs are being tested. It's also quite possible that a product which doesn't work for 999 people will work for one person in a thousand, due to their unique body chemistry. For the other 999, though, they might spend thousands of dollars buying one product after another, with nothing to show for it but a drained bank account. They experience no more benefit than if they had simply given themselves time for their brain to adjust to the new phantom sounds by using coping techniques such as meditation, masking, and yoga.

There are certainly supplements that have been used to calm tinnitus symptoms and have been shown to provide some benefit to more than just a few people. Chapter 58, "Popular Supplements for Tinnitus," lists 12 of those most likely to help. If your head is roaring, even the smallest bit of relief can make a big difference. But if you're looking for a cure in a bottle, stop looking. Do not waste your money. **Do not reward these charlatans who profit from the misfortune of others.** Instead, spend your hard-earned money on activities that will take your mind off your tinnitus, even if only for a few minutes. Invest your time in authentic treatments like audio notch therapy, Acoustic CR® Neuromodulation, tinnitus retraining therapy, meditation, and brain training. That will give you a much better chance of adapting to your tinnitus than a bottle of pills ever will. You're better off if you don't stress your body with substances that provide no benefit and could possibly cause unwanted side effects, or negative reactions with other supplements or medications you might be taking.

In this chapter, I'll focus on one product as an example of the con artists who only care about profiting from your suffering. Any time you search online for a tinnitus remedy, it's almost certain that this product will come up in your search results. The product contains no ingredients. Instead, it's an instruction manual of a "unique 5-step method" you need to follow that will supposedly cure your tinnitus. The author claims that he developed this cure over 14 years, supported by over 45,000 hours of intense clinical research. First of all, 45,000 hours is equal to eight hours a day, every single day, for 5,625 days. That's more than 15 years. The author doesn't acknowledge any partners in this research, so we have to assume he did all the research himself. Nor does he state where the research lab is. He has published no white papers or abstracts to prove up his claimed results from clinical trials. In fact, the person who wrote the book is promoting it under a false name. The author is actually from Israel, and has published his so-called "unique 5-step method" using a common American name.

The predator who created this product cares so little about truth in advertising that he doesn't even bother to fact check his own website. In one instance, he says that 95% of people who try conventional methods to treat their tinnitus end up with worse tinnitus. In the next instance, he claims it's 92% of people. Either way, that statement is blatantly false! The only reason he cites such a false statistic is to scare people into thinking they had better buy his product or their tinnitus will get worse. The truth is that for most people, whether they do nothing, a little or a lot to treat their tinnitus, it will eventually get better to some degree. But as I said, he's a predator, and he preys on desperate people. To make matters worse, his product appears in almost every single tinnitus search online, because he has identified many of the keywords associated in searching for tinnitus and bought domains using those keywords. When you click on a link, thinking you're going to an informative site about tinnitus, it's set up to automatically redirect you to his product website. Once you're there, he assumes you'll read the information he's peddling, and no doubt many will buy the product. To someone unfamiliar with tinnitus, what he presents may sound convincing. It's still hogwash.

For an in-depth exposé of the book which claims that tinnitus can be cured with this magical 5-step program, I recommend that you visit Duane's Blog. Please note that the writer of this blog article uses very strong language in describing his feelings about this book and its author. Many people with chronic and intrusive tinnitus would use the same (or worse) language to express their anger at this scam artist. I do not know Duane and have no affiliation with him. However, it's obvious that he conducted extensive research into this charlatan and his bogus product. He has written a lengthy, indisputable point-by-point criticism of it. You can find it by doing a search for "Duane's Blog" + "Tinnitus Miracle." I believe it's of great benefit to the tinnitus community to pass along what he learned. I encourage everyone to read his exposé and share it with others as well. Scam artists deserve to be shunned.

The best advice concerning scams is to steer clear of any product that claims to be a cure. Believe me, if someone invented a cure for tinnitus, they would be interviewed on all the talk shows. They would be nominated and likely receive the Nobel Prize in Physiology or Medicine. It would be a scientific breakthrough as significant to the human race as that of the 2015 winners, William C. Campbell and Satoshi Ōmura. Campbell and Ōmura helped to develop a novel therapy of fighting infections caused by roundworm parasites, a debilitating affliction that can be found throughout the world. Tinnitus is also a debilitating affliction found throughout the world. A genuine cure for tinnitus would make headlines, receiving instant national and global attention.

One deceitful tactic used by scam artists is to claim that medical science has no interest in curing tinnitus, and that their product is being ignored by the medical community because it's so effective. This is the same claim used by predators who peddle fraudulent cancer cures. Please don't let any tinnitus snake oil marketer convince you that that their product has some sort of secret formula that makes it special, or that medical science doesn't want a cure because they make more money treating tinnitus than curing it. That simply isn't true, and it's an insult to researchers who are dedicated to finding a way to stop the phantom sounds once and for all.

Having said all that, if there is a research-based product with a combination of ingredients that a manufacturer claims can help ease the symptoms of tinnitus, that's perfectly acceptable. Chances are those ingredients will help some people, and maybe help you as well. Testimonials and reviews can be bought and posted on a product website, but I would suggest that you read them anyway and judge for yourself if they seem trustworthy. Make sure the manufacturer has a solid money-back guarantee, and gives you enough time to try the product to determine if it's effective. A reputable manufacturer should be willing to offer at least a 30-day money-back guarantee. How much you're willing to pay will be based on your budget, but tinnitus relief products usually cost from $12 to $50 for a one-month supply. Look at the ingredients list of whatever you're considering, and search online for information about each ingredient. Sometimes there's one main ingredient that is touted as being beneficial for tinnitus, and the rest of the ingredients are added to make it seem like a more complicated potion. That's done to convince you how unique that product is. Take the time to know what you're buying. Hope for the best, but be prepared for no change in your tinnitus with these types of products.

SECTION IX

FOOD AND DRINK

69
CAFFEINE, SUGAR, SALT, AND ADDITIVES

When you first get tinnitus, one of the common bits of well-meaning advice you're likely to hear is that you need to reduce or eliminate your caffeine intake. The reason for this is because caffeine, and especially excess caffeine, can elevate anxiety in some people. This in turn increases the perception of tinnitus. In addition, medical researchers have known for a long time that caffeine stimulates the central nervous system and has an effect on the inner ear. You'll remember from Chapter 22, "How We Hear Sound," that the inner ear is where the cochlea and the ultra delicate hair cells are located. The inner ear is critical to the sense of hearing and is often where the trouble with tinnitus begins, so it makes sense to protect it as much as possible and avoid overstimulating it.

So, the bad news is, too much caffeine can negatively affect the inner ear. The good news is, for most people, totally giving up caffeine isn't necessary. Eliminating caffeine has not been proven to be effective at reducing or eliminating tinnitus. If you enjoy your morning cup of java energy, there's no need to deprive yourself out of fear that you're going to make your tinnitus worse. In fact, studies show coffee contains ingredients which are actually good for your overall health. Drinking two 8-ounce cups of coffee every day reduces your chance of getting liver cancer by 40 percent, it decreases your risk of heart failure by 11 percent, and it can reduce your risk of getting type II diabetes by 11 percent. For those who enjoy their alcoholic beverages, regular coffee consumption can cut the risk of acquiring cirrhosis of the liver by 22 percent. Decaf coffee has also been shown to reduce the risk of liver disease; therefore, the researchers cannot state with certainty that it's the caffeine itself which makes the difference. It hasn't been determined yet which specific ingredients are responsible for the health benefits, but coffee is known to contain powerful antioxidants which are essential for scavenging free radicals that can cause cellular damage. It's good to get your antioxidants from fruits and vegetables, but Americans are so fond of coffee that it's actually the number 1 source of antioxidants in the American diet.

Recent studies have shown that women who drink coffee have a lower risk of getting tinnitus. Brigham and Women's Hospital in Boston, Massachusetts, conducted an 18-year study of 65,000 nurses and came to a surprising conclusion. Regardless of age, women with a daily caffeine intake of 450 to 600 milligrams were 15 percent less likely to develop tinnitus than women whose daily consumption of caffeine was 150 to 300 milligrams. One cup of coffee contains approximately 100 milligrams of caffeine. So in other words, four-and-a-half to six cups of coffee per day created an unusual protective effect compared to drinking one-and-a-half to three cups per day. One researcher specifically noted that the results were surprising, considering that caffeine has potential negative effects on the inner ear. As of yet there has been no specific reason identified for the difference in tinnitus susceptibility between the two groups of women.

If you're pregnant, your doctor has probably already advised you to keep your caffeine intake to less than 200 milligrams per day, which is equivalent to about two 8-ounce cups. Caffeine goes into the amniotic fluid by way of the placenta and enters the baby's bloodstream. It takes much longer for a baby in utero to metabolize caffeine than an adult human. It's better to follow precautions and limit your caffeine intake. Decaf coffee may not give you the same energy boost, but higher quality brands offer exceptional decaf varieties that taste just as good. Keep in mind, though, that decaf coffee still contains between 2 and 12 milligrams of caffeine per 8-ounce cup.

Tea and soft drinks also contain caffeine, so add that to your daily tally if you're trying to keep your caffeine intake below a certain level. In the early 2000s there was a flurry of bad press about Red Bull, a potent energy drink, when several young people in unrelated incidents died after consuming a considerable quantity. The deaths were initially blamed on taurine being added to the Red Bull, but that wasn't the case. Instead, other factors combined with the caffeine were responsible. The irony is that taurine had been added by the Red Bull manufacturers as a safety measure against caffeine overdose. When measuring your caffeine intake, be mindful of caffeine that's been added to soft drinks to increase the energy buzz. Too much caffeine can have a negative effect on your tinnitus, but it's the excess amount of caffeine that's the culprit. In moderation, caffeine won't affect most people with tinnitus. You can look up your favorite drinks on the chart, "Caffeine Content of Popular Drinks," provided by the National Soft Drink Association and published on www.math.utah.edu.

Experiment and find out whether drinking coffee with or without caffeine makes a difference in how you feel and how it affects your tinnitus. You might be pleasantly surprised to discover that it has absolutely no effect at all. It's nice to know that drinking coffee isn't the bad habit we once believed it to be. You no longer need to feel restricted to decaf at your favorite cafe. When you're at your table with your cup of coffee and inhaling the heavenly aroma, you'll be able to relax and enjoy the flavor, with one less worry about your tinnitus. Be careful, though, about drinking coffee in the late evening. Because caffeine is a stimulant for the central nervous system, it can cause more disruption to your sleep than it did in the past, due to the already hyperactive neurons in your brain. Instead, think about making a cup of non-caffeinated tea near bedtime, perhaps a soothing tea made with chamomile and lavender. Chamomile is one of the best herbs for inducing restful sleep, and lavender promotes drowsiness with a sense of well-being. Celestial Seasonings is well-known for their Sleepytime tea, with chamomile as the main ingredient, and their Sleepytime Extra tea includes valerian, a gentle and safe way to calm the nervous system and help you to fall asleep.

If you're a chocaholic, you've probably already heard the news about the antioxidant benefits of dark chocolates. A study from the University of San Diego showed that daily consumption of 1.7 ounces of dark chocolate over a 15-day period resulted in improved HDL levels (a cholesterol marker), and lower blood sugar levels. White chocolate had the opposite effect of raising blood sugar levels, which causes blood flow in the skin to slow down, an undesirable reaction. The differences were attributed to the rich antioxidants contained in dark chocolate. Joe Vinson, Ph.D., is a professor at the University of Scranton who specializes in studying antioxidants. He advises that if you're going to give in to the temptation to eat fat and sugar, do it in combination with antioxidants. Lucky for you, dark chocolate fits that bill.

Unfortunately, you can't get around the fact that dark chocolate is made with an abundance of sugar. For many people with tinnitus, sugar can be a trigger that increases tinnitus severity. Like caffeine, this is something you'll want to experiment with. When determining a safe amount of chocolate to eat, be sure to start off slowly with maybe 1 ounce of chocolate, then see how you feel within an hour and how you feel the next day. If all goes well, and if your diet allows, you can treat yourself to more chocolate. Until you know your tinnitus tolerance, limit how much dark chocolate you eat to 1 or 2 ounces a day. A typical chocolate bar is 1.7 ounces, so that will give you an idea of how much is too much. Remember that excess sugar and fat aren't good for you under any circumstances. Just because dark chocolate is loaded with antioxidants isn't a green light to eat more than a reasonable amount.

Sugar has become the number 1 offender in the average diet, so let's take a look at refined sugar and why you might want to limit your intake. Most people with moderate to severe tinnitus will tell you that sugar aggravates their tinnitus. One theory is that excess sugar promotes the release of adrenalin. The purpose of adrenalin is to prepare you for fight or flight. All your nerve impulses are on high alert and you become sensitive to nerve impulses that normally lie beneath your conscious attention. This includes the nerve impulses responsible for you perceiving your tinnitus. Sugar is also a known inflammatory agent. It is directly tied to insulin production. Insulin is a hormone produced by the pancreas that allows your body to metabolize glucose. It may surprise you to know that roughly 70 percent of your immune cells are located in your digestive system. When you eat too much sugar, from whatever source, it can upset the balance of insulin in your body and trigger an inflammation alert. Inflammation has been linked to tinnitus because it can cause an increase in vasoconstriction (blood vessel narrowing), so that the capillaries to the inner ear don't receive adequate blood flow. This may help to explain why tinnitus can spike after consuming food high in sugar.

One little-known fact about excess sugar consumption is that high amounts of sugar increase the number of advanced glycation end-products (AGEs). An AGE is a protein that binds to a glucose molecule. The result is a damaged cross-linked protein. This is important when you look at factors for reducing tinnitus or keeping it from worsening. Your genetic makeup determines where in your body these advanced glycation end-products will occur. Scientists are looking at the possibility that AGEs can adversely affect the hair cells of the inner ear. Studies have already shown that diabetics with poor glycemic control have a greater extent of hearing loss than diabetics with good glycemic control. AGEs have not been ruled out as being partly responsible for the greater extent of hearing loss.

Refined sugar has been demonized for causing all sorts of human ailments. Countless studies have proven a link between excess sugar consumption and many disorders and diseases. Among these are obesity, heart disease, high blood pressure, kidney disease, fibromyalgia, chronic fatigue syndrome, ADHD, and of course diabetes. It might satisfy your sweet tooth, but sugar isn't good for your body and it certainly isn't good for your brain. I won't add any more than I've already written, because the information about the detrimental effects of sugar is widely available in libraries, at bookstores, and online.

White flour is another culprit in the inflammatory process. White flour is a simple carbohydrate, which means it is quickly absorbed into the bloodstream. You get a rapid rise in blood sugar, which requires your pancreas to produce large amounts of insulin. In fact, white flour is just one step away from the same damaging effects as processed white sugar. It turns into glucose once your digestive enzymes go to work on it. If your tinnitus volume or intrusiveness consistently increases after you eat white bread or any product with added sugar, or if your tinnitus gets worse within two to four hours of eating a meal, make an appointment with your healthcare practitioner for a blood glucose test. This could be a sign that your body is not metabolizing sugars efficiently. Glucose metabolism abnormalities can cause or contribute to tinnitus.

Studies have shown increased levels of glutamate in the prefrontal area of people who have type 1 diabetes. If you have any form of hyperglycemia (high blood glucose), you are more susceptible to glutamate damaging the neurons in your brain, particularly the prefrontal area. This can lead to depression as well as impaired cognitive function. It's possible that changing your diet or how you schedule your meals could improve your tinnitus symptoms in addition to improving the health of your prefrontal cortex. As a side benefit, you might find your mood lifting and your thought processes becoming more clear. Incidentally, hyperglycemia has also been shown to cause damage to the hippocampus, which has already been discussed regarding its importance to neurogenesis.

It's difficult to muster the self-control to resist carbohydrates and foods which contain sugar. After all, humans have been genetically programmed from the time of our primitive ancestors to crave carbohydrates and sweet food. These were important fuels back in those days, and much more scarce. Food processing techniques have become increasingly sophisticated and manipulative, with manufacturers adding excess sugar simply to satisfy our natural cravings and induce us to buy more of their products. Carbohydrates and sweets have now gone far beyond the useful role of fuel and instead have become indulgences that we don't monitor as well as we should. If you have a sweet tooth, try cutting back on your sugar consumption little by little, and see if your tinnitus improves. Instead of a whole slice of cake or pie, reduce it to half a slice. Instead of a tablespoon of jam on bread, use two teaspoons. Add stevia, a healthier alternative, to your coffee or tea and keep the sugar bowl closed. Xylitol is also a great sugar substitute. It's used in many chewing gum products, as well as candies, toothpastes, and mouthwash. **Please keep any product containing Xylitol away from dogs.** Even small amounts can rapidly lead to severe hypoglycemia, resulting in liver failure and death.

Caffeine and sugar are addictive, especially in excess, and can be very difficult to live without once your body has become accustomed to a regular supply. Taper off gradually until your consumption is at a reasonable level. There are experts who advocate for total elimination of sugar from the daily diet. Unfortunately, that's just asking too much of the average person, especially in our sugar-heavy environment. It's perfectly natural to have occasional cravings for something sweet, or to enjoy a few cups of coffee throughout the day, but keep in mind that a healthy body is not addicted to any substance. As a bonus, the healthier you are, the more likely you are to get restful sleep, which will help to lower your anxiety and raise your ability to cope with tinnitus. Whenever you're tempted to get a candy bar, or add an extra teaspoon of sugar to something, remind yourself that the price of that momentary sweetness is the possibility of aggravated neurotoxicity which contributes to tinnitus. It's simply not worth it.

Salt intake can be linked to tinnitus in people who have hypertension, usually referred to as high blood pressure. Hypertension is a serious disease which is more common than most people would believe, affecting nearly 1 in 3 American adults. It's known as a "silent killer," because you can have it and yet experience no warning signs or obvious symptoms. Anyone can develop high blood pressure, including children, so it's very important to have your blood pressure checked on a regular basis. To learn more about healthy blood pressure levels, see the article "Understanding Blood Pressure Readings" on the American Heart Association website, www.heart.org.

Blood pressure is the measure of the force of blood as it circulates in the body and pushes against the walls of blood vessels. Higher blood pressure means your heart must work harder to keep the blood circulating. High salt intake tends to increase blood pressure. This is because your body tries to keep a balance between sodium and fluid levels. As you increase salt intake, your body retains more water. This increases blood volume and can potentially raise your blood pressure beyond normal safe limits. Even though salt in and of itself is not a cause of tinnitus, the consumption of excess salt which raises blood pressure can make your tinnitus more noticeable. The onset of tinnitus in an otherwise healthy person may actually be a warning sign of otherwise asymptomatic hypertension.

One of the best things you can do to reduce excess salt intake is to stop buying processed foods, which are laden with salt. The salt is added to enhance flavor, but also to extend shelf life. That's right, food manufacturers add salt as a preservative so the food will last longer. Not only that, salt absorbs moisture, thus adding weight to the product. If much of your diet is based on processed foods, you are probably eating far more sodium than you realize. The average American gets 11% of their daily sodium intake from table salt; the remainder is in the processed foods they eat.

The human body needs salt to maintain a natural balance of fluids, to help nerves transmit information, and to help with muscle contraction and relaxation. The recommended daily intake for adolescents and adults is 2,300 milligrams per day or less. Start paying attention to the labels on processed foods, and keep a tally for a week to see how much extra sodium you're consuming that you're probably not even aware of. Have your blood pressure checked by your healthcare provider and get their guidance on the safest level of sodium intake for you.

It seems we can't go a week without being told by some experts about something we shouldn't eat, only to find out later that equally qualified experts have a totally opposite opinion. Unlike other health suggestions, reducing salt intake has remained a constant piece of advice for decades from healthcare organizations. You can gradually adjust your diet to where you rarely add salt to food. There are many wonderful non-salt seasonings that can enhance the flavor of food, and you'll never miss the salt. A favorite of many consumers is Trader Joe's 21 Seasoning Salute, a blend of spices that adds just the right touch of flavor to food. Try substituting that for your usual sprinkle of salt, or visit your local spice store and begin experimenting to make your own special blend. If you have tinnitus linked to high blood pressure, eliminating salt whenever possible may help to improve both conditions.

70
INTERMITTENT FASTING

When people think of fasting, they tend to think of it in negative terms like hunger pangs, feeling deprived, having brain fog, and lacking energy. That's because fasting is associated with eating nothing at all for a period of at least 24 hours, and in some extreme diets up to three days at a time. I have always been skeptical of fasting diets, and believed that severe restriction of food on a regular basis is taking a risk of destabilizing one's metabolism. My attitude changed, however, after watching a fascinating BBC documentary called "Eat, Fast & Live Longer." The documentary features Dr. Michael Mosley, who set out on a quest for a diet that would not only help him to lose weight, but one which he could live with for the rest of his life and not feel constantly deprived, nor be burdened with ceaseless calorie counting or restricting carbohydrates, fats, or proteins. In addition, he wanted a diet that would protect not just the health of his body, but his brain health as well.

It sounds like magical thinking, doesn't it? What kind of diet is going to let you basically eat what you want, shed excess weight, and help to keep your brain healthy, too? The secret (which really isn't a secret at all) is to incorporate a minimal level of fasting into your eating habits. The result of Dr. Mosley's research and testing of various diets with himself as the subject led him to the conclusion that intermittent fasting would help anyone achieve those goals. You may have heard of his 5:2 diet. It's based on the principle of fasting two nonconsecutive days a week, and the other five days you eat what you want. No calorie restrictions and no forbidden foods five days every week. The fasting days aren't total fasting. An adult woman on the 5:2 diet is allowed 500 calories per day, and an adult man is allowed 600 calories. Keep in mind that if you're only eating 500 or 600 calories, you should choose your food wisely because your body still needs good nutrients for optimal performance.

So what does this have to do with tinnitus? The "Eat, Fast & Live Longer" documentary was recommended by a member of Tinnitus Talk who said it had definitely improved her tinnitus. Because of her positive experience, I watched the documentary with more than casual interest.

Many people with tinnitus, myself included, have never been able to pin down anything in our diets which we can definitely say worsens our tinnitus, except for the usual suspects of too much salt, too much caffeine, too much sugar, and possibly excess MSG from over-indulging in processed foods. In watching the documentary, I wanted to know what specifically about the 5:2 diet could improve tinnitus. At 46:29 on the video, I found the answer: neurogenesis is increased with fasting. You can start at that point on the video for a quick overview. However, I recommend watching the entire documentary to learn about different fasting diets and their pros and cons. If you simply want to understand the basics of the scientific studies that support the theory that fasting is good for brain health, begin watching at 43:00 on the timeline, which leads up to the neurogenesis explanation.

Dr. Mattson, a neuroscientist featured in the "Eat, Fast & Live Longer" documentary, gave a TEDx talk at Johns Hopkins University about fasting and its effects on the brain. You can watch the video of that TEDx talk, "Why fasting bolsters brain power" on YouTube. Dr. Mattson explains in detail the benefits of fasting and why it's good for most people to introduce fasting into their diet.

Unfortunately, neither Dr. Mosley nor Dr. Mattson address the issue of how fasting affects tinnitus, but that's not unusual. Neuroscientists are generally more concerned with finding a cure or improved treatment methods for neurodegenerative diseases such as Alzheimer's, Parkinson's, epilepsy, and ALS (also known as Lou Gehrig's disease). Tinnitus does not rank high on their list of priorities.

In April 2016, I began my own version of the 5:2 diet. I chose to follow a 1:1 diet because it's easier for me to stick to a schedule of every other day instead of just two days a week. Getting rid of a few pounds was a nice thought, but my aim was not to lose weight. My one and only goal was to increase neurogenesis and hopefully increase the volume of grey matter in my brain. You'll recall that people with tinnitus have significantly reduced volume of grey matter in their prefrontal cortex and hippocampus. If I could restore grey matter simply by fasting every other day, and perhaps in doing so decrease the tinnitus volume and intrusiveness, I was certainly willing to give it a try.

After a year of following the 1:1 diet, I switched to a 4:3 plan. Fasting days are Mondays, Wednesdays, and Fridays. Throughout the entire time of being on this diet, I never felt deprived on the fasting days. I eat well because I focus on protein and a bit of carbs, and use only the good fats in my diet as much as possible. My energy level hasn't suffered, nor has fasting caused any negative changes in my sleep, despite sometimes being a bit hungry at bedtime. On the non-fasting days, I eat what I want but still try to limit my sugar intake.

As for my tinnitus, it has definitely reduced in volume. The days of intrusive tinnitus are less frequent. I have more days where it recedes far into the background, especially if I'm focused on work, involved in conversation, or watching a movie. Although it can still intrude, it's certainly better than it was in the past. In other words, the volume is nowhere near the level it was when it started in April 2014, and it's even better than it was when I first began fasting.

Another difference is that my tinnitus sounds less like a screech, squeal, or cicada swarm, and more like a high-pitched radiator hiss with a slight ebb and flow characteristic. The high-pitched whine is still present in my head to some degree, and maybe it always will be. However, it's been a very long time since I had a day filled with blasting tinnitus on a 9 out of 10 scale. I'm grateful for the relief.

I want to emphasize that along with intermittent fasting, I've also been utilizing Acoustic CR® Neuromodulation (ACRN) sound therapy since the first week of March 2016. I began to experience improvement with the ACRN therapy within six weeks, but the improvement accelerated when I drastically slashed carbohydrates from my meals in the first two weeks of the 1:1 diet. Because I'm addicted to carbs, either psychologically or physically, it was too difficult for me to stay on such a low carbohydrate diet. I think it's important that no matter what kind of fasting regimen you choose, it should be a way of eating that you can comfortably follow for the rest of your life. Any diet which leaves you feeling constantly deprived is not going to work long-term.

For those who are interested in the weight loss aspect, I lost about 16 pounds within three months, a steady reduction rather than a drastic drop. If you can manage the self-discipline of calorie restriction two days a week, you will likely lose weight and possibly gain some improvement in your tinnitus.

There have been no fMRI (functional magnetic resonance imaging) studies of my brain. There's no way to really know how much, if at all, the grey matter in my hippocampi or prefrontal cortex has increased. I believe that fasting has proven beneficial in reducing the severity of my tinnitus, although I don't know how big a role it played since I was also using the ACRN sound therapy and exercising more. The scientific evidence that intermittent fasting increases neurogenesis is fairly strong, so I hope you will be encouraged to try it. Give it at least three months to see if it makes a difference.

There are many intermittent fasting diets to choose from: eight-hour fast, 12-hour fast, three-day fast, mini-fast, 5:2 fast and its variations, et cetera. You can search for the keywords "intermittent fasting" and find information on the Internet, or peruse your local bookstore to see which one of those diets best matches your lifestyle. As always, check with your healthcare practitioner before altering your diet to include fasting. For obvious reasons, pregnant women should not fast. Anyone with a chronic or serious medical condition, such as diabetes, or a heart or thyroid problem, certainly should not attempt fasting without medical supervision.

71
KETOGENIC DIET

The ketogenic diet was first developed in the 1920s for the treatment of pediatric epilepsy that failed to respond to medication and conventional treatment. The goal is to keep the body in a state of ketosis. Technically speaking, ketosis is a form of starvation mode for your body where you have an increase in the number of ketone bodies in your blood. Usually our body's energy is supplied via blood glucose. In ketosis, the energy is supplied by the ketones. The ketogenic diet is high in fat, very low in carbohydrates, with enough protein to sustain nourishment, adequate weight, and bodily repair. The success rate for improvement in pediatric epilepsy patients is high: number of seizures were reduced by 50% in half of the patients on the diet, and an astonishing 90% reduction in number of seizures in a third of the patients. Keep in mind that these numbers reflect improvement in cases of refractory epilepsy; that is, epilepsy that does not respond to other modes of treatment.

2500 years ago, Hippocrates said, "Tinnitus is the little brother of epilepsy." Hippocrates was right on the money with his observation. Both epilepsy and tinnitus exhibit unusual and erratic electrical activity in the brain. Whenever a treatment appears to improve the condition of epilepsy, those in the tinnitus community want to know if the same treatment can be used to reduce or eliminate their tinnitus. As an interesting sidenote, ADHD, another neurological disorder, is more prevalent in epileptics and in people who have tinnitus than in people who have neither epilepsy nor tinnitus. A 2006 study performed on Long-Evans rats noted that the ketogenic diet not only improved the symptoms of epilepsy, but also helped to decrease the hyperactivity level associated with ADHD. All the studies I found online were limited to observing the effects of a ketogenic diet when epilepsy and ADHD were both present. I found no studies which determined any benefits of a ketogenic diet in subjects with tinnitus and ADHD.

Despite a lack of specific research, there have been anecdotal reports of the ketogenic diet being useful as a treatment for tinnitus. Let's take a look at the basics of the ketogenic diet and why it might help.

The ketogenic diet slashes carbohydrates from your eating regimen. For most people, this means reducing carb intake to 50 or 60 net grams per day. In comparison, 225 to 325 is the normal recommended total carbs for someone on a 2,000 calories per day diet. To calculate net carbs, subtract the total fiber gram count from the total carbohydrate gram count, as fiber is not absorbed or utilized as caloric energy. For example, a serving of lentils (one cup) contains 12.3 grams of carbs and 4.3 grams of fiber, so the net carbs would be 8 grams. One cup of uncooked spinach contains 1.1 grams of carbs and 0.4 grams of fiber. Its net carb count is 0.7 grams.

Protein grams are not as restricted as carbs, but they do need to be counted accurately. Proteins usually comprise 20 to 25% of calories in a ketogenic diet, compared to 5% of calories from carbs. Adult men generally need 56 grams of protein per day; adult women need 46 grams, or up to 71 grams per day if pregnant or breastfeeding.

The ketogenic diet emphasizes high amounts of fat in the diet, from 70 to 75% of your caloric intake. We're talking about the good fats here, the monounsaturated fats and polyunsaturated fats. Monounsaturated fats are contained in avocados, olives, and natural peanut butter (nothing added), to name a few. Some of the best polyunsaturated fats are omega-3 fatty acids. These are found in fish such as salmon and lake trout, and in vegetarian sources like walnuts, spinach and kale. Other good fats are those with medium chain triglycerides (MCTs) such as coconut oil. Foods containing saturated fats are allowed when eaten in moderate amounts, but there is controversy about their pros and cons. Among the most popular foods containing saturated fats are chocolate, butter, cream, and coconut.

The foods to completely strike off your list are those containing trans fats. If you read a food label with either the words "hydrogenated oil" or "partially hydrogenated oil," put it back on the shelf. You can avoid a lot of trans fats by simply not adding any processed foods to your shopping cart. "Choosing Healthy Fats," published on www.HelpGuide.org, offers more detailed information about the different types of fat in our food sources. Eliminating trans fats from your diet is a positive step for your health, whether you decide to try the ketogenic diet or not.

There is emerging evidence that a ketogenic diet produces favorable effects in the brain. From the standpoint of controlling tinnitus, the most important of these effects is that ketones have been shown to inhibit the ability of hippocampal neurons to load up on glutamate. This is from the study, "The ketogenic diet: metabolic influences on brain excitability and epilepsy." You'll recall from Chapter 21, "Meet Your Neurotransmitters," that glutamate is an excitatory neurotransmitter. Too much glutamate results in neurotoxicity and hyperexcited neurons. Ketones also appear to have a beneficial effect on the inhibitory neurotransmitter GABA. Elevated ketones have been shown to increase the amount of GABA in nerve synapses, which helps the brain to calm down. In laboratory animals, as well as in some (but not all) epilepsy patients, the combination of inhibiting glutamate and increasing GABA has the effect of reducing seizures and being neuroprotective. More studies need to be done as there is still not enough data to reach positive conclusions.

Elevated ketones might be part of the reason why people on this diet tend to report that they feel better and their moods are lighter. If GABA is having a greater influence on the brain because there's less glutamate, then the inhibitory action of GABA will naturally promote a sense of calm and ease. One small but significant study suggests that the ketogenic diet protects dopamine-producing brain cells. As mentioned before, dopamine is known as the feel-good neurotransmitter. It makes sense that keeping a sufficient level of dopamine in one's system will lead to feeling good emotionally.

A potential downside of a high fat diet is its effect on neurogenesis. Studies conducted on mice have shown that a high fat diet consisting of omega-6 and omega-3 polyunsaturated fats decreases the production of brain-derived neurotrophic factor (BDNF) when the diet extends beyond 72 hours. Mice are commonly used in research because their biological systems closely resemble those of humans. If this study applies to humans, then it could possibly be detrimental for someone with tinnitus to lower their BDNF level, since BDNF is essential for promoting neurogenesis. Other studies also indicate that a ketogenic diet may significantly affect normal brain activity as well as limiting synaptic plasticity. You will recall that synapses are the narrow gaps between the neurons over which neurotransmitters send chemical or electrical signals. Synaptic plasticity refers to the changes in structure and function of the synapse, the process by which information is stored in the central nervous system.

In contrast to the studies just mentioned, other studies have shown that consumption of MCT fats in a ketogenic diet improves cognition and memory. This would seem to contradict a decrease in neurogenesis or negative effects on synaptic plasticity. The difference may lie in whether the high fat diet is mostly comprised of omega-6 and omega-3 polyunsaturated fats, or whether MCT fats are the primary source of fat. Without going into specifics, it would be difficult to maintain a diet high in MCTs. A good summary of MCTs is in the article, "The Benefits of Medium Chain Triglycerides," published on www.VeryWell.com. The article includes some important cautionary advice for anyone considering upping their intake of MCTs.

Theoretically, any diet which includes restricting carbohydrate intake to 50 milligrams or less per day will put your body into a state of nutritional ketosis. In other words, no matter how you arrange your intake of proteins and fats, if you eat less than 50 grams of carbs each day, you are technically on a ketogenic diet. The Paleo diet, which focuses on whole foods and excludes processed or cultivated foods (grains, for example), can be modified to induce ketosis. You can read more about this in "The Paleo Guide to Ketosis," published on www.PaleoLeap.com. Basically you would limit starchy foods like potatoes and instead choose cruciferous vegetables such as broccoli and other low carb vegetables. The VeryWell website lists delicious veggies that will add very little to your carb count. These vegetables include mushrooms, asparagus, salad greens, onions, artichokes, tomatoes, peppers, and cabbage. The website article is "Vegetables You Can Enjoy Guilt-Free on a Low Carb Diet."

In my opinion — and again, I'm not a healthcare practitioner — the main reason for improvement that anyone with tinnitus might experience with the ketogenic diet has less to do with the fat and protein intake and is most likely attributable to the severe restriction of carbs. During the digestive process, carbohydrates turn to glucose in your system. This causes a rise in insulin to handle the glucose. After the insulin is released, the glucose level drops. In response to your blood sugar level dropping, glutamate is increased. Glutamate is an excitatory neurotransmitter necessary for cognitive function by helping the nerve cells to communicate effectively, and it also plays a role in the formation of memory. Too much glutamate leads to hyperactivity of the neurons and can result in excitotoxicity which damages those neurons. For example, people with hyperglycemia are particularly susceptible to glutamate toxicity due to inefficient glucose control. With the ketogenic diet, less carbs equals less glucose which in turn equals less insulin release. This results in less glutamate being released, and therefore reduced neuronal excitement and potential damage. Again, that's my opinion. As I indicated in the prior chapter, a drastic reduction in carbs did seem to reduce my tinnitus somewhat, but it was too strict a regimen for me to follow.

When you're deciding which carbs to include or exclude from your diet, you need to consider their glycemic index, which is the rate of how quickly they raise blood sugar levels. Low glycemic foods take longer to digest, so the rise in blood sugar is gradual, whereas high glycemic foods can create a spike in blood sugar. For more detailed guidance on which carbs are best to keep your blood sugar level (and glutamate) under control, read "Carbohydrates and Blood Sugar," published by the Harvard School of Public Health on www.hsph.harvard.edu.

Remember that diabetics are more likely to have hearing loss. In Chapter 69, "Caffeine, Sugar, Salt, and Additives," I mentioned advanced glycation end-products and their possible link to inner ear hair cell damage. This may tie in with the theory that high blood glucose levels, along with a corresponding elevation of glutamate, can cause chemical changes to the blood vessels and nerves of the inner ear. Since hearing loss is a strong factor in tinnitus, it's important not to stress your system with an overload of carbohydrates. Even if you decide the ketogenic diet isn't right for you, try limiting your carb intake for a while, especially high glycemic index carbs, and see what happens. The American Diabetes Association article, "Understanding Carbohydrates," provides valuable information on what kinds of carbs are best for keeping blood glucose levels under control, and how to determine your optimal daily intake.

Although some components of the ketogenic diet may help reduce tinnitus, overall it probably isn't the best choice you can make. Because of the severe carb restriction, it can be a difficult diet to follow for more than a few months. In children, there are long-term effects of the ketogenic diet which can include a risk of stunted growth and increased risk of bone fractures. Adults are more likely to experience complications such as constipation, decreased level of micronutrients, and increased levels of cholesterol and triglycerides. There is also a potential risk of gall bladder problems. Women may experience irregularities in their menstrual cycles, possibly affecting fertility. The ketogenic diet should not be undertaken by anyone with a known serious medical condition. Diabetics in particular should avoid this diet altogether, as ketones are related to a decrease in production of insulin.

There is currently no conclusive proof whether the ketogenic diet is either good or bad for brain health, especially since the primary focus has been on pediatric epilepsy and not on the recent emphasis of a ketogenic diet for weight loss. There have been limited studies conducted on potential benefits of the ketogenic diet for Parkinson's disease, Alzheimer's, and Amytrophic Lateral Sclerosis (ALS). The results are cautiously optimistic, and more studies are planned to determine the feasibility of the ketogenic diet for those and other neurodegenerative disorders.

Countless websites offer in-depth information about the ketogenic diet. For example, www.KetoDietApp.com/blog has helpful articles and a clear presentation. There is a handy keto calculator on the website www.MyDreamShape.com to help you apportion your daily calories into carbohydrates, proteins, and fats. If you're a vegan or vegetarian, there are far fewer websites to help you get started with the ketogenic diet. I found one helpful article, "The Ketogenic Diet and Vegetarianism: Can They Coexist," on www.MyHealthWire.com, which offers some guidelines regarding how to follow the fat and protein requirements and still abstain from eating meat and animal-derived products.

If you want to try the ketogenic diet for a few weeks to see if it improves your tinnitus, be sure to do so under the supervision of a healthcare practitioner. It's possible you may have an underlying condition which can worsen with this diet, and you need to be especially aware of potential serious complications if you have any heart problems. Even if your health is good and you have no chronic medical conditions requiring a doctor's supervision, there can be side effects in addition to those previously noted. These can include sluggishness, fatigue, headaches, frequent urination, and more, especially in the first two weeks. Long-term effects may include thyroid problems, bone density loss, kidney stones, and Vitamin C deficiency. You might experience mood disorders, as the ketogenic diet could eventually alter the balance of your neurotransmitters. A good summary of the downside is in the article, "Ketogenic Diet Side Effects," published on www.News-Medical.net. Be mindful that there are experts who recommend against the ketogenic diet for adults. In fact, The National Institute for Health and Clinical Excellence in the UK specifically advises against managing epilepsy in adults with this type of diet.

A note of caution: When you read online articles praising the benefits of a ketogenic diet, keep in mind that many websites have a vested interest in encouraging you to try the ketogenic diet, either because they sell recipe plans or books or consultation services. Look for objective sources such as the Mayo Clinic's "Epilepsy - Diagnosis & Treatment" page to get a more conservative but objective view. Medically-oriented websites tend to focus on discussing the ketogenic diet for pediatric epilepsy, Alzheimer's, Parkinson's disease and other neurological disorders. They usually do not address the weight loss or other promoted aspects of the diet.

SECTION X

CLOSING THOUGHTS

72
YOU CAN BE BOTH REALISTIC
AND HOPEFUL

Whether tinnitus is mild, moderate, or severe, people usually want to know, will this go away? The best way to answer that is to say it's possible, but the longer you've had it, the less likely it is that it will disappear completely. If you have tinnitus for six months or longer, it's generally considered to be chronic. That's when you need to face the fact that tinnitus is going to be with you for the rest of your life. However, that doesn't mean it's going to keep the same characteristics, and it certainly doesn't mean you're going to perceive it at the same level of volume or intensity. I cannot stress enough that tinnitus usually does get better in time. Your brain eventually adapts to the noise, and, if you keep your focus off the tinnitus, the sound will move into the background of your awareness. You will discover one day that you didn't hear your tinnitus for a minute, maybe five minutes, maybe even an hour. Then, as soon as you noticed you weren't hearing it — boom! — you hear it again. The trick to becoming the master of your tinnitus instead of the other way around is to pay as little attention to it as you can. I know what some of you are thinking, "How can I possibly ignore it? It's so loud!!"

My tinnitus was often so severe during the first eight months, I sometimes thought I would lose my mind. In April 2018, I will reach my four-year anniversary with tinnitus and am feeling more hopeful than ever. I still have one or two days a week when it's harder to concentrate on work because the tinnitus is somewhat difficult to ignore, but there are certainly many more days now of moderate or mild tinnitus. I believe the improvement is not simply due to the passing of time. Things didn't really begin to change for the better until I began using sound enrichment, ACRN, and intermittent fasting. I've also recently started the Back to Silence method again. It sounds like a lot, but you'd be surprised how easy it is to gradually make several different therapies a part of your everyday life. Just choose the ones that feel right to you, and go from there.

Michael J. Fox is a well-known and popular actor who was diagnosed with young-onset Parkinson's disease when he was 30 years old. He is passionate about helping people learn how to live with Parkinson's, and has spoken about the difference between acceptance and resignation. He wants people to know that no matter what they are dealing with, that it's important first of all to accept that things are what they are. But that doesn't mean you need to be resigned to your fate, so to speak. It means accept it, then find a way to live with it, to get through it. Although most cases of tinnitus are not as debilitating as Parkinson's, his message still applies. With tinnitus, you need to have hope and patience as you work toward improving it, while still accepting that you may never be entirely rid of it.

The interesting thing is that chronic tinnitus has been known to suddenly disappear. It's rare but not unheard of for someone who has had it for six months, a year, two years, or even 10 years, that their tinnitus simply stops. This can happen when physical problems that caused the tinnitus have been corrected, the most common of these being TMJ problems. When someone stops taking certain ototoxic medications, the tinnitus can stop. But spontaneous remission in someone with chronic tinnitus remains a mystery. No wonder people with severe tinnitus are reluctant to give up hope that their tinnitus will disappear, or maybe fade away gradually to where they never notice it. My impression from reading online stories is that this kind of outcome is more likely when tinnitus is idiopathic in origin; that is, no one really knows what caused it. It's apparently less likely to happen if the tinnitus is due to extreme acoustic trauma or in the case of severe hearing loss, because both of those are more closely associated with damaged or dead hair cells. However, the brain is an unpredictable thing. There's no way to know for certain what will happen in any individual case of tinnitus.

I covered in an earlier chapter how David Letterman's tinnitus began, and how William Shatner and Leonard Nimoy got tinnitus when an explosion occurred on the set of Star Trek while filming the episode "Arena." Letterman and Shatner talk about their personal experience with tinnitus on the YouTube video, "David Letterman with William Shatner - March 1996." (Warning: this video seems to be preset at high volume, so adjust your volume downward before watching.) Their discussion about tinnitus begins at timeline 1:18. Shatner and Letterman sometimes make light of the subject in this video clip, because obviously they don't want to bring down the mood of the audience. However, the sincerity of their discussion highlights how serious the condition has been for both of them. The show took place in March of 1996, and Shatner refers to tinnitus as a hearing disorder. Since that time, of course, science is looking at tinnitus as being more of a brain disorder.

The condition is no longer a critical issue for either of them, as they have both learned how to cope with their tinnitus. Just imagine how difficult it must have been for Shatner to memorize his lines with a constant sound in his head, or for Letterman to stay upbeat and informed so he and his guests could entertain audiences night after night. Using their lives as an example, you can feel confident that the odds are on your side. It's important to maintain a positive attitude and avoid spiraling into negative thinking patterns, and to make a genuine effort to keep your body and mind healthy. In time, you will be able to get back into your life and function as well as you always have.

Take a look at the Pinterest board "Famous People with Hearing Loss and Tinnitus." You'll be surprised how many well-known people have one or both afflictions. The next time you see one of your favorite actors in a movie, someone like Gerard Butler who has had tinnitus since childhood, let it be a reminder that tinnitus is not an insurmountable obstacle to pursuing your dreams.

One of the best things I read on the Tinnitus Talk forum was a post that said, "Your brain will become hardened to the tinnitus in time." That statement has given me a lot of hope and comfort over the past three and a half years. As difficult as it may be to imagine at the beginning, your tinnitus more than likely will eventually either decrease in severity or you will discover that you aren't as obsessed with it as you were in the first few months or the first year. However, if you're constantly feeling stressed or overwhelmed by your tinnitus, it may be too difficult to simply wait and see what happens. You need to take steps so that you have control over your tinnitus and not the other way around. Whatever you decide to do, I sincerely hope that what you have learned from reading *Living With Tinnitus* will help you to calm your tinnitus and live a full and happy life again.

SECTION XI

APPENDIX

ABOUT THE AUTHOR

Laura Cole has 30+ years experience as a professional researcher, editor, and proofreader covering a broad range of subjects, from common business contracts to complex product liability litigation. Laura lives in the mountains of eastern Oregon, where she enjoys hiking with her rescue dog Zoe and spending time with her friends.

Website: www.livingwitht.com
Follow me on Twitter: https://twitter.com/livingwitht

If you received value from this book in any way, I'd like to ask you for a favor: would you be kind enough to leave a review for this book on Amazon? You'll be helping me as the author, but, even more important, you'll be helping others who may be struggling with tinnitus and looking for answers.

Thank you!

RESOURCES

The categories listed here are a summary of resources regarding tinnitus, hearing loss, hyperacusis, and related matters. Also listed are some products that have been suggested as useful by people in the tinnitus community. Some of these are mentioned in the main text of this book. They are included here so you can quickly browse through and follow up on anything of particular interest.

Please note that anything listed here does not constitute a recommendation, nor can I verify the accuracy of information presented on any website or video.

Apps:
1. Decibel 10th - for iPhone and iPad, measures decibel levels
2. Decibel Meter Pro - for iPhone and iPad, measures decibel levels
3. f.lux - automatically adjust the screen to match your environment lighting, for Windows, iPhone, iPad, Mac, Linux, and Android devices
4. myNoise - for Android devices, sound generator app with soundscapes from the myNoise website
5. myNoise - for iPhone, iPad, and iPod touch, sound generator app with soundscapes from myNoise website
6. Sleep Cycle alarm clock - for iPhone, iPad, Android, an app which analyzes your sleep patterns and awakens you during your lightest sleep phase
7. Sound Meter - for Android devices, measures decibel levels
8. Tinnitus Balance by Phonak - create your own library of personalized sounds and music, available for both iPhone and Android
9. Tinnitus Calmer - sound therapy with relaxation exercises, from Beltone

Hearing aids:
Widex Zen - hearing aid with therapeutic sounds.

Medical-based information:
1. BHI Noise Guide - "Your Guide to Prevention of Hearing Loss From Noise," a PDF file regarding hearing loss and noise exposure
2. Drugs.com - features a drug index, pill identifier, and interactions information. Includes Tinnitus Support Group for Q&A relating to tinnitus
3. Examine - "independent, unbiased, and objective source" for supplements information
4. Marijuana Doctors - information regarding medical marijuana
5. Science Direct - "scientific, technical and medical research." Input your search term in the Keywords field for the subject of your interest.
6. The International Tinnitus Journal - professional publications on tinnitus

Miscellaneous:
1. BrainHQ - brain training exercises
2. Cronometer - keep track of data regarding your nutrition, health, and fitness
3. Loop - Automatically loops YouTube videos so they continuously repeat
4. myNoise.net - streaming audio with extensive selection of exceptional quality sound generators (soundscapes) for masking, sound enrichment, concentration, and more
5. Neural Symphony - sound generator on myNoise website specifically designed to calm tinnitus

Organizations:
1. American Audiology Online - educational courses for those who want to pursue professional-level knowledge of tinnitus, hyperacusis, and other hearing-related disorders
2. American Speech-Hearing-Language Association - tinnitus information
3. American Tinnitus Association - informative up-to-date articles about tinnitus and hyperacusis. Membership includes subscription to *Tinnitus Today* magazine.

4. British Tinnitus Association - information about tinnitus and hyperacusis
5. American Tinnitus Practitioners - helpful for locating someone to treat tinnitus
6. hear-it - extensive information on hearing loss and tinnitus, featuring articles, hearing tests, and samples of what tinnitus and hearing loss sound like

Products:
1. 2breathe - Sleep inducer
2. Bose noise-cancelling headphones
3. Eargasm High Fidelity - earplugs which maintain full spectrum of sound
4. Gamma Ray Flexlite - blue light blocking glasses for computer reading
5. Puro Sound - headphones and earbuds designed for children
6. Quiet vacuum cleaners - to reduce noise exposure, helpful for anyone with hearing sensitivity
7. Sleepytime Extra - soothing herbal tea with chamomile and valerian, from Celestial Seasonings
8. Sound machines - for sound therapy and as a sleeping aid
9. V-moda - earplugs and other products for musicians
10. Voyager Focus UC headset - noise cancelling Bluetooth stereo headset
11. Wireless Bluetooth speakers - streams audio from your smartphone for higher quality sound enrichment

Support forums:
1. The Hyperacusis Network - for those suffering from hyperacusis, hypersensitive hearing, phonophobia, misophonia, tinnitus, as well as auditory disorders associated with Ménière's and autism
2. Tinnitus Talk - information and support for people with auditory disorders including tinnitus, hyperacusis, hearing loss, and ear pain. (Also visit their companion website, www.tinnitushub.com, and their Facebook page, https://www.facebook.com/TinnitusHub. Follow them on Twitter, @tinnitushub.)

Videos (on YouTube):

1. "Acoustic CR Neuromodulation Tinnitus Treatment" - an overview of ACRN sound therapy presented by The Tinnitus Clinic
2. "Back to Silence" - innovative tinnitus therapy which focuses on the emotional reaction to tinnitus instead of monitoring and describing the tinnitus
3. "British Tinnitus Association - Sounds of Tinnitus" - simulation of tinnitus sounds created by an electronic music synthesizer. Please turn volume down before listening; many of these sounds are extremely unpleasant. Sounds begin at 0:50 on the timeline.
4. "Eat, Fast & Live Longer BBC Documentary" - a healthier body and mind with the 5:2 diet, including the promotion of neurogenesis. The focus on neurogenesis begins at timeline 46:29.
5. "Excitotoxins: The Taste That Kills" - 2011 presentation by neurosurgeon Russell Blaylock about food additives, such as MSG and aspartame, and their role in neurotoxicity
6. "Remodeling Sensory and Motor Circuits in the Brain: New Insights from Hearing Loss and Tinnitus," 2011 presentation by Richard Salvi, Center for Hearing & Deafness University at Buffalo. Dr. Salvi begins addressing tinnitus at timeline 14:20.
7. "The Exact Moment I Got Tinnitus" - a warning video from Jacob Everett on the danger of firing weapons without ear protection
8. "The Noise" - Michael Berardi shows a typical day of living with severe tonal tinnitus, with some encouraging words
9. "Tinnitus - Can you hear that?" - a video aimed at young adults to encourage ear protection. The tinnitus level demonstrated is in the mild to moderate range.
10. "Tinnitus: Ringing in the Brain" - informative presentation by leading expert Josef Rauschecker
11. "Tinnitus Talk: Sounds of Tinnitus" - a short video with examples of tinnitus as experienced around the world
12. Vyanah channel on YouTube, relaxing music for meditation and yoga
13. "What NOT to do with tinnitus" - advice by Julian Cowan Hill
14. "William Shatner speaks about his tinnitus" - presented by the American Tinnitus Association

15. "Music star Will.i.am speaks about his Tinnitus - 2011 Interview" - will.i.am of the Black Eyed Peas shares what it's like to have both tinnitus and attention deficit disorder

---

I learned a lot about tinnitus from the members of Tinnitus Talk. If you need emotional support right away, or if you have a question you want answered without searching high and low on the Internet, I highly recommend you visit this forum. You don't have to join to read the comments, but you will need to register if you want to participate. Registration is easy, and it's free. Tinnitus Talk is a place where you'll find people who are more than willing and able to help you get through both the initial and ongoing experience of dealing with tinnitus, hyperacusis, hearing loss, Ménière's disease, and ear pain. The members have been in your shoes and they understand exactly what you are going through. Tinnitus Talk is also a wonderful resource for friends and family members who want to learn more and are looking for ways to show support when someone they care about is struggling with auditory-related disorders.

GLOSSARY

Acoustic Coordinated Reset® Neuromodulation (ACRN) - Sound therapy consisting of specific repetitive frequency tones and strategically-timed gaps of silence to remap the brain. It utilizes brain plasticity as a means of correcting the hyperactive neurons which cause tinnitus.

Acoustic event - An incident of sound loud enough and/or lasting a sufficient period of time to potentially damage the auditory system.

Acoustic trauma - An incident of exposure to an extreme decibel level, resulting in temporary or permanent damage to one or more components of the auditory system.

Acute - The initial stage of a condition when it first appears. Acute tinnitus may arise and then disappear after a short period of time. If the symptoms persist long enough, the condition is considered to be chronic.

Adrenalin - A stress hormone secreted by the adrenal gland, which contributes to the "fight or flight" response to perceived danger; also called epinephrine.

Afferent - Leading towards a part; for example, an afferent nerve that carries a message to the central nervous system.

Agonist - A molecule that promotes the same effect on a post-synaptic neuron as a compatible neurotransmitter; for example, a GABA agonist enhances the effect of the neurotransmitter GABA.

Alpha waves - The brain waves associated with calm, relaxation, daydreaming, and creative thinking. People with tinnitus tend to have lower than normal alpha wave activity.

Amygdala – Almond-shaped mass of cells located deep within the temporal lobe of the brain, one in each hemisphere. It is involved in motivation, emotions, and the storage of memories.

Antagonist - A substance that blocks or suppresses the action of another substance; the opposite of an agonist.

Antioxidant - Substances which bind with and help to counteract the effects of oxidants (free radicals) that can cause cellular damage.

Anxiolytic - A medication, herb, or other substance which reduces anxiety and promotes calm.

Ataxia - Unable to control one's muscles, especially in the extremities.

A distinct sign of ataxia is an abnormal gait. Some inner ear disorders can cause ataxia.

Audiologist - A medical professional who specializes in hearing and balance disorders.

Auditory cortex - Located in the temporal lobe, the auditory cortex processes information received through hearing. This includes pitch and volume, which allows the listener to process and understand different sounds.

Audio notch therapy - Sound therapy wherein a notch of tinnitus-matching frequencies is removed from an audio file. Listening to notched audio causes surrounding normal neurons to be stimulated and thereby send inhibitory signals to misfiring dysfunctional neurons.

Barotrauma - Injury caused by increased pressure in surrounding air or water; barotrauma can be limited to the ear, or may affect the entire body.

Baseline - The usual volume and characteristics of your tinnitus when you are at rest in an environment with only ambient sound and no other external sound input.

Blood lactate - Lactate acid appears in the blood when metabolic demands outweigh available oxygen to body tissues. High performance exercise can raise blood lactate above resting levels.

Brain - The organ of the central nervous system which is contained within the skull. It contains specialized areas for different functions and is the center of thought and movement in the human body.

Brain-derived neurotrophic factor - Protein derived from the brain which nourishes brain cells and contributes to neurogenesis. Low levels of blood plasma BDNF have been shown to correlate with tinnitus severity.

Brain plasticity - Changes in the brain which occur as a result of new experiences, changes in behavior, or injury. Among these changes are differences in volume of gray matter and rewiring of neural connections. (Related to *neuroplasticity*.)

Brown noise - Sound with more energy at the lower frequencies, such as the low roar of a waterfall.

Bruxism - Grinding of the teeth, usually in one's sleep, but can occur without conscious awareness during waking hours.

Cerebellum - The part of the brain which controls coordination of movement, balance, and muscle tone, among other functions. The cerebellum is being studied as a potential generator of tinnitus.

Chronic - A condition which persists over a long period of time, generally with little to no improvement or a very slow process of improvement.

Chronification - The shifting over time of pain or negative stimuli from nociceptive to emotional circuits. Chronification occurs when the brain perceives pain via an emotional circuit rather than the normal response of pain receptors.

Cochlea - The snail-shaped spiral tube in the middle ear; among other components, it contains the hair cells that convert sound waves to neural signals.

Cortisol - Stress hormone secreted by the adrenal glands. It is responsible for regulating and modulating bodily changes in response to stress.

Cycling tinnitus - Tinnitus which changes in intensity over the course of days in either a random or predictable pattern.

Decibel - The measuring unit for relative intensity of sound.

Delta waves - The slowest brain waves, associated with trance and deep sleep. People with tinnitus tend to have higher than normal delta wave activity.

Eardrum - Common name for the tympanic membrane, the thin tissue separating the ear canal from the middle ear. The eardrum is critical to transmitting sound wave vibrations to the inner ear.

Efferent - Leading away from a part; for example, an efferent nerve that carries an impulse away from the central nervous system.

Electrode - For medical purposes, a conductor through which an electrical current can be measured by a monitoring device. Electrodes are either connected to a bodily surface, such as the scalp, or implanted.

Epilepsy - Neurological disorder whereby misfiring of the brain's electrical system causes physical seizures, ranging from mild to severe. Approximately 125,000 Americans are diagnosed with epilepsy each year.

Excitatory - Producing a stimulating effect; for example, causing a neuron to fire.

Excitotoxin - A substance which causes excessive stimulation of neurons to such a degree that they can be damaged or die.

Fleeting tinnitus - An isolated but sometimes repetitive occurrence of increased tinnitus volume accompanied by the impression of diminished or muffled hearing.

Fluctuating tinnitus - Tinnitus which changes in characteristics and/or intensity over the course of a day.

Frequency - The number of waveforms a sound source produces in one second. 1 hertz equals 1 waveform per second. The pitch of a sound rises as its frequency increases (more waveforms per second).

Frontal lobe - The part of the brain involved in executive functions such as decision-making, and the expression of personality. This area is also referred to as the frontal cortex or prefrontal cortex.

GABA - Gamma aminobutyric acid, an inhibitory neurotransmitter. Insufficient GABA in the auditory system is thought to be one component responsible for persistent tinnitus.

Glutamate - Excitatory neurotransmitter which facilitates the transmission of electrical signals between nerve cells.

Glutamate storm - A release of excess glutamate by stressed hair cells in response to events such as acoustic trauma or infection. This causes overstimulation of inner ear nerve cells, resulting in their damage or death. Brain cells are also susceptible to a glutamate storm from head injury or stroke.

Glutamatergic - Related to the neurotransmission of glutamate. A glutamatergic substance assists in the modulation of glutamate.

Glutathione - Molecule produced by the liver, consisting of L-cysteine, glycine, and L-glutamate. Glutathione is considered to be a powerful antioxidant as well as playing a role in stimulating the immune system.

Grey noise - Random noise with equal loudness throughout all its frequencies. (May also be spelled as "gray noise.")

Habituation - A state of mind where you no longer have a negative emotional response to your tinnitus. Habituation sometimes leads to no longer being aware of the tinnitus.

Hair cells - Sensory receptors located on the basilar membrane of the cochlea which respond to vibrations caused by sound waves and transmit electrical impulses to the acoustic nerve. These receptors have stereocilia which resemble hairs that stick out, thus the name "hair cell."

Hippocampus - Structure within the limbic system, located in the temporal lobe of the cerebral cortex. The hippocampus is critical to learning and memory, and is affected by mental states such as anxiety, PTSD, bipolar disorder, and depression.

Hyperacusis - An increased and usually painful sensitivity to sound, with or without accompanying hearing loss.

Inhibitory - Producing a calming or suppressive effect.

Intermittent tinnitus - Tinnitus which spontaneously appears and lasts from a few seconds to a few hours, then disappears.

Ketones - Alternative fuel made in the liver through the breakdown of fats. Ketones are formed when the body doesn't have enough sugar or glucose to fuel metabolism.

Lateral inhibition - The ability of neurons to inhibit the activity of neighboring neurons. Audio notch therapy is a tinnitus treatment which relies on lateral inhibition of misfiring neurons.

Light therapy - The treatment of seasonal affective disorder (SAD) or other conditions by exposure to light which is brighter than indoor light but not as bright as direct sunlight.

Limbic system - The area of the brain considered to be our emotional and motivational center, consisting of the hypothalamus, thalamus, hippocampus, and amygdala, as well as the fornix, cingulate gyrus, and mammillary bodies.

Loudness matching - A hearing test designed to measure the volume of one's tinnitus.

Masking - Therapy whereby one listens to a neutral or pleasant soundscape to shift the brain's focus away from tinnitus.

Meditation - The practice of training the mind, usually through focused attention, in order to create a change in consciousness, induce calm, and enhance awareness.

Ménière's disease - A dysfunction of fluids of the inner ear resulting in problems with balance, and may include hearing loss and tinnitus.

Modulation - To control or adjust the level; for example, tianeptine is an antidepressant that modulates the glutamatergic system.

Monosodium glutamate (MSG) - An artificially processed flavor enhancer which is considered to be an excitotoxin by many in the health community.

Motility - The ability to move spontaneously.

NMDA receptor - A neuron receptor which is activated by the excitatory neurotransmitter glutamate.

Neurogenesis - The process by which new neurons are generated.

Neuroimaging - Images of the brain produced by non-invasive procedures such as magnetic resonance imaging (MRI) and positron-emission tomography (PET).

Neuron - An impulse-conducting cell which is the basic unit of the nervous system. A neuron is commonly referred to as a nerve cell.

Neuroplasticity - The potential of the brain to reorganize and adapt by changing its neural pathways. (Related to *brain plasticity*.)

Neurotransmitter - Brain chemicals that promote communication between the brain and body. They are the messengers that relay signals between neurons (nerve cells).

Nociception - The encoding and processing of harmful stimuli in the nervous system.

Norepinephrine - A neurotransmitter and hormone released in response to stress. It is secreted by the adrenals and nerve endings in the parasympathetic nervous system. Also called noradrenaline.

Notched audio therapy - Removing a frequency range from music or colored noise (white, pink, violet, etc.), with the goal of inhibiting hyperactive neurons from firing that are responsible for producing the sounds of tinnitus.

Objective tinnitus - Tinnitus caused by an anatomical disorder such as vascular abnormality or Eustachian tube dysfunction, and which can be heard by a listener other than the person experiencing the tinnitus.

Oscillation - A back and forth or ebb and flow pattern of movement.

Otolaryngologist - A medical professional specializing in diseases and disorders of the ear, nose, and throat, as well as related structures of the head and neck.

Ototoxic - Capable of causing harm to the auditory system, especially the nerve supply to the ear. Two common ototoxic effects are hearing loss and tinnitus.

Oxidative stress - The imbalance between the presence of reactive oxygen species (ROS), which can cause damage at the cellular level, and the body's ability to detoxify the ROS or repair the damage.

Panic - A feeling of overwhelming fear which can provoke an agitated emotional response and/or irrational behavior.

Pink noise - Sound which contains all the frequencies audible to the human ear, with emphasis on the lower frequencies. It has a constant energy across all octaves.

Post-synaptic neuron - The nerve cell on the receiving end of an electrical impulse. Post-synaptic neurons contain receptors for neurotransmitters.

Post-traumatic stress disorder - A mental health issue which results from a traumatizing event; PTSD can be a constant state but is typically intermittent and triggered by a reminder of the initial event.

Prednisone - Corticosteroid drug which, if administered within a short period of time following a severe acoustic event, may help lessen the damage to the auditory system.

Prefrontal cortex - The area of the brain involved in executive functions such as decision-making, and the expression of personality. Also referred to as the frontal lobe or frontal cortex.

Presbycusis - Irreversible age-related hearing loss, most noticeable in the higher frequencies.

Pre-synaptic neuron - The nerve cell on the transmitting end of an electrical impulse. Pre-synaptic neurons send neurotransmitters across the synapse to receptors on the post-synaptic neuron.

Progenitor cell - A cell that arises from a stem cell and develops into a specialized cell; for example, a neuronal progenitor cell develops into a nerve cell.

Psychoactive - Affecting the mind or mental processes; for example, thinking or memory.

Pulsatile tinnitus - The sensation of hearing the rhythm of one's heartbeat pulsing in the ear, generally producing a whooshing sound.

Reactive tinnitus - Tinnitus which increases in intensity when a person is exposed to an acoustic event that is perceived as exceedingly loud, annoying, and/or stress-inducing.

Receptor - A molecule on or within a cell which is designed to be activated by a specific substance; for example, GABA receptors are designed to respond specifically to the neurotransmitter GABA.

Residual inhibition - Reduced perception of tinnitus when a sound similar to one's tinnitus or matching one's tinnitus frequency is heard.

Sensorineural hearing loss (SNHL) - Hearing loss due to damage to the inner ear (the cochlea and its resident hair cells), or damage to the nerve pathways from the inner ear to the brain.

Serotonin - An inhibitory neurotransmitter which affects or helps to regulate mood as well as bodily functions such as digestion, sexual desire, blood clotting, and bone density.

Somatic tinnitus - Tinnitus which arises from a joint and/or muscular problem in the body; also, tinnitus which can be modulated by moving the jaw, neck, head, or shoulders into various positions.

Sound enrichment - The constant presence of soothing or masking sounds in one's environment as a means of keeping the brain's focus attuned to the sounds, with less attention directed to the tinnitus.

Sound generator - A device which plays audio to mask tinnitus as part of sound therapy. Sound generators can be solo devices such as MP3 players, or incorporated within hearing aids.

Sound therapy - The use of soundscapes or specially modified audio to gradually desensitize the user to their tinnitus. Sound therapies such as ACRN and audio notch therapy are designed to reduce the severity of the tinnitus itself.

Sound wave - Vibrations which pass through an object or a medium such as air or water, being interpreted as sound via the auditory system.

Spike - A sudden and sometimes unexplainable marked increase in tinnitus volume, which can last for minutes, hours, days, or weeks.

Streaming - Visual and/or audio data from the Internet which is transmitted in a continuous flow.

Subjective tinnitus - Tinnitus which can only be heard by the person experiencing the tinnitus.

Sudden sensorineural hearing loss (SSNHL) - An acute and sudden episode of hearing loss which requires immediate medical attention.

Synapse - A gap between neurons through which nerve signals are passed via the release of neurotransmitters.

Temporomandibular joint disorder - Dysfunction of the jaw joint and/or surrounding facial muscles that can lead to somatic tinnitus; often abbreviated as TMJ.

Tinnitus - Phantom sounds produced by the auditory system and/or brain which are not present in the environment, but are heard as real sounds in the ears, head, or both.

Tinnitus Handicap Inventory - A subjective questionnaire for measuring degree of tinnitus severity and perceived distress.

Tinnitus Retraining Therapy - A management therapy developed by Dr. Pawel Jastreboff which incorporates sound enrichment to address the auditory system, as well as personal counseling to address fears and anxiety associated with tinnitus.

Tonotopic - Occupying a space according to frequency. For example, different sound frequencies are assigned to a specific location in the brain. This is referred to as a tonotopic map of the auditory cortex in the temporal lobe of the brain.

Traumatic brain injury - An impact from an external force or high velocity acceleration/deceleration of the head which causes brain dysfunction.

Vertigo - The sensation of one's surroundings spinning around while you are standing still, which can result in difficulty maintaining balance.

Violet noise - Also called purple noise. A sound with its energy increasing at the higher frequencies. Each successive octave contains as much energy as the four preceding octaves.

White noise - Sound which contains an equal amount of high frequencies to low frequencies. It is popular for masking because it cuts through background noise.

REFERENCE LINKS

For ease of reference, links referenced in each chapter are listed below.

Chapter 2 - What Is Tinnitus?

Whooshers
http://whooshers.com

Chapter 3 - Tinnitus Sounds and Volume

"British Tinnitus Association" - Sounds of Tinnitus (video)
https://www.youtube.com/watch?v=2mV-Z54fiBo

Online Audiogram Hearing Test
http://www.audiocheck.net/testtones_hearingtestaudiogram.php

Noise Level Chart, dB Levels of Common Sounds
http://www.noisehelp.com/noise-level-chart.html

Chapter 6 - Tinnitus is Everywhere

"Classification and Epidemiology of Tinnitus"
https://www.ncbi.nlm.nih.gov/pubmed/12856294

Chapter 7 - Tinnitus Has Many Origins

"Stress and prevalence of hearing problems in the Swedish working population"
https://bmcpublichealth.biomedcentral.com/articles/
10.1186/1471-2458-11-130

"Tinnitus Evaluation and Management Considerations for Persons with Mild Traumatic Brain Injury"
http://www.asha.org/Articles/Tinnitus-Evaluation-and-Management-Considerations-for-Persons-with-Mild-Traumatic-Brain-Injury/

"Tinnitus and disorders of the temporo-mandibular joint and neck"
https://www.tinnitus.org.uk/tinnitus-and-tmj

"Neck Exercises - Topic Overview"
http://www.webmd.com/pain-management/tc/neck-exercises-topic-overview

"Olive Oil Ear Wax"
http://www.home-remedies-for-you.com/articles/1094/diseases-and-ailments/olive-oil-ear-wax.html

Chapter 8 - Salicylates and NSAIDS

The FailSafe Diet
http://www.failsafediet.com/the-rpah-elimination-diet-failsafe/salicylate-content-of-foods/

"What Is a Salicylate Allergy?"
http://www.webmd.com/allergies/salicylate-allergy

Chapter 9 - Mycins, Micins, and Chemotherapy

Drugs.com
https://www.drugs.com

WebMD
http://www.webmd.com

Chapter 11 - Decibels and Safe Levels

Sound Meter
https://play.google.com/store/apps/details?id=com.gamebasic.decibel

Decibel 10th
https://itunes.apple.com/us/app/decibel-10-db-sound-meter-spl-noise-level-fft/id448155923?mt=8

Seahawks vs. Packers game
https://www.youtube.com/watch?v=AZrr7wjb8ZE

Chapter 12 - Why Me?

Noise Addicts - "Hearing Test - Can You Hear This?"
http://www.noiseaddicts.com/2009/03/can-you-hear-this-hearing-test/

Science Forum - "Cool Hearing test"
https://www.youtube.com/watch?v=h5l4Rt4Ol7M

"Music Star Will.i.am speaks about his Tinnitus - 2011 Interview"
https://www.youtube.com - Search for video title (direct link to video not available)

Chapter 14 - How It Begins

"The Exact Moment I Got Tinnitus" - video by Jacob Everett
https://www.youtube.com/watch?v=kjMLtbzoE6A

Chapter 16 - Thoughts of Suicide

OHSU Ear, Nose and Throat Tinnitus Program
http://www.ohsu.edu/xd/health/services/ent/services/tinnitus-clinic/index.cfm/

The Telegraph: "Coroner slams delay over tinnitus sufferer who stabbed himself to death"
http://www.telegraph.co.uk/news/health/news/9198029/Coroner-slams-delays-over-tinnitus-sufferer-who-stabbed-himself-to-death.html

"I have tinnitus and I want to die" - YouTube video about Gaby Olthuis, from a journalist's firsthand account of Gaby's decision to end her life
https://www.youtube.com/watch?v=HGcUJ2Dg3uo

"Tinnitus Short Film - 24.7.52.10." - YouTube video by Zoe Cartwright, a young woman who lives with both deafness and tinnitus
https://www.youtube.com/watch?v=BN1xIXye6s4

Tinnitus Talk - online support forum - compassionate and knowledgeable help from forum members around the world
https://www.tinnitustalk.com

Chapter 17 - How Tinnitus Affects You

"Stress - Portrait of a Killer" - National Geographic documentary
https://www.youtube.com/watch?v=eYG0ZuTv5rs

Chapter 19 - Tinnitus Handicap Inventory

PDF download on Living With Tinnitus website
http://livingwitht.com/thi

Starkey Research & Clinical Blog, "The Tinnitus Handicap Inventory (THI): A Quick and Reliable Method for Measuring Tinnitus Outcomes"
http://blog.starkeypro.com/the-tinnitus-handicap-inventory-thi-a-quick-and-reliable-method-for-measuring-tinnitus-outcomes/

THI References:
Dr. Andrew McCombe
http://www.entpartnership.co.uk/Consultants/AndrewMcCombe/Default.aspx
Dr. David Baguley
http://www.neuroscience.cam.ac.uk/directory/profile.php?dmb29
Dr. Laurence McKenna
https://www.uclh.nhs.uk/OurServices/Consultants/Pages/DrLaurenceMcKenna.aspx

Chapter 20 - The Pain of Hyperacusis

"When even soft noises feel like a knife to the eardrums"
https://www.statnews.com/2016/02/18/noise-induced-ear-pain/

Tinnitus Talk Hyperacusis & Ear Pain forum
https://www.tinnitustalk.com/forums/support.55/

The Hyperacusis Network
http://www.hyperacusis.net

Chapter 21 - Meet Your Neurotransmitters

"Light Therapy"
http://www.webmd.com/a-to-z-guides/light-therapy

"Dr. Russell Blaylock: Excitotoxins - The Taste That Kills"
https://www.youtube.com/watch?v=tTSvlGniHok

Chapter 24 - The Brain Creates Tinnitus

"In search of tinnitus, that phantom ringing in the ears"
https://www.sciencedaily.com/releases/2015/04/150423125858.htm

Chapter 26 - Brain Waves and Tinnitus

"Modulatory effects of aromatherapy massage intervention on electroencephalogram, psychological assessments, salivary cortisol and plasma brain-derived neurotrophic factor"
http://www.sciencedirect.com/science/article/pii/S0965229914000582

Essential Glutathione: The Mother of all Antioxidants
http://drhyman.com/blog/2010/05/19/glutathione-the-mother-of-all-antioxidants/

OmHarmonics - binaural beats meditation
http://www.omharmonics.com

Chapter 27 - Alcohol and Marijuana

"What Is the Endocannabinoid System and What Is Its Role?"
https://www.leafly.com/news/science-tech/what-is-the-endocannabinoid-system

"The Best Strains for Tinnitus"
https://www.leafly.com/search?q=tinnitus&lat=45.323&lon=-118.2027

"Cannabis Science 101: The Physics and Chemistry of the Joint"
https://www.leafly.com/news/science-tech/cannabis-science-101-the-physics-and-chemistry-of-the-joint

"Smoke vs. Stack: Why Edible Marijuana Is Stronger Than Smoking"
http://www.thedailybeast.com/smoke-vs-snack-why-edible-marijuana-is-stronger-than-smoking

"State Marijuana Laws in 2017 Map"
http://www.governing.com/gov-data/state-marijuana-laws-map-medical-recreational.html

Chapter 30 - Hearing Aids

Muse, Halo 2, and Sound Lens hearing aids for tinnitus
http://www.starkey.com/hearing-aids/technologies/tinnitus

Tinnitus Balance Portfolio - hearing aid, app, and sound generator combo
https://www.phonak.com/com/en/hearing-aids/tinnitus-treatment.html

Waterfall sound generator for masking tinnitus
https://mynoise.net/NoiseMachines/waterfallNoiseGenerator.php

Pretty Hearing Aids on Pinterest
https://www.pinterest.com/stephtara/pretty-hearing-aids/

"Hearing Aid Buying Guide" by Consumer Reports
http://www.consumerreports.org/cro/hearing-aids/buying-guide.htm

Budget-friendly hearing aids sold online
http://www.hearingdirect.com/us/

Chapter 31 - Masking

Texas High Def - YouTube channel featuring masking sounds for tinnitus
https://www.youtube.com/user/TexasHighDef

Relaxing White Noise - YouTube channel featuring masking sounds for tinnitus
https://www.youtube.com/user/RelaxingWhiteNoise

Cat Purr - soothing sound generator
https://mynoise.net/NoiseMachines/catPurrNoiseGenerator.php

B-17 Flying Fortress - a sound generator to take you back in time
https://mynoise.net/NoiseMachines/propellerNoiseGenerator.php

Audio Jammer - unique sound generator for masking and protecting conversations
https://mynoise.net/NoiseMachines/audioJammerNoiseGenerator.php

"How to Use Sound Machines" - Dr. Pigeon's overview of how to use sound generators
https://mynoise.net/howToUseSoundMachines.php

Chapter 32 - Sound Enrichment

myNoise Screencasts - video tutorials for using the myNoise website
https://mynoise.net/screencasts.php

myNoise app for iPhone, iPad and iPod touch
https://itunes.apple.com/us/app/mynoise/id813099896?mt=8

myNoise app for Android devices
https://play.google.com/store/apps/details?id=com.mynoise.mynoise&hl=en

"Tinnitus Calmer" app - sound therapy with relaxation exercises, from Beltone
https://www.beltone.com/apps/tinnitus-calmer-app.aspx

Chapter 33 - Meditation

Vyanah - YouTube channel featuring music for meditation
https://www.youtube.com/channel/UCu_14PpxWo-m1PWGhpxZoVQ

Chapter 34 - Sleeping

Rain Noise - the most popular sound generator for those who love the sound of rain
https://mynoise.net/NoiseMachines/rainNoiseGenerator.php

Distant Thunder - rain and gentle thunder
https://mynoise.net/NoiseMachines/thunderNoiseGenerator.php

BrainHQ - brain training website
https://www.brainhq.com

Sleep Loss Infographic - negative effects on the brain from lack of sleep
http://blog.brainhq.com/wp-content/uploads/
2015/09/89a2209b16e829ceec4a62663d501684.png

"Sleeping Disorder Statistics" - the toll on human life caused by sleep deprivation
http://www.statisticbrain.com/sleeping-disorder-statistics/

"CPAP Therapy for Obstructive Sleep Apnea" - WebMd article
http://www.webmd.com/sleep-disorders/sleep-apnea/continuous-positive-airway-pressure-cpap-for-obstructive-sleep-apnea

"Have sleep apnea? You might have hearing loss, too" - how sleep apnea affects hearing
http://www.healthyhearing.com/report/52200-Have-sleep-apnea-you-might-have-hearing-loss-too

Chapter 35 - Methods for Better Sleep

f.lux - adjusts the lighting of your screen
https://justgetflux.com

Gamma Ray Flexlite - glasses to block blue ray light
https://www.amazon.com/Comfortable-Computer-Reducing-Eyestrain-Eyeglasses/dp/B00BQ7KBV4

Memory foam mattress toppers
https://www.overstock.com/Bedding-Bath/Memory-Foam/457/dept.html

2breathe - FDA-approved device to aid in relaxation for sleep
http://2breathe.com

Sleep Cycle alarm clock - app which awakens you during your lightest sleep phase
https://www.sleepcycle.com

Sleep Cycle alarm clock - "How does it work?"
https://www.sleepcycle.com/how-it-works

Chapter 37 - Yoga

Yogis Anonymous - online yogi classes, subscription $15/month
https://yogisanonymous.com

Asanas (poses):
Sphinx asana - beginner
https://www.yogajournal.com/poses/sphinx-pose

Cat asana - beginner
https://www.yogajournal.com/poses/cat-pose

Cow face asana - intermediate
https://www.yogajournal.com/poses/cow-face-pose

Balancing Table Pose - beginner
https://www.verywell.com/hands-and-knees-balance-3567081

Downward Facing Dog - beginner
https://www.yogajournal.com/poses/downward-facing-dog

Plank asana - beginner
https://www.verywell.com/how-to-do-plank-pose-3567104

Warrior asana - beginner
http://www.wikihow.com/Do-the-Warrior-Pose-in-Yoga

Chapter 38 - Realistic But Positive Attitude

"Positive thinking: Stop negative self-talk to reduce stress" - Mayo Clinic
stress management article
http://www.mayoclinic.org/healthy-lifestyle/stress-management/in-depth/positive-thinking/art-20043950

Chapter 39 - Stay Busy

"Adventures in the Land of Illness" - from the blog of author Sam
Harris
https://www.samharris.org/blog/item/adventures-in-the-land-of-illness

"Five Steps to Finding Your Passion" - Susan Biali, M.D., Psychology Today
https://www.psychologytoday.com/blog/prescriptions-life/201205/five-steps-finding-your-passion

Udemy - online learning
https://www.udemy.com

Chapter 41 - Aromatherapy

Mountain Rose Herbs aromatherapy products
https://www.mountainroseherbs.com/catalog/aromatherapy

"Essential Oil Skin Patch Testing" - how to do a skin patch test
https://www.aromaweb.com/articles/essential-oil-skin-patch-test.asp

"Essential Oils: Poisonous When Misused" - National Capital Poison Center
http://www.poison.org/articles/2014-jun/essential-oils

Chapter 42 - Audio Notch Therapy

"Listening to tailor-made notched music reduces tinnitus loudness and tinnitus-related auditory cortex activity" - published by National Center for Biotechnology Information
https://www.ncbi.nlm.nih.gov/pmc/articles/PMC2824261/

"Frequently Asked Questions" - AudioNotch website
http://www.audionotch.com/faq

Chapter 43 - Audio Notch - Do It Yourself Guide

"Find your tinnitus tone" - frequency matcher tool
http://www.audionotch.com/app/tune/

"ACRN Tinnitus Protocol" - frequency matcher tool
http://generalfuzz.com/acrn

Audacity - audio software for recording and editing
http://www.audacityteam.org

Audacity installation tutorials on YouTube
https://www.youtube.com/results?search_query=install+audacity

"What Data Compression Does to Your Music"
http://www.soundonsound.com/techniques/what-data-compression-does-your-music

Chapter 44 - The Colors of Noise

"Grey Noise" - article explaining the properties of grey noise
https://www.techopedia.com/definition/27898/gray-noise

"White Rain" - white noise sound generator
https://mynoise.net/NoiseMachines/whiteRainNoiseGenerator.php

"Impulse Noise" - brown noise sound generator
https://mynoise.net/NoiseMachines/impulseNoiseGenerator.php

"Waterfall Noise" - pink noise sound generator
https://mynoise.net/NoiseMachines/waterfallNoiseGenerator.php

"White Noise & Co." - grey noise sound generator
https://mynoise.net/NoiseMachines/whiteNoiseGenerator.php

"Ten Hours of Ambient Sound - Blue Noise" - blue noise video
https://www.youtube.com/watch?v=WSCU_t3o7KI

"Ten Hours of Violet Noise - Ambient Sound" - violet noise video
https://www.youtube.com/watch?v=GYZy5f92FpQ

"Grey Brown Violet and Pink Noise for Ten Hours" - combination noise video
https://www.hindawi.com/journals/bmri/2015/569052/

Chapter 45 - Acoustic CR Neuromodulation

"Acoustic Coordinated Reset Neuromodulation in a Real Life Patient Population with Chronic Tonal Tinnitus" - BioMed Research International
https://www.hindawi.com/journals/bmri/2015/569052

Acoustic CR Neuromodulation: Do It Yourself Guide - General Fuzz
https://www.tinnitustalk.com/threads/acoustic-cr®-neuromodulation-do-it-yourself-guide.1469/page-6

Acoustic CR Neuromodulation: Do it Yourself Guide - complete Tinnitus Talk thread
https://www.tinnitustalk.com/threads/acoustic-cr-neuromodulation-do-it-yourself-guide.1469

Chapter 46 - ACRN - Do It Yourself Guide

General Fuzz ACRN generator
http://www.generalfuzz.net/acrn/

Audacity - recording and editing software
http://www.audacityteam.org

YouTube tutorials on how to install Audacity
https://www.youtube.com/results?search_query=install+audacity

"Fix Audacity not recording!" - YouTube tutorial
https://www.youtube.com/watch?v=SI7xyuKbAKk

YouTube tutorials on how to fix Audacity not recording
https://www.youtube.com/results?search_query=audacity+not+recording

"What Data Compression Does To Your Music"
http://www.soundonsound.com/techniques/what-data-compression-does-your-music

Donate to General Fuzz
http://generalfuzz.net/donate.php

Chapter 47 - Back to Silence Method

"Back to Silence" - Terry's video explaining the method
https://www.youtube.com/watch?v=wNjDBOJfMfY

"Putting Feelings Into Words Produces Therapeutic Effects In The Brain"
https://www.sciencedaily.com/releases/2007/06/070622090727.htm

Chapter 48 - Back to Silence Q&A

"Back to Silence" - message thread on Tinnitus Talk support forum
https://www.tinnitustalk.com/threads/back-to-silence.7172/

Chapter 49 - Cognitive Behavioral Therapy

"What is Cognitive Behavioral Therapy?"
https://www.verywell.com/what-is-cognitive-behavior-therapy-2795747

"In Depth: Cognitive Behavioral Therapy"
https://psychcentral.com/lib/in-depth-cognitive-behavioral-therapy/

"Dr. Hubbard's Tinnitus Story"
https://www.cbtfortinnitus.com/dr-hubbards-story/

Chapter 50 - Hypnotherapy

"Hypnosis in Dentistry"
https://www.youtube.com/watch?v=ErKU1rPQqmY

"Can You Be Hypnotized? The Lemon Test"
https://www.youtube.com/watch?v=x7wr_y-ThPs

Skype - audio/visual Internet communication
www.skype.com

Chapter 51 - Self-Hypnosis for Sleep

"Soothing words do more than pills to calm anxious patients, study shows"
https://www.asahq.org/about-asa/newsroom/news-releases/2015/10/soothing-words-do-more-than-pills-to-calm-anxious-patients

"Healing Trees"
https://mynoise.net/NoiseMachines/isabelleKnightHypnosisTalkGenerator.php

Chapter 52 - Low-Level Laser Therapy

Konftec LLLT device for tinnitus
http://www.konftec.com/html/ko_product_tinnitus.htm

"Low-Level Laser Therapy (LLLT) for Tinnitus"
https://www.tinnitustalk.com/threads/low-level-laser-therapy-lllt-for-tinnitus-%E2%80%94-experiences-dr-wilden-etc.295/

"Is LLLT for Tinnitus by Dr. Wilden a Scam?"
https://www.tinnitustalk.com/threads/is-lllt-for-tinnitus-by-dr-wilden-a-scam.14079

Chapter 53 - Mozart Therapy and The Tomatis Effect

"The Mozart effect in patients suffering from tinnitus"
http://www.tandfonline.com/doi/abs/10.3109/00016489.2012.684398

"Mozart Classical Piano Study Music & Alpha Waves: Ultimate Concentration, Mozart K.448 Study Music" - music video with binaural beats embedded
https://www.youtube.com/watch?v=CiaV_4KQJcQ

"Mozart - Sonata for Two Pianos in D, K.448" - music video
https://www.youtube.com/watch?v=tT9gT5bqi6Y

"Beethoven's Für Elise,"
https://www.youtube.com/watch?v=Lkcvrxj0eLY

The Tomatis Effect
http://www.tomatis.com/en/tomatis-method/its-function.html

"The Listening Centre successfully treats: Tinnitus"
http://www.listeningcentre.co.uk/tinnitus.php

Eric Jordan studies
http://www.soundtherapyperth.com/research/tinnitus.php

"Rafaele Joudry Interview - Tinnitus Relief" - video
https://www.youtube.com/watch?v=NePxKfJu2V8

Aural Scan - sound generator
https://mynoise.net/NoiseMachines/auralScannerNoiseGenerator.php

Misophonia - auditory system dysfunction
http://www.misophonia.com/symptoms-triggers/

Chapter 54 - Neurofeedback

"Neurofeedback for treating tinnitus"
http://www.sciencedirect.com/science/article/pii/S0079612307660464

"Meta-Analysis of EEG Biofeedback in Treating Epilepsy"
http://www.eeginfo.com/research/epilepsy_main.jsp

BRAINtellect
https://braintellect.com

NeurOptimal
https://neuroptimal.com/home-neurofeedback/

BrainMaster Technologies, Inc.
http://brainmaster.com

RESPeRATE
http://www.resperate.com

Chapter 55 - Neurogenesis

"Neurogenesis In Adult Brain: Association With Stress and Depression"
https://www.sciencedaily.com/releases/2008/08/080831114717.htm

"Physical Exercise Habits Correlate with Gray Matter Volume of the Hippocampus in Healthy Adult Humans"
https://www.nature.com/articles/srep03457

"Various levels of plasma brain-derived neurotrophic factor in tinnitus patients"
https://www.researchgate.net/publication/221781294_Various_levels_of_plasma_brain-derived_neurotrophic_factor_in_patients_with_tinnitus

"Adult hippocampal neurogenesis and its role in Alzheimer's disease."
https://molecularneurodegeneration.biomedcentral.com/articles/10.1186/1750-1326-6-85

"New Blood Test May Detect Traumatic Brain Injury"
https://psychcentral.com/news/2015/08/02/new-blood-test-may-detect-traumatic-brain-injury/88415.html

Chapter 56 - Tips to Increase BDNF

"Don't Feed Your Head"
https://hub.jhu.edu/magazine/2012/summer/dont-feed-your-head

5:2 Diet
https://thefastdiet.co.uk

"Eat, Fast, and Live Longer BBC Documentary"
https://www.youtube.com/watch?v=Ihhj_VSKiTs

"Foods highest in Total Omega-3 fatty acids"
http://nutritiondata.self.com/foods-000140000000000000000.html

"What is Ultraviolet (UV) Radiation?"
https://www.cancer.org/cancer/skin-cancer/prevention-and-early-detection/what-is-uv-radiation.html

"Neck Massage: Do It While You View It"
https://www.youtube.com/watch?v=duSNnBnqFts

Chapter 58 - Popular Supplements for Tinnitus

"Ginkgo and blood thinners"
http://medherb.com/Materia_Medica/Ginkgo_and_blood_thinners.htm

Nootropic supplements, including idebenone
https://www.smartdrugsforthought.com

In-depth review of idebenone
https://examine.com/supplements/idebenone

Chapter 59 - Prescription Drugs

"The efficacy of medication on tinnitus due to acute acoustic trauma"
https://www.ncbi.nlm.nih.gov/pubmed/11318462

Clonazepam (Klonopin) information
https://www.drugs.com/clonazepam.html

User reviews on Xanax for tinnitus
https://www.drugs.com/comments/alprazolam/for-tinnitus.html

BenzoBuddies - forum dedicated to information about benzodiazepines
http://www.benzobuddies.org/forum/index.php

"Benzodiazepines: How They Work and How to Withdraw"
http://www.benzo.org.uk/manual/bzcha01.htm

Chapter 61 - Residual Inhibition

"Hush Tinnitus Sound Therapy Experiences?"
https://www.tinnitustalk.com/threads/hush-tinnitus-sound-therapy-experiences.2470/

"Experimental Tinnitus Sound Treatment"
https://www.youtube.com/watch?v=ibWYcDSbcwg

Chapter 63 - What to Expect With TRT

"Test your hearing today - free online hearing test"
http://www.starkey.com/online-hearing-test

Chapter 65 - Train the Brain - Exercises

Epic Puzzles - puzzle app
http://amzn.to/2Apvqq7

Classic Words - scrabble app
http://amzn.to/2Aqf5l7

Sharp Brains brain teasers
https://sharpbrains.com/blog/2008/05/26/brain-games-and-teasers-top-50/

"What is BrainHQ" - video
https://vimeo.com/190944852

"Research Opened Door to Restoring Brain Damaged Function"
https://www.ucsf.edu/news/2016/06/403136/michael-merzenich-wins-2016-kavli-prize-neuroscience

"Adult Neurogenesis in the Hippocampus"
https://mindsparke.com/adult_neurogenesis_hippocampus.php

Chapter 67 - Other Treatments

"My Trip to Bangkok: Stem Cell Treatment [Journal],"
https://www.tinnitustalk.com/threads/my-trip-to-bangkok-stem-cell-treatment-journal.1884

"What Is The Hypothalamus?"
https://www.thoughtco.com/hypothalamus-anatomy-373214

"HIFU (High Intensity Focused Ultrasound) Surgery"
https://www.tinnitustalk.com/threads/hifu-high-intensity-focused-ultrasound-surgery.276/

SoniModul Clinic
https://sonimodul.ch/home/about-us/therapeutic-offer/

"Stop telling people there is no cure for tinnitus!"
https://www.youtube.com/watch?v=TFgu0q2otE

Chapter 68 - Scams

"Tinnitus Miracle is Bullshit"
http://fixedgear808.blogspot.com/2015/03/tinnitus-miracle-is-bullshit.html

Chapter 69 - Caffeine, Sugar, Salt and Additives

"Caffeine Content of Popular Drinks"
http://www.math.utah.edu/~yplee/fun/caffeine.html

"Understanding Blood Pressure Readings"
http://www.heart.org/HEARTORG/Conditions/HighBloodPressure/KnowYourNumbers/Understanding-Blood-Pressure-Readings_UCM_301764_Article.jsp#.WXFD7caZM6g

Chapter 70 - Intermittent Fasting

"Eat, Fast & Live Longer BBC Documentary"
https://www.youtube.com/watch?v=Ihhj_VSKiTs

"Why fasting bolsters brain power: Mark Mattson at TEDx Johns Hopkins University"
https://www.youtube.com/watch?v=4UkZAwKoCP8

Chapter 71 - Ketogenic Diet

"Choosing Healthy Fats"
https://www.helpguide.org/articles/healthy-eating/choosing-healthy-fats.htm

"The ketogenic diet: metabolic influences on brain excitability and epilepsy"
https://www.ncbi.nlm.nih.gov/pubmed/23228828

"The Benefits of Medium Chain Triglycerides"
https://www.verywell.com/the-benefits-of-medium-chain-triglycerides-90054

"The Paleo Guide to Ketosis"
https://paleoleap.com/paleo-guide-to-ketosis/

"Vegetables You Can Enjoy Guilt-Free on a Low Carb Diet."
https://www.verywell.com/low-carb-vegetables-list-2242530

"Carbohydrates and Blood Sugar"
https://www.hsph.harvard.edu/nutritionsource/carbohydrates/carbohydrates-and-blood-sugar/

"Understanding Carbohydrates"
http://www.diabetes.org/food-and-fitness/food/what-can-i-eat/understanding-carbohydrates

KetoDiet Blog
https://ketodietapp.com/Blog

"The Real Keto Calculator"
http://www.mydreamshape.com/keto-calculator

"The Ketogenic Diet and Vegetarianism: Can They Coexist?"
http://www.myhealthwire.com/news/breakthroughs/895

"What Are Ketosis Side Effects?"
http://www.wisegeekhealth.com/what-are-ketosis-side-effects.htm#didyouknowout

"Epilepsy" - Mayo Clinic
http://www.mayoclinic.org/diseases-conditions/epilepsy/diagnosis-treatment/treatmenttxc-20117241

Chapter 72 - You Can Be Both Realistic and Hopeful

"David Letterman with William Shatner - March 1996"
https://www.youtube.com/watch?v=yCdx8aueK9I

"Famous People with Hearing Loss and Tinnitus"
https://www.pinterest.com/TinnitusHub/famous-people-with-hearing-loss-and-tinnitus/

BIBLIOGRAPHY

"15 Ways to Get Tinnitus." Sanuthera, Inc. (Accessed 2016.) http://www.sanuthera.com/15-ways-to-get-tinnitus/

AboutNeurofeedback, "Neurofeedback F.A.Q.." (Accessed 2017.) http://www.aboutneurofeedback.com/neurofeedback-info-center/faq/

Adjamian, Peyman, Deborah A. Hall, Alan R. Palmer, et al., "Neuroanatomical abnormalities in chronic tinnitus in the human brain." *Neuroscience and Biobehavioral Reviews*, Volume 45, September 2014. http://www.sciencedirect.com/science/article/pii/S0149763414001389

Aetna, "Tinnitus Treatments." June 13, 2017. http://www.aetna.com/cpb/medical/data/400_499/0406.html

Aguiar, Jr., Aderbal S., Adalberto A. Castro, Eduardo L. Moreira, et al., "Short bouts of mild-intensity physical exercise improve spatial learning and memory in aging rats: Involvement of hippocampal plasticity via AKT, CREB and BDNF signaling." *Mechanisms of Aging and Development*, Volume 132, Issues 11-12, November-December 2011. http://www.sciencedirect.com/science/article/pii/S0047637411001564

Ahuja, Navneet, Wutyi Thwe Myat, Alexandra Cervantes, Natasha Zahn, "Amygdala Hijack." (Accessed 2016.) http://neurosciencefundamentals.unsw.wikispaces.net/The+limbic+System

AIT Institute, "Sound Sensitivity: A Summary of Probable Causes of Hypersensitivity to Sound (Hyper acute hearing)." *The Sound Connection* newsletter. (Accessed 2017.) https://www.aitinstitute.org/sound_sensitivity_causes.htm

Alcohol MD, "The Neurobiology of Addiction." http://www.alcoholmd.com/dependancy.htm

Aldhafeeri, F.M., I. Mackenzie, T. Kay, et al., "Neuroanatomical correlates of tinnitus revealed by cortical thickness analysis and diffusion tensor imaging." *Neuroradiology* (2012) 54: 883. https://doi.org/10.1007/s00234-012-1044-6

Allen, Jane E., "Tinnitus Drives Sufferers to Distraction, Desperation." ABC News Medical Unit, November 28, 2011. http://abcnews.go.com/Health/Depression/tinnitus-suicide/story?id=15003057

ALS Association, "Disease Mechanisms." (Accessed 2017.) http://www.alsa.org/research/about-als-research/glutamate.html

Alvarez-Bullya, Arturo, Jose Manuel Garcia-Verdugo, "Neurogenesis in Adult Subventricular Zone." *The Journal of Neuroscience*, Volume 22, Number 3, February 1, 2002 http://www.jneurosci.org/content/22/3/629

Alzheimer's Association, "Alzheimer's Disease and the Brain, More Brain Changes." (Accessed 2017.) https://www.alz.org/braintour/healthy_vs_alzheimers.asp

American Academy of Audiology, "Motivational Interviewing: Something to Consider When Fitting Hearing Aids to Patients with Tinnitus?" September 20, 2016. https://www.audiology.org/news/motivational-interviewing-something-consider-when-fitting-hearing-aids-patients-tinnitus

American Academy of Otolaryngology - Head and Neck Surgery, "Hyperacusis: An Increased Sensitivity to Everyday Sounds." (Accessed 2017.) http://www.entnet.org/content/hyperacusis-increased-sensitivity-everyday-sounds

American Academy of Otolaryngology – Head and Neck Surgery, "Tinnitus Patient Health Information." 2017. http://www.entnet.org/content/tinnitus

American Academy of Pediatrics, "Noise: A Hazard for the Fetus and Newborn." October 1997, Volume 100, Issue 4. http://pediatrics.aappublications.org/content/100/4/724.full

American Cancer Society, "How Do I Protect Myself from UV Rays?" (Accessed 2017.) https://www.cancer.org/cancer/skin-cancer/prevention-and-early-detection/uv-protection.html

American Cancer Society, "What is Ultraviolet (UV) Radiation?" (Accessed 2017.) https://www.cancer.org/cancer/skin-cancer/prevention-and-early-detection/what-is-uv-radiation.html

American Diabetes Association, "Understanding Carbohydrates." (Accessed 2017.) http://www.diabetes.org/food-and-fitness/food/what-can-i-eat/understanding-carbohydrates/

American Foundation for Suicide Prevention, "Suicide Statistics." (Accessed 2017.) https://afsp.org/about-suicide/suicide-statistics/

American Hearing Research Foundation, "High Doses of AntiOxidants May Help Prevent Hearing Loss." (Accessed 2017.) http://american-hearing.org/high-antioxidants/

American Heart Association, "Understanding Blood Pressure Readings." October 19, 2017. http://www.heart.org/HEARTORG/Conditions/HighBloodPressure/KnowYourNumbers/Understanding-Blood-Pressure-Readings_UCM_301764_Article.jsp#.WevQX0yZM6g

American Nutrition Association, "Free Glutamic Acid (MSG): Sources And Dangers." *Nutrition Digest*, Volume 38, Number 2, 2000. http://americannutritionassociation.org/newsletter/free-glutamic-acid-msg-sources-dangers

American Nutrition Association, "Review of: Excitotoxins: The Taste that Kills." *Nutrition Digest*, Volume 38, Number 2. (Accessed 2016.) http://americannutritionassociation.org/newsletter/review-excitotoxins-taste-kills

American Society of Anesthesiologists, "Soothing words do more than pills to calm anxious patients, study shows." October 27, 2015. https://www.asahq.org/about-asa/newsroom/news-releases/2015/10/soothing-words-do-more-than-pills-to-calm-anxious-patients

American Speech-Language-Hearing Association, "Causes of Hearing Loss in Children." (Accessed 2017.) https://www.asha.org/public/hearing/Causes-of-Hearing-Loss-in-Children/

American Speech-Language-Hearing Association, "State Insurance Mandates for Hearing Aids." (Accessed 2016.) http://www.asha.org/advocacy/state/issues/ha_reimbursement/

American Speech-Language-Hearing Association, "The Audiogram." (Accessed 2016.) http://www.asha.org/public/hearing/Audiogram/

American Tinnitus Association, "Demographics." (Accessed 2016.) https://www.ata.org/understanding-facts/demographics

American Tinnitus Association, "Emotion Processing in the Brain Changes with Tinnitus Severity." (Accessed 2016.) https://www.ata.org/news/news/emotion-processing-brain-changes-tinnitus-severity

American Tinnitus Association, "Impact of Tinnitus." (Accessed 2016.) https://www.ata.org/understanding-facts/impact-tinnitus

American Tinnitus Association, "Measuring Tinnitus." (Accessed 2016.) https://www.ata.org/understanding-facts/measuring-tinnitus

American Tinnitus Association, "Symptoms." (Accessed 2016.) https://www.ata.org/understanding-facts/symptoms

American Tinnitus Association, "Two Types of Tinnitus in the Brain." (Accessed 2016.) https://www.ata.org/news/news/two-types-tinnitus-brain

Ananda Apothecary, "Aromatherapy Research: Essential Oils Alter Brainwaves When Inhaled." (Accessed 2016.) https://www.anandaapothecary.com/archive/aromatherapy-research-essential-oils

Bibliography

Anari, Mart, Alf Axelsson, Anette Eliasson, Lennart Magnusson, "Hypersensitivity to Sound. Questionnaire data, audiometry and classification." *Scandinavian Audiology*, February 1999. https://www.ncbi.nlm.nih.gov/pubmed/10572967

Anderson, James, "Chronic Pain Remodels Brain Region for Emotion." ReliaWire, December 22, 2015. https://reliawire.com/chronic-pain-emotion/

Anft, Michael, "Don't feed your head." *Johns Hopkins Magazine*, Summer 2012. http://hub.jhu.edu/magazine/2012/summer/dont-feed-your-head/

Arbor Teas, "The Difference Between Decaffeinated Tea and Caffeine-Free." (Accessed 2017.) https://www.arborteas.com/tea-caffeine/

Ashton, DM, FRCP, C. Heather, "Benzodiazepines: How They Work and How to Withdraw." Benzo, August 2002. https://www.benzo.org.uk/manual/bzcha01.htm

Attanasio, Giuseppe, Giulia Cartocci, Edoardo Covelli, et al., "The Mozart effect in patients suffering from tinnitus." *Acta Oto-Laryngologica*, November 2012. https://www.ncbi.nlm.nih.gov/pubmed/23025336

attheedgeofscience (Member), "My Trip to Bangkok: Stem Cell Treatment [Journal]." Tinnitus Talk, August 18, 2013. https://www.tinnitustalk.com/threads/my-trip-to-bangkok-stem-cell-treatment-journal.1884

AudioNotch, "Frequently Asked Questions." (Accessed 2017.) http://www.audionotch.com/faq

aurelientt (Member), "Neurofeedback for Tinnitus." Tinnitus Talk, March 15, 2013. https://www.tinnitustalk.com/threads/neurofeedback-for-tinnitus.1205/

Bailey, Regina, "Amygdala. Fear and the Amygdala." ThoughtCo, August 17, 2017. http://biology.about.com/od/anatomy/p/Amygdala.htm

Bailey, Regina, "Hypothalamus Activity and Hormone Production." ThoughtCo, July 28, 2017. https://www.thoughtco.com/hypothalamus-anatomy-373214

Bainbridge, K.E., H.J. Hoffman, C.C. Cowie, "Diabetics twice as likely to have hearing loss." *Annals of Internal Medicine*, Volume 149, Number 1, July 2008. http://annals.org/aim/fullarticle/741637/does-diabetes-affect-hearing

Balkenhol, Tobias, Elisabeth Wallhäusser-Franke, Wolfgang Delb, "Psychoacoustic tinnitus loudness and tinnitus-related distress show different associations with oscillatory brain activity." PubMed, 2013. https://www.ncbi.nlm.nih.gov/pubmed/23326394

Balthazar (Member), "Creatine and Tinnitus." Tinnitus Talk, January 5, 2014. https://www.tinnitustalk.com/threads/creatine-and-tinnitus.9083/

Banga, Shrey, "Can you go deaf from a loud sound beyond the hearing frequency?" Quora, December 31, 2012. https://www.quora.com/Can-you-go-deaf-from-a-loud-sound-beyond-the-hearing-frequency

Barcott, Bruce, "Cannabis Science 101: The Physics and Chemistry of the Joint." Leafly. March 5, 2016. https://www.leafly.com/news/science-tech/cannabis-science-101-the-physics-and-chemistry-of-the-joint

Barlow, MD, PhD, Carrolee, Steven D. Targum, MD, "Hippocampal Neurogenesis, Can it be a Marker for New Antidepressants?" *Psychiatry*, Volume 4, Number 5, May 2007. http://www.ncbi.nlm.nih.gov/pmc/articles/PMC2922342/

Bauer, Carol A., Kurt Wisner, Lauren T. Sybert, Thomas J. Brozoski, "The cerebellum as a novel tinnitus generator." *Hearing Research*, Volume 295, January 2013. http://www.sciencedirect.com/science/article/pii/S0378595512000676

Bauman, Ph.D., Neil, "The Ototoxicity of Drugs Ending in '-mycin' (and '-micin')." Hearing Loss Help. December 29, 2015. http://hearinglosshelp.com/blog/the-ototoxicity-of-drugs-ending-in-mycin-and-micin/

BBC News, Health, "Mozart 'can cut epilepsy.'" April 2, 2001.
http://news.bbc.co.uk/2/hi/health/1251839.stm

Beck, Gabriel, R. Joseph, "Limbic System: An Introduction: Hypothalamus, Septal Nuclei, Amygdala, Hippocampus, Emotion and the Unconscious Mind." BrainMind. 2015.
http://brainmind.com/BrainLecture4.html

Becvarovski, MBBS, FRACS, Zoran, "Sensorineural Hearing Loss in Children." St. George Ear-Nose-Throat. (Accessed 2017.) http://www.ent.com.au/index.php/information-for-doctors/otology/sensorineural-hearing-loss-in-children

Bergner, Paul, "Ginkgo and blood thinners." Medical Herbalism, 2001.
http://medherb.com/Materia_Medica/Ginkgo_and_blood_thinners.htm

Berke, Jamie, "Ototoxicity and Hearing Loss." VeryWell, April 29, 2017.
https://www.verywell.com/cause-of-hearing-loss-ototoxicity-1049380

Better Health, "Tinnitus." Tinnitus Association Victoria, July 2012.
https://www.betterhealth.vic.gov.au/health/conditionsandtreatments/tinnitus

Biali, MD, Susan, "Five Steps to Finding Your Passion." Psychology Today, May 8, 2012. https://www.psychologytoday.com/blog/prescriptions-life/201205/five-steps-finding-your-passion

Billeke, P., Aboitiz, F., "File: Brain areas that participate in social processing." Wikimedia. https://commons.wikimedia.org/wiki/File:Brain_areas_that_participate_in_social_processing.jpg

billie48 (Member), "From Darkness to Light, How I Recovered from Tinnitus & Hyperacusis." Tinnitus Talk, January 17, 2014. https://www.tinnitustalk.com/threads/from-darkness-to-light-how-i-recovered-from-tinnitus-hyperacusis.3148/

Billings, Katie, '16, "The Future of Depression Treatment: The Neurogenesis Theory." Dartmouth Undergraduate Journal of Science, February 17, 2014, http://dujs.dartmouth.edu/2014/02/the-future-of-depression-treatment-the-neurogenesis-theory/#.V3Uq2KJWsih

Biology Stack Exchange, "What exactly is Tinnitus?" April 3, 2014. http://biology.stackexchange.com/questions/16327/what-exactly-is-tinnitus/16379#16379

Biology Stack Exchange, "Why do adults lose hearing at high frequencies?" January 2015. http://biology.stackexchange.com/questions/27822/why-do-adults-lose-hearing-at-high-frequencies

Blaise, J. Harry, David N. Ruskin, Jessica L. Koranda, Susan A. Masino, "Effects of a ketogenic diet on hippocampal plasticity in freely moving juvenile rats." Physiological Reports, Volume 3, Issue 5, May 2015. http://onlinelibrary.wiley.com/doi/10.14814/phy2.12411/full

Blaszczak-Boxe, Agata, "People with Tinnitus May Process Emotions Differently." Live Science, July 2, 2014. http://www.livescience.com/46645-tinnitus-brain-process-emotions-amygdala.html

Borsook, D., Moulton, E.A., Schmidt, K.F., Becerra, L.R., "File: schematic of cortical areas involved with pain processing and fMRI.jpg." Wikimedia. https://commons.wikimedia.org/wiki/File:Schematic_of_cortical_areas_involved_with_pain_processing_and_fMRI.jpg

Brain Health & Puzzles, "An Introduction to Your Brain's Frontal Lobe." (Accessed 2017.)
http://www.brainhealthandpuzzles.com/frontal_lobe.html

Brain Health & Puzzles, "Brain Parts and Function." (Accessed 2016.)
http://www.brainhealthandpuzzles.com/brain_parts_function.html

BrainMaster Technologies, "Neurofeedback in a Nutshell." (Accessed 2017.)
http://brainmaster.com/what-is-neurofeedback/

Brain Power, "Vinpocetine." http://www.brainpower.org/research/vinpocetine.html

Brain State Technologies, "Brainwave Optimization." (Accessed 2016.)
http://brainwaveoptimization.com

Bibliography

Brain Stimulation Clinic, "Transcranial Direct Current Stimulation." (Accessed 2017.) http://www.transcranialbrainstimulation.com/

BRAINtellect, "How It Works." (Accessed 2017.) https://braintellect.com/how-does-it-work/

Brainwave Optimization, "What is Brainwave Optimization?" (Accessed 2017.) http://brainwaveoptimization.com

Branchi, Igor, Ivana D'Andrea, Marco Fiore, et al, "Early social enrichment shapes social behavior and nerve growth factor and brain-derived neurotrophic factor levels in the adult mouse brain. *Biology Psychiatry*, Volume 60, Number 7, October 1, 2006. http://www.ncbi.nlm.nih.gov/pubmed/16533499

Breus, Ph.D., Michael J., "Sleep Habits: More Important Than You Think." WebMD. (Accessed 2017.) https://www.webmd.com/sleep-disorders/features/important-sleep-habits#1

Briggs, Bill, "Hearing loss the most prevalent injury among returning veterans." Northern Virginia Resource Center, May 22, 2014. http://www.nvrc.org/2014/05/hearing-loss-the-most-prevalent-injury-among-returning-veterans/

British Tinnitus Association, "Drugs and Tinnitus." (Accessed 2017.) https://www.tinnitus.org.uk/drugs

British Tinnitus Association, "Ear wax removal and tinnitus." (Accessed 2016.) http://www.tinnitus.org.uk/ear-wax-removal-and-tinnitus

British Tinnitus Association, "Hearing aids and tinnitus." (Accessed 2016.) http://www.tinnitus.org.uk/hearing-aids-and-tinnitus

British Tinnitus Association, "Sound therapy (sound enrichment)." (Accessed 2017.) https://www.tinnitus.org.uk/sound-therapy

British Tinnitus Association, "Tinnitus and disorders of the temporo-mandibular joint (TMJ) and neck." (Accessed 2016.) https://www.tinnitus.org.uk/tinnitus-and-tmj

Browning, Duane, "Tinnitus Miracle is Bullshit!" Duane's Blog, March 21, 2015. http://fixedgear808.blogspot.com/2015/03/tinnitus-miracle-is-bullshit.html

Bruno, Karen, "Hard to Hear: Cisplatin Can Cause Hearing Loss for Men With Testicular Cancer." September 23, 2016. https://www.curetoday.com/publications/cure/2016/genitourinary-2016/hard-to-hear-cisplatin-can-cause-hearing-loss-for-men-with-testicular-cancer

Brynie, Ph.D., Faith, "Music Therapy for Tinnitus." Psychology Today, January 3, 2010. https://www.psychologytoday.com/blog/brain-sense/201001/music-therapy-tinnitus

Buddie, "Benzos, Tinnitus, and Neuromodulation." BenzoBuddies Community Forum, April 24, 2014. http://www.benzobuddies.org/forum/index.php?topic=106121.0

Bushak, Lecia, "The Brain Of An Introvert Compared To That Of An Extrovert: Are They Really Different?" August 21, 2014. http://www.medicaldaily.com/brain-introvert-compared-extrovert-are-they-really-different-299064

California Ear Research, "Hair Cell Regeneration Research." (Accessed 2016.) http://www.californiaearinstitute.com/ear-disorders-hair-cell-regeneration-research-california-ear-institute-bay-area.php

Campbell, MS, RD, LDN, CDE, Amy, "Intermittent Fasting: Not So Fast." Diabetes Self-Management, August 12, 2013. http://www.diabetesselfmanagement.com/blog/intermittent-fasting-not-so-fast/

Cant Sleep, "Chamomile." (Accessed 2016.) http://www.cantsleep.org/aids/chamomile.html

Capsule Depot, "Differences Between Vegetarian and Gelatin Capsules." (Accessed 2016.) http://www.capsuledepot.com/differences-between-vegetarian-and-gelatin-capsules/

Carpenter-Thompson, Jake, Schmidt, Sara, McAueley, Edward, Husain, Fatima T., "Increased Frontal Response May Underlie Decreased Tinnitus Severity." PLoS ONE 10(12): e0144419. https://doi.org/10.1371/journal.pone.0144419

Carol (Member), "Hush Tinnitus Sound Therapy Experiences?" Tinnitus Talk, November 12, 2013. https://www.tinnitustalk.com/threads/hush-tinnitus-sound-therapy-experiences.2470/

Carollo, Kim, "Getting Relief From Tinnitus May Be Mind Over Matter." ABC News, July 22, 2011. http://abcnews.go.com/Health/mind-body-intervention-holds-promise-alleviating-tinnitus-symptoms/story?id=14126165

Carroll, Ph.D., Jeff, "Hope for Veterans with Military Service-Induced Tinnitus." Defense Media Network, April 2014, http://www.defensemedianetwork.com/stories/hope-for-veterans-with-military-service-induced-tinnitus/

Carroll, Linda, "'It's going to get worse': Nearly 30 percent of teens have hearing damage." TODAY, June 7, 2016. http://www.nbc15.com/content/news/Its-going-to-get-worse-Nearly-30-percent-of-teens-have-hearing-damage-382118261.html

Cassani, Monica, "GABA/glutamate system and how it might work with benzodiazepines and Lamictal." Beyond Meds, May 24, 2010. https://beyondmeds.com/2010/05/24/gabaglutamate-system-benzos-lamictal/

Castro, Joseph, "What Is Pink Noise?" Live Science, July 29, 2013. http://www.livescience.com/38464-what-is-pink-noise.html

Cavalheiro, Esper A., John W. Olney, "Glutamate Antagonists: Deadly liaisons with cancer." Proceedings of the National Academy of Sciences of the United States of America, May 22, 2001. http://www.ncbi.nlm.nih.gov/pmc/articles/PMC33400/

Cell Press, "In search of tinnitus, that phantom ringing in the ears." ScienceDaily. *ScienceDaily*, April 23, 2015. https://www.sciencedaily.com/releases/2015/04/150423125858.htm

Center for Hearing and Communication, "Common Environmental Noise Levels." (Accessed 2016.) http://chchearing.org/noise/common-environmental-noise-levels/

Centers for Disease Control and Prevention, "Fact Sheets - Alcohol and Caffeine." June 9, 2017. https://www.cdc.gov/alcohol/fact-sheets/caffeine-and-alcohol.htm

Centers for Disease Control and Prevention, "High Blood Pressure Frequently Asked Questions (FAQs)." (Accessed 2017.) http://www.cdc.gov/bloodpressure/faqs.htm#2

Cerebrum Function, "Cerebellum Function." (Accessed 2016.) http://cerebrumfunction.net/cerebellum-function/

Cerebrum Function, "Cerebrum function definition." (Accessed 2016.) http://cerebrumfunction.net/cerebrum-function-definition/

Cerebrum Function, "Lobe functions in the cerebrum." (Accessed 2016.) http://cerebrumfunction.net/lobe-functions-in-the-cerebrum/

Cerner Moltum, "Clonazepam." Drugs, September 28, 2016. https://www.drugs.com/clonazepam.html

Champ, Dr. Colin, "The Ketogenic Diet and Vegetarianism: Can They Co-Exist?" Health Wire, October 15, 2014. http://www.myhealthwire.com/news/breakthroughs/895

Chartrand, Ph.D., BC-HIS, "Tinnitus Loudness Perception in Precipitous HF Losses." Audiology Online, April 18, 2005. http://www.audiologyonline.com/articles/tinnitus-loudness-perception-in-precipitous-1035

Chaudhari, Nirupa, Hui Yang, Cynthia Lamp, et al., "The Taste of Monosodium Glutamate: Membrane Receptors in Taste Buds." *The Journal of Neuroscience*, Volume 16, Number 12, June 15, 1996. http://www.jneurosci.org/content/16/12/3817.full

Bibliography

Chen, C.R., R. Tan, W.M. Qu, et al., "Magnolol, a major bioactive constituent of the bark of *Magnolia officinalis*, exerts antiepileptic effects via the GABA/benzodiazepine receptor complex in mice." *British Journal of Pharmacology*, Volume 164, Issue 5, November 2011. https://www.ncbi.nlm.nih.gov/pubmed/21518336

Cherry, Kendra, "Can We Reverse Brain Cell Loss?' VeryWell, October 5, 2017. https://www.verywell.com/adult-neurogenesis-can-we-grow-new-brain-cells-2794885

Cherry, Kendra, "What Is Cognitive Behavioral Therapy?" VeryWell, July 12, 2017. https://www.verywell.com/what-is-cognitive-behavior-therapy-2795747

Cherry, Kendra, "What is the Role of the Hippocampus?" VeryWell, September 26, 2017. https://www.verywell.com/what-is-the-hippocampus-2795231

Cherry, Kendra, "When and Why Does Habituation Occur?" VeryWell, October 9, 2017. https://www.verywell.com/what-is-habituation-2795233

Church, William H., Ryan E. Adams, Livia S. Wyss, "Ketogenic diet alters dopaminergic activity in the mouse cortex." *Neuroscience Letters*, Volume 571, June 13, 2014. http://www.sciencedirect.com/science/article/pii/S030439401400319X

Circadian Sleep Disorders Network, "Treatments for Delayed Sleep Phase and Non-24." (Accessed 2017.) https://www.circadiansleepdisorders.org/treatments.php

Clason, Debbie, "Have sleep apnea? You might have hearing loss, too." Healthy Hearing, June 27, 2014. http://www.healthyhearing.com/report/52200-Have-sleep-apnea-you-might-have-hearing-loss-too

Cleveland Clinic, "Age Related Hearing Loss." (Accessed 2016.) http://my.clevelandclinic.org/health/diseases_conditions/hic_What_is_Presbycusis

Cohen, Joyce, "Want a Better Listener? Protect Those Ears." *The New York Times*, March 1, 2010. http://www.nytimes.com/2010/03/02/health/02baby.html

Cohen, Joyce, "When even soft noises feel like a knife to the eardrums." STAT, February 18, 2016. http://www.statnews.com/2016/02/18/noise-induced-ear-pain/

Cohn, MD, Thomas, "Is Your Chronic Pain an Addiction?" Minnesota Physical Medicine Blog, January 8, 2016. http://mnphysicalmedicine.com/2016/01/08/chronic-pain-an-addiction/

College Site, "Types of Brainwaves." (Accessed 2016.) http://www.collagesite.org/causeof/brainwaves.htm#Alpha

Collingwood, Jane, (Reviewed by John M. Grohol, Psy.D.), "The Power of Music to Reduce Stress." PsychCentral, 2016. http://psychcentral.com/lib/the-power-of-music-to-reduce-stress/

Collins, BSc, BCM, Simone, "Sound Therapy Research: Tinnitus." Sound Therapy Perth, October 2, 2014. http://www.soundtherapyperth.com/research/tinnitus.php

Consumer Reports, "Hearing Aid Buying Guide." February 2017. http://www.consumerreports.org/cro/hearing-aids/buying-guide.htm

Contestabile, Antonio, Silvia Sintoni, Barbara Monti, "Histone Deacetylase (HDAC) Inhibitors as Potential Drugs to Target Memory and Adult Hippocampal Neurogenesis." *Current Psychopharmacology*, Volume 1, Issue 1, 2012. http://www.eurekaselect.com/96064/article

Cool, Lisa Collier, "Are Male and Female Brains Different?" WebMD. (Accessed 2017.) http://www.webmd.com/brain/features/how-male-female-brains-differ#1

Corbett, Ian, "What Data Compression Does to Your Music." Sound On Sound, April 2012. http://www.soundonsound.com/sos/apr12/articles/lost-in-translation.htm

Core Spirit, "Background on Sound Therapy Research." (Accessed 2016.)
http://www.corespirit.com/background-sound-therapy-research/

Cotman, Carl W., Jennifer S. Kahle, Stephan E. Miller, et al., "Excitatory Amino Acid
Neurotransmission." 2000. https://www.acnp.org/g4/GN401000007/Default.htm

Cox, Ashley, "The Science Behind Heartbreak." Science 2.0, November 14, 2008.
www.science20.com/variety_tap/science_behind_heartbreak-33900

Crummer, M.D., Richard W., Ghinwa A. Hassan, M.D., "Diagnostic Approach to Tinnitus."
American Family Physician, January 1, 2004 (69).
http://www.aafp.org/afp/2004/0101/p120.html

CVAX Magazine, "Information on the chemotherapy medication Cisplatin." (Accessed 2016.)
http://cisplatin.org

daedalus (Member), "HIFU (High Intensity Focused Ultrasound) Surgery." Tinnitus Talk,
February 21, 2012. https://www.tinnitustalk.com/threads/hifu-high-intensity-
focused-ultrasound-surgery.276/

Daftary, Aditya, Abraham Shulman, Arnold M. Strashun, et al., "Benzodiazepine receptor
distribution in severe intractable tinnitus." The International Tinnitus Journal, 2004.
https://www.researchgate.net/publication/8336256_Benzodiazepine_receptor_
distribution_in_severe_intractable_tinnitus

Dangerous Decibels, "Decibel Exposure Time Guidelines, How loud is too loud?" http://
dangerousdecibels.org/education/information-center/decibel-exposure-time-guidelines/

Day, MD, John, "10 Ways to Boost Brain Function With BDNF." March 1, 2015.
http://drjohnday.com/10-ways-to-boost-brain-function-with-bdnf/

Daya, Shabir, "The Multiple Benefits of Taurine." Victoria Health.
https://www.victoriahealth.com/editorial/the-multiple-benefits-of-taurine

Deans, MD, Emily, "Autism and Ketogenic Diets." Psychology Today, April 8, 2011.
https://www.psychologytoday.com/blog/evolutionary-psychiatry/201104/autism-and-
ketogenic-diets

Deans, MD, Emily, "Yoga (ba) GABA, Evidence that yoga can enhance anxiety-killing
neurotransmitters in the brain." Psychology Today, March 15, 2013.
https://www.psychologytoday.com/blog/evolutionary-psychiatry/201303/yoga-ba-gaba

DeNoon, Daniel J., "The Truth About Vitamin D: Can You Get Too Much Vitamin D?" WebMd.
(Accessed 2017.) http://www.webmd.com/osteoporosis/features/the-truth-about-
vitamin-d-can-you-get-too-much-vitamin-d

De Ridder, Dirk, Elsa van der Loo, Karolien Van der Kelen, et al., "Theta, alpha and beta
burst transcranial magnetic stimulation: brain modulation in tinnitus."
International Journal of Medical Sciences, Volume 4, Number 5, October 2007.
http://www.medsci.org/v04p0237.htm

Dhamma, "Vipassana Meditation." (Accessed 2016.) http://www.dhamma.org/en-US/index

Doc Gautham's Neuro Centre, "Brain Waves." (Accessed 2017.)
www.docgautham.com/causes/brain_waves

Doheny, Kathleen, "Choose Dark Chocolate for Health Benefits." WebMD, April 4, 2012.
https://www.webmd.com/diet/news/20120424/pick-dark-chocolate-health-benefits#1

Dohrmann, Katalin, Nathan Weisz, Winfried Schlee, et al., "Neurofeedback for treating tinnitus."
Progress in Brain Research, Volume 166, 2007.
https://www.ncbi.nlm.nih.gov/pubmed/17956812

Donaldson, Gloria, "What Will Happen To Your Body When You Stop Exercising." Lifehack. (Accessed 2017.) http://www.lifehack.org/323427/what-will-happen-your-body-when-you-stop-exercising

Donovan, John, "How to Sleep Easier With Your CPAP Machine." WebMD. (Accessed 2017.) http://www.webmd.com/sleep-disorders/sleep-apnea/continuous-positive-airway-pressure-cpap-for-obstructive-sleep-apnea

Drozdowski, Ted, "It Might Get Loud: The 10 Loudest Rock Bands of All Time." Gibson, February 18, 2014. http://www.gibson.com/News-Lifestyle/Features/en-us/10-Loudest-Rock-Bands.aspx

Drugs, "User Reviews for Alprazolam." (Accessed 2016.) https://www.drugs.com/comments/alprazolam/for-tinnitus.html

Duggal, Neel, (Reviewed by Timothy J. Legg, PMHNP-BC), "Attention Deficit Hyperactive Disorder (ADHD): The Role of Dopamine." June 10, 2016. https://www.healthline.com/health/adhd/adhd-dopamine#overview1

Dvorsky, George, "Playing Scrabble Changes the Way You Use Your Brain." Gizmodo, October 1, 2015. https://gizmodo.com/playing-scrabble-changes-the-way-you-use-your-brain-1734003624

Educational Healthcare Resources, "The Ventricles of the Brain." (Accessed 2016.) http://teachmeanatomy.info/neuro/vessels/ventricles

Educational Healthcare Resources, "The Vestibulocochlear Nerve (CN VIII)." (Accessed 2017.) http://teachmeanatomy.info/head/cranial-nerves/vestibulocochlear/

Edwards, Lin, "Study suggests reliance on GPS may reduce hippocampus function as we age." Medical XPress, November 18, 2010. https://medicalxpress.com/news/2010-11-reliance-gps-hippocampus-function-age.html

Ehrlich, NMD, Steven D., "Aromatherapy." University of Maryland Medical Center, August 9, 2011. http://www.umm.edu/health/medical/altmed/treatment/aromatherapy

Ehrlich, NMD, Steven D., "Lemon Balm." University of Maryland Medical Center, January 2, 2015. http://umm.edu/health/medical/altmed/herb/lemon-balm

Ehrlich, NMD, Steven H. "Valerian." University of Maryland Medical Center, June 26, 2014. http://umm.edu/health/medical/altmed/herb/valerian

Eíríu-Eolas, "Vagus nerve stimulation - Tinnitus: Latest Research Results May Help to 'eliminate the source of the tinnitus.'" January 21, 2011. https://eiriu-eolas.org/2011/01/21/vagus-nerve-stimulation-tinnitus-latest-research-results-may-help-to-"eliminate-the-source-of-the-tinnitus"/

Enzor, MBiol, Laura, "What is Norepinephrine? - Effects, Function & Definition." Study. (Accessed 2016.) http://study.com/academy/lesson/what-is-norepinephrine-effects-function-definition.html

EOC Institute, "Meditation Boosts Anti-Anxiety Neurotransmitters: Serotonin & GABA." (Accessed 2017.) https://eocinstitute.org/meditation/8-reasons-meditation-best-natural-anxiety-relief-technique/#codeword2

erik (Member), "Light Therapy In Treatment of Tinnitus." Tinnitus Talk, July 4, 2012. https://www.tinnitustalk.com/threads/light-therapy-in-treatment-of-tinnitus.470/#post-2879

EurekAlert!, American Association for the Advancement of Science, "Quiet that ringing in the brain." June 23, 2015. http://www.eurekalert.org/pub_releases/2015-06/uoc-qtr062315.php

European College of Neuropsychopharmacology, "Neurogenesis in Adult Brain: Association With Stress And Depression." September 2, 2008. https://www.sciencedaily.com/releases/2008/08/080831114717.htm

Examine, "Idebenone." (Accessed 2016.) https://examine.com/supplements/idebenone

Examine, "Magnolia officinalis." (Accessed 2016.)
https://examine.com/supplements/magnolia-officinalis/

Examine, "Melissa officinalis." (Accessed 2016.)
https://examine.com/supplements/Melissa+officinalis/

Examine, "Theanine." (Accessed 2016.) http://examine.com/supplements/Theanine/

Fan, Shelly, "The fat-fueled brain: unnatural or advantageous?" *Scientific American*,
October 1, 2013. https://blogs.scientificamerican.com/mind-guest-blog/
the-fat-fueled-brain-unnatural-or-advantageous/

Farlet, Pete, "Research Opened Door to Restoring Brain Damaged Function." University of
California San Francisco News Center, June 2, 2016. https://www.ucsf.edu/news/
2016/06/403136/michael-merzenich-wins-2016-kavli-prize-neuroscience

Feller, Stephen, "Researchers find gene network that repairs nervous system." February 19,
2016. https://www.upi.com/Health_News/2016/02/19/Researchers-find-gene-network-
that-repairs-nervous-system/5571455914957/

Fernandez, Alvaro, "20 Must-Know Facts to Harness Neuroplasticity and Improve Brain Health."
The Creativity Post, June 22, 2016. http://www.creativitypost.com/science/20_must_know_
facts_to_harness_neuroplasticity_and_improve_brain_health

Fernandez, Alvaro, "Test Your Brain with these Brain Teasers, Games and Illusions."
SharpBrains, May 26, 2008.
https://sharpbrains.com/blog/2008/05/26/brain-games-and-teasers-top-50/

Fornaro, Michele, Matteo Martino, "Tinnitus psychopharmacology: A comprehensive review of
its pathomechanisms and management." Neuropsychiatric Disease and Treatment, 2010.
https://www.ncbi.nlm.nih.gov/pmc/articles/PMC2898164/

Fotuhi, Majid, Dr., "Can you grow your hippocampus? Yes, here's how, and why it matters."
SharpBrains. November 4, 2015. http://sharpbrains.com/blog/2015/11/04/can-you-grow-
your-hippocampus-yes-heres-how-and-why-it-matters/

Fountain, Henry, "Suppressing Tinnitus With Music Therapy." The New York Times, January 4,
2010. http://www.nytimes.com/2010/01/05/science/05obhear.html?ref=science

Gabriel, Linda, "Brain Wave Basics - What You Need to Know about States of Consciousness."
Thought Medicine. (Accessed 2016.) http://thoughtmedicine.com/2011/06/brain-wave-
basics-what-you-need-to-know-about-states-of-consciousness/

Gagnon, Louise, "Light, laser therapy may stimulate hair growth." Dermatology Times,
April 1, 2014. http://dermatologytimes.modernmedicine.com/dermatology-times/content/
tags/dermatology/light-laser-therapy-may-stimulate-hair-growth?page=full

Galen Carol Audio, "The Relationship of Voltage, Power, Loudness and Decibels." (Accessed
2017.) https://www.gcaudio.com/tips-tricks/the-relationship-of-voltage-loudness-power-
and-decibels/

Gall, Dr. James, "Tinnitus Causes." http://tinnitus.net/tinnitus-causes.php

Gan, Ling, Emily England, Jeong-Yeh Yang, et al., "A 72-hour high fat diet increases transcript
levels of the neuropeptide galanin in the dorsal hippocampus of the rat."
BMC Neuroscience, August 11, 2015.
https://bmcneurosci.biomedcentral.com/articles/10.1186/s12868-015-0188-9

Gandel, Cathie, "Paying for Your Hearing Aid." AARP, April 2016. http://www.aarp.org/health/
conditions-treatments/info-05-2011/paying-for-hearing-aids.html

Gandel, Cathie, "Why Do Hearing Aids Cost So Much?" AARP, October 3, 2016. http://www.aarp.org/health/conditions-treatments/info-2016/hearing-aid-costs-prices-cs.html

Garvin, Karen S., "Magnesium & Sensitive Hearing." Livestrong, October 3, 2017. https://www.livestrong.com/article/529672-magnesium-sensitive-hearing/

Gary, Claudia, "Tinnitus: The Thief of Silence." Vietnam Veterans of America, March/April 2013. http://vvaveteran.org/33-2/33-2_tinnitus.html

Gena (Member), "Benzos." Tinnitus Talk, February 16, 2016. https://www.tinnitustalk.com/threads/benzos.13605/#post-164966

Georgetown University Medical Center. "Imaging reveals how brain fails to tune out phantom sounds of tinnitus." ScienceDaily. *ScienceDaily*, June 23, 2010. https://www.sciencedaily.com/releases/2010/06/100623123338.htm

Georgetown University Medical Center. "Neuroscientists uncover brain abnormalities responsible for tinnitus and chronic pain." ScienceDaily. *ScienceDaily*, September 23, 2015. http://www.sciencedaily.com/releases/2015/09/150923133521.htm

Giese, Maria, Eva Unternaehrer, Serge Brand, et al., The Interplay of Stress and Sleep Impacts BDNF Level." *Public Library of Science ONE*, October 16, 2013. http://journals.plos.org/plosone/article?id=10.1371/journal.pone.0076050

Gillaspy, Rebecca, "Pineal Gland, Functions, Melatonin & Circadian Rhythm." Study, http://study.com/academy/lesson/pineal-gland-functions-melatonin-circadian-rhythm.html

Godiyal, Sandeep, "Anthocyanin-rich foods you should be eating." Natural News, October 17, 2013. http://www.naturalnews.com/042540_anthocyanins_antioxidants_healthy_foods.html

Goldstein, Ph.D., Barbara, Abraham Shulman, MD, "Tinnitus - Hyperacusis and the Loudness Discomfort Level Test - A Preliminary Report." *International Tinnitus Journal*, Volume 2, Number 1, 1996. http://www.tinnitusjournal.com/articles/tinnitus--hyperacusis-and-the-loudness-discomfort-level-test--a-preliminary-report.pdf

GoodTherapy, "Acetylcholine." August 4, 2015. http://www.goodtherapy.org/blog/psychpedia/acetylcholine

Goto, Fumiyuki, Juri Saruta, Sho Kanzaki, et al., "Various levels of plasma brain-derived neurotrophic factor in patients with tinnitus." *Neuroscience Letters*, February 2012. https://www.researchgate.net/publication/221781294_various_levels_of_plasma_brain-derived_neurotrophic_factor_in_patients_with_tinnitus

Governing, "State Marijuana Laws in 2017 Map." (Accessed 2017.) http://www.governing.com/gov-data/state-marijuana-laws-map-medical-recreational.html

Gradiavita, "The 'awakened mind' - the optimally functioning brain." (Accessed 2016.) http://gradiavita.com/en/gehirnwellen/

Grant1 (Member), "Marijuana/Cannabis and Tinnitus." Tinnitus Talk, September 9, 2013. https://www.tinnitustalk.com/threads/marijuana-cannabis-and-tinnitus.1993/

Grant, Bob, "One-Man Tinnitus Map." The Scientist, April 26, 2015. http://www.the-scientist.com/?articles.view/articleNo/42823/title/One-Man-Tinnitus-Map/

Green, Tara, "Does green tea have caffeine? Seven things you need to know." Natural News, November 23, 2011. http://www.naturalnews.com/034227_green_tea_caffeine.html

Grohol, Psy.D., John M.,"Clinical factors of tinnitus influence perceived loudness and annoyance." PsychCentral, April 30, 2016. https://psychcentral.com/news/archives/2006-12/jaaj-cfo121406.html

Guest contributor, "What is the Hippocampus?" ReliaWire, April 4, 2012. http://reliawire.com/hippocampus/

Gunnars, BSc, Kris, "10 Evidence-Based Health Benefits of Intermittent Fasting." Healthline, August 16, 2016. https://authoritynutrition.com/10-health-benefits-of-intermittent-fasting/

Gunnars, BSc, Kris, "10 Proven Health Benefits of Turmeric and Curcumin." Healthline, June 9, 2017. https://authoritynutrition.com/top-10-evidence-based-health-benefits-of-turmeric/

Hagg, Theo, "From Neurotransmitters to Neurotrophic Factors to Neurogenesis." Neuroscientist, Volume 15, Issue 1, February 2009. http://www.ncbi.nlm.nih.gov/pmc/articles/PMC2722065/

Hahn, Dr. Adam, "Tinnitus Is the Most Common Injury for Veterans of Afghanistan and Iraq." Smile Columbia Dentistry, November 20, 2013. https://www.tmjtreatmentsc.com/tinnitus-common-injury-veterans-afghanistan-iraq/

Hain, M.D., Timothy C., "Tinnitus Defined." Dizziness-and-balance, September 17, 2016. http://www.dizziness-and-balance.com/disorders/hearing/tinnitus.htm

Hamilton Spectator, "McMaster team pinpoints source of tinnitus." (Accessed 2016.) http://www.thespec.com/news-story/2177153-mcmaster-team-pinpoints-source-of-tinnitus/

Hanus, Bill, "Acoustic Trauma - How to Avoid It." Gun Dogs Online. (Accessed 2017.) http://www.gundogsonline.com/Article/acoustic-trauma-how-to-avoid-it-Page1.htm

Harris, Sam, "Adventures in the Land of Illness." Sam Harris Blog, May 26, 2014. https://www.samharris.org/blog/item/adventures-in-the-land-of-illness

Harris, Tom, "How Hearing Works, Fluid Wave." HowStuffWorks. (Accessed 2016.) http://health.howstuffworks.com/mental-health/human-nature/perception/hearing4.htm

Harris, Tom, "How Hearing Works, Hair Cells." HowStuffWorks. (Accessed 2016.) http://health.howstuffworks.com/mental-health/human-nature/perception/hearing5.htm

Harvard Medical School, "Blue light has a dark side." Harvard Health Letter, September 2, 2015. http://www.health.harvard.edu/staying-healthy/blue-light-has-a-dark-side

Harvard Medical School, Department of Neurobiology, "Dancing and the Brain." (Accessed 2017.) http://neuro.hms.harvard.edu/harvard-mahoney-neuroscience-institute/brain-newsletter/and-brain-series/dancing-and-brain

Hashmi, J.A., M.N. Baliki, L. Huang, et al., "Shape shifting pain: chronification of back pain shifts pain representation from nociceptve to emotional circuits." Brain, September 2013. https://www.ncbi.nlm.nih.gov/pubmed/23983029

Hasson, Dan, Töres Theorell, Martin Benka Wallén, et al, "Stress and prevalence of hearing problems in the Swedish working population." http://bmcpublichealth.biomedcentral.com/articles/10.1186/1471-2458-11-130

Hattan, Ph.D., David G., "FALSE: Aspartame - Sweet Poison." USFDA, Division of Health Effects Evaluation, June 8, 2015. http://www.snopes.com/medical/toxins/aspartame.asp

Hauptmann, Christian, Armin Ströbel, Mark Williams, et al., "Acoustic Coordinated Reset Neuromodulation in a Real Life Patient Population with Chronic Tonal Tinnitus." BioMed Research International, Volume 2015, January 11, 2015. https://www.hindawi.com/journals/bmri/2015/569052

Hazell, Jonathan, "Environmental Sound Enrichment." 2015. http://tinnitus.org/sound-enrichment/

Heagberg, Kat, "This is Your Brain on Yoga." Yoga International, January 15, 2014. https://yogainternational.com/article/view/this-is-your-brain-on-yoga

HealthAliciousNess, "Top 10 Foods Highest in Saturated Fat." September 12, 2017. https://www.healthaliciousness.com/articles/foods-highest-in-saturated-fat.php

Health Line, "Can Hops Help You Sleep?" (Accessed 2017.)
http://www.healthline.com/health/can-hops-get-me-to-sleep#Otheruses4

Hearing and Speech Center, "Tinnitus FAQ - What Is Biofeedback?" (Accessed 2017.)
https://www.hearingspeech.org/services/audiology-services/tinnitus/

Hear-It, "Gender a factor in the side effects of tinnitus." (Accessed 2017.)
http://www.hear-it.org/Gender-a-factor-in-the-side-effects-of-tinnitus

Hear-It, "Hearing aids stimulate brain activity." (Accessed 2016.)
http://www.hear-it.org/hearing-aids-stimulate-brain-activity

Hear-It, "Sudden Hearing Loss - SSNHL." (Accessed 2016.)
http://www.hear-it.org/Sudden-Hearing-Loss

Hearing Direct, "Hearing Aid Types." (Accessed 2016.)
http://www.hearingdirect.com/us/pages/Hearing-Aid-Types.html

Hearing Health Foundation, "Hearing Loss & Tinnitus Statistics." (Accessed 2017.)
https://hearinghealthfoundation.org/hearing-loss-tinnitus-statistics/

Hearing Health Foundation, "What is Tinnitus." (Accessed 2017.)
https://hearinghealthfoundation.org/tinnitus-resources

Hearing Loss Association of America, "Basic Facts About Hearing Loss." (Accessed 2016.)
http://hearingloss.org/content/basic-facts-about-hearing-loss

Hearing Science, "Natural Nutrients for Better Hearing Health." February 13, 2017.
http://www.hearing-science.com/2017/02/13/natural-nutrients-better-hearing-health/

Hedlin, M., "Diet and Neurogenesis." Huntington's Outreach Project for Education, at Stanford,
July 1, 2011. http://web.stanford.edu/group/hopes/cgi-bin/hopes_test/diet-and-
neurogenesis/

Heller, A.J., "Classification and epidemiology of tinnitus." *Otolaryngologic Clinics of North
America*, April 2003. http://www.ncbi.nlm.nih.gov/pubmed/12856294

Henry1492 (Member), "Is LLLT for Tinnitus by Dr. Wilden a Scam?" Tinnitus Talk, March 10,
2016. https://www.tinnitustalk.com/threads/is-lllt-for-tinnitus-by-dr-wilden-a-scam.14079/

Heuser Hearing Institute, "Tinnitus." (Accessed 2017.)
https://thehearinginstitute.org/clinic/clinical-services/tinnitus/

Heyman, Elsa, François-Xavier Gamelin, Maaike Goekint, et al., "Intense exercise increases
circulating endocannabinoid and BDNF levels in humans--possible implications for reward
and depression. *Psychoneuroendocrinology*, Volume 37, Number 6, June 2012.
http://www.ncbi.nlm.nih.gov/pubmed/22029953

Hidden Hearing, "What is Tinnitus?" (Accessed 2017.)
https://www.hiddenhearing.ie/hearing-loss/what-is-tinnitus

Honkura, Yohei, Hirotaka Matsuo, Shohei Murakami, et al., "NRF2 Is a Key Target for Prevention
of Noise-Induced Hearing Loss by Reducing Oxidative Damage of Cochlea." *Scientific
Reports*, January 18, 2016. http://www.nature.com/articles/srep19329

Hopkins, Sharon, "Olive Oil Ear Wax." Home Remedies for you. (Accessed 2016.)
http://www.home-remedies-for-you.com/articles/1094/diseases-and-ailments/
olive-oil-ear-wax.html

Hubbard, Dr. Bruce, "Dr. Hubbard's Tinnitus Story." CBT for Tinnitus. (Accessed 2017.)
http://www.cbtfortinnitus.com/dr-hubbards-story/

Huelke, Donald F., Jamie L. Moore, Timothy W. Compton, et al., "Hearing loss and automobile
airbag deployments." *Accident Analysis & Prevention*, November 1999, Volume 31,
Issue 6. http://www.sciencedirect.com/science/article/pii/S0001457599000329

Humphries, Courtney, "Regenerating Teeth, and Maybe Other Body Parts, with Light." MIT Technology Review, May 30, 2014. https://www.technologyreview.com/s/527701/regenerating-teeth-and-maybe-other-body-parts-with-light/

Hyman, MD, Mark, "Essential Glutathione: The Mother of all Antioxidants." Dr. Hyman Blog. (Accessed 2016.) http://drhyman.com/blog/2010/05/19/glutathione-the-mother-of-all-antioxidants/

I who love music (Member), "Back to Silence." Tinnitus Talk, December 7, 2014. https://www.tinnitustalk.com/threads/back-to-silence.7172/

Integrated Supplements, "Creatine - A Possible Weapon Against Tinnitus And Noise-Induced Hearing Loss." January 4, 2010. http://integratedsupplements.typepad.com/integrated_supplements_bl/2010/01/creatine-a-possible-weapon-against-tinnitus-and-noiseinduced-hearing-loss.html

International Neuromodulation Society, "Neuromodulation, or Neuromodulatory Effect." http://www.neuromodulation.com/neuromodulation-defined

Jankowiak, MD, Janet, "Too Much Sugar May Cause Brain Decay." Neurology, Volume 63, Number 4, August 24, 2004. http://www.neurology.org/content/63/4/E9.full

Jenkins, MD, FRCP, J.S., "The Mozart effect." Journal of the Royal Society of Medicine, April 2001. https://www.ncbi.nlm.nih.gov/pmc/articles/PMC1281386/

Jefferson Philadelphia University + Thomas Jefferson University, "Jefferson First Hospital in City to Offer New, Non-Invasive Tinnitus Treatment." (Accessed 2016.) http://www.jefferson.edu/university/jmc/departments/otolaryngology/centers/balance_hearing/news_tinnitus.html

Ji, Guangchen, Volker Neugebauer, "CB1 augments mGluR5 function in medial prefrontal cortical neurons to inhibit amygdala hyperactivity in an arthritis pain model." European Journal of Neuroscience, February 2014. http://europepmc.org/articles/PMC4288820

jibs (Member), "Acoustic CR® Neuromodulation: Do It Yourself Guide." Tinnitus Talk, April 24, 2013. https://www.tinnitustalk.com/threads/acoustic-cr-neuromodulation-do-it-yourself-guide.1469/

Jikomes, Nick, "What is the Endocannabinoid System and What is Its Role?" Leafly. (Accessed 2016.) https://www.leafly.com/news/science-tech/what-is-the-endocannabinoid-system

Jockers, Dr. David, "Reduce inflammation and stop tinnitus." Natural News, January 16, 2011. http://www.naturalnews.com/031021_tinnitus_inflammation.html

joe (Member), "Hyperbaric Oxygen Therapy." Tinnitus Talk, January 18, 2012. https://www.tinnitustalk.com/threads/hyperbaric-oxygen-therapy.211/

joe (Member), "Low-Level Laser Therapy (LLLT) for Tinnitus - Experiences (Dr. Wilden, etc)." Tinnitus Talk. (Accessed 2016.) https://www.tinnitustalk.com/threads/low-level-laser-therapy-lllt-for-tinnitus-%E2%80%94-experiences-dr-wilden-etc.295/

Johns Hopkins Medical Institutions. "Ears Ringing? Cells In Developing Ear May Explain Tinnitus." ScienceDaily. ScienceDaily, November 5, 2007. http://www.sciencedaily.com/releases/2007/10/071031152922.htm

Johns Hopkins Medicine, "Transcranial Direct Current Stimulation." (Accessed 2017.) http://www.hopkinsmedicine.org/psychiatry/specialty_areas/brain_stimulation/tdcs.html

Johnson, Cort, "Breaking the BDNF Blues: Dr. Courtney Craig D.C. on Natural Ways to Raise BDNF Levels in Chronic Fatigue Syndrome." Pro Health, June 18, 2014. http://www.prohealth.com/library/showarticle.cfm?libid=18998

Johnson, Cort, "Magnetic Effect: New Brain Technology Reduces Pain in Fibromyalgia." ProHealth, April 8, 2014. http://www.prohealth.com/library/showArticle.cfm? libid=18871&site=articles

Joslin Diabetes Center, "Joslin Study Links High Glutamate Levels in Brain with Depression, Low Cognitive Function." August 3, 2009. http://www.joslin.org/news/ joslin_study_links_high_glutamate_levels_in_brain_with_depression.html

Jon Wayne (Member), "Tinnitus Pitch and Loudness Matching." Tinnitus Talk, January 27, 2012. https://www.tinnitustalk.com/threads/tinnitus-pitch-and-loudness-matching.242/

Kahlbrock, Nina, Nathan Weisz, "Transient reduction of tinnitus intensity is marked by concomitant reductions of delta band power." BioMed Central Biology, January 16, 2008. https://bmcbiol.biomedcentral.com/articles/10.1186/1741-7007-6-4

Kaidanovich-Beilin, Oksana, Danielle S. Cha, Roger S. McIntyre, "Metabolism and the Brain." The Scientist, December 1, 2012. http://www.the-scientist.com/?articles.view/articleNo/33338/title/Metabolism-and-the-Brain/

Kalish, Nancy, "Hearing Loss Prevention: Loud Noises We Hear Daily." Huffington Post, March 2015. http://www.huffingtonpost.com/2013/02/07/hearing-loss-loud-noises-noise-levels_n_2632499.html

Kaltenbach, James, "Insights on the origins of tinnitus: An overview of recent research." Hearing Journal, Volume 62, Issue 2, February 2009. http://journals.lww.com/thehearingjournal/ Fulltext/2009/02000/Insights_on_the_origins_of_tinnitus__An_overview.5.aspx

Karlidag, Turgut, Şinasi Yalçin, Ahmet Öztürk, et al., "The role of free oxygen radicals in noise induced hearing loss: effects of melatonin and methylprednisolone." Auris Nasus Larynx, Volume 29, Issue 2, April 2002. http://www.sciencedirect.com/science/article/pii/S0385814601001377

Keiley, Lynn, "Avoid Salt and Reduce Your Blood Pressure." Mother Earth News, June/July 2007. http://www.motherearthnews.com/natural-health/avoid-salt-reduce-blood-pressure.aspx

Keller, PhD, Simona, Marco Sarchiapone, MD, Federica Zarilli, PhD, et al., "Increased BDNF promoter methylation in the Wernicke area of suicide subjects." Archives of General Psychiatry, Volume 67, Number 3, 2010. https://jamanetwork.com/journals/jamapsychiatry/fullarticle/210623

Kennard, Jerry, "How Much Alcohol Is It Safe for Men to Drink?" VeryWell, February 21, 2017. http://menshealth.about.com/od/lifestyle/a/alcohol_intake.htm

Keville, Kathi, "Aromatherapy Stress Relief." HowStuffWorks. (Accessed 2016.) https://health.howstuffworks.com/wellness/natural-medicine/aromatherapy/ aromatherapy-stress-relief.htm

Keville, Kathi, "History of Aromatherapy." HowStuffWorks. (Accessed 2016.) https://health.howstuffworks.com/wellness/natural-medicine/aromatherapy/ history-of-aromatherapy.htm

Khan Academy, "Overview of the functions of the cerebral cortex." (Accessed 2016.) https://www.khanacademy.org/test-prep/mcat/behavior/biological-basis-of-behavior-ner/v/ overview-of-the-functions-of-the-cerebral-cortex

Killgore, William D.S., Elizabeth A. Olson, Mareen Weber, "Physical Exercise Habits Correlate with Gray Matter Volume of the Hippocampus in Healthy Adult Humans." Scientific Reports 3, December 12, 2013. http://www.nature.com/articles/srep03457

Kimpton, Jessica, "The Brain Derived Neurotrophic Factor and Influences of Stress in Depression." *Psychiatria Danubina*, Volume 24, 2012. http://www.hdbp.org/psychiatria_danubina/pdf/dnb_vol24_sup1/dnb_vol24_sup1_169.pdf

King, Ph.D., Michael W., "Brief Overview of Human Nervous System - Introduction to Neurotransmitters." (Accessed 2016.) themedicalbiochemistrypage.org/nerves.php

Kirkwood, David, "Researchers regenerate hair cells in deafened mice and improve their hearing." Hearing Health & Technology Matters, January 15, 2013. http://hearinghealthmatters.org/hearingnewswatch/2013/researchers-regenerate-hair-cells-in-deafened-mice-and-improve-their-hearing/

Knight, Isabelle, "Healing Trees." myNoise. (Accessed 2017.) https://mynoise.net/NoiseMachines/isabelleKnightHypnosisTalkGenerator.php

Knobloch, Marlen, Sebastian Jessberger, "Metabolism and Neurogenesis." *Current Opinion in Neurobiology*, Volume 42, February 2017. http://www.sciencedirect.com/science/article/pii/S0959438816302264

KnowMental, "Neurotransmitters: Serotonin Gaba Dopamine and Acetylcholine." (Accessed 2016.) http://knowmental.com/neurotransmitters-serotonin-gaba-dopamine-acetylcholine/

Koch, Sarah-Neena, "Hyperlinked Site Outline for MyBrainNotes.com." (Accessed 2016.) http://mybrainnotes.com/brain-anatomy-information.html

Koch, Sarah-Neena, "Sub-Cortical Brain Structures, Stress, Emotions, and Mental Illness." MyBrainNotes. (Accessed 2016.) http://mybrainnotes.com/memory-brain-stress.html

Kraus, K.S., S. Mitra, Z. Jimenez, et al., "Noise trauma impairs neurogenesis in the rat hippocampus." *Neuroscience*, June 2, 2012. http://www.ncbi.nlm.nih.gov/pubmed/20206235

Kronberg, Martin T., "Sulfite intolerance: A cause of tinnitus?" *Bioscience Hypotheses*, Volume 1, Issue 4, 2008. http://www.sciencedirect.com/science/article/pii/S1756239208000785

Krucik, MD, MBA, George (Reviewed by), "What Causes Ringing in Ears? 14 possible conditions." Healthline. (Accessed 2016.) http://www.healthline.com/symptom/ringing-in-ears

Kumar, Parvathy, Musthafa Essa, Samir Al-Adawi, "Omega-3 fatty acids could alleviate the risks of traumatic brain injury - a mini review." *Journal of Traditional and Complementary Medicine*, Volume 4, Number 2, April 2014. http://www.ncbi.nlm.nih.gov/pubmed/24860731

Landis, Ph.D., Bernard, Erica Landis, "Is biofeedback effective for chronic tinnitus? An intensive study with seven subjects." *American Journal of Otolaryngology*, Volume 13, Issue 6, November-December 1992. https://www.ncbi.nlm.nih.gov/pubmed/1443390

Lechtenberg, Richard, Abraham Shulman, "Benzodiazepines in the treatment of tinnitus." *The Journal of Laryngology & Otology*, Volume 98, 1984. https://www.researchgate.net/publication/232019268_Benzodiazepines_in_the_treatment_of_tinnitus

Lee, Augustine C., Donald A. Godfrey, "Cochlear Damage Affects Neurochemistry in the Central Auditory System." *Frontiers in Neurology*, November 19, 2014. http://europepmc.org/articles/PMC4237057

Lee, Matthew, "Foods That Help Hearing." Livestrong, July 18, 2017. https://www.livestrong.com/article/450373-foods-that-help-hearing/

Bibliography

Lehmann, Alexandre, Marc Schönwiesner, "Selective Attention Modulates Human Auditory Brainstem Responses: Relative Contributions of Frequency and Spatial Cues." *Public Library of Science ONE*, Volume 9, Issue 1, January 2014. http://www.academia.edu/14531594/Selective_Attention_Modulates_Human_Auditory_Brainstem_Responses_Relative_Contributions_of_Frequency_and_Spatial_Cues

Lichtman, Professor, Jeff, "What is synaptic plasticity?" Cold Spring Harbor Laboratory, DNA Learning Center. (Accessed 2016.) https://www.dnalc.org/view/2057-What-is-synaptic-plasticity-.html

Licinio, Julio, Ma-Li Wong, "Brain-derived neurotrophic factor in stress and affective disorders." *Molecular Psychiatry*, Volume 7, Number 6, 2002. http://www.nature.com/mp/journal/v7/n6/full/4001211a.html

Life Extension, "Hearing Loss and Tinnitus, How Hearing Loss Occurs." (Accessed 2016.) http://www.lifeextension.com/protocols/eye-ear/tinnitus/Page-04

Lijie, Liu, Pei Shen, Tingting He, et al., "Noise-induced hearing loss impairs spatial learning/memory and hippocampal neurogenesis in mice." Scientific Reports, February 4, 2016. https://www.nature.com/articles/srep20374

linearb (Member), "DIY Neurofeedback?" Tinnitus Talk, March 6, 2015. https://www.tinnitustalk.com/threads/diy-neurofeedback.8500/

Liou, Stephanie "Brain-derived neurotrophic factor (BDNF)." Huntington's Outreach Project for Education, at Stanford, June 26, 2010. http://web.stanford.edu/group/hopes/cgi-bin/hopes_test/brain-derived-neurotrophic-factor-bdnf/

Lisa88 (Member), "Intermittent Fasting for Tinnitus Relief." Tinnitus Talk, March 31, 2016. https://www.tinnitustalk.com/threads/intermittent-fasting-for-tinnitus-relief.14490/

Liu, Yuan F., Jinwei Hu, Matthew Steelman, O'neil W. Guthrie, "The Epworth Sleepiness Scale in the Assessment of Sleep Disturbance in Veterans with Tinnitus." *International Journal of Otolaryngology*, Volume 2015, December 19, 2014. https://www.hindawi.com/journals/ijoto/2015/429469/

Love, CNT, Amy, "Excitotoxins, MSG and its hidden names." Real Food Whole Health, 2011. http://www.realfoodwholehealth.com/2011/05/excitotoxins-msg-and-hidden-names/

Lutas, Andrew, Gary Yellen, "The ketogenic diet: Metabolic influences on brain excitability and epilepsy." *Trends in Neurosciences*, Volume 36, January 2013. https://www.ncbi.nlm.nih.gov/pubmed/23228828

Maguire, MD, Melissa (Contributor), "The Mozart Effect and epilepsy." Epilepsy Action, August 2015. https://www.epilepsy.org.uk/sites/epilepsy/files/info/references/Mozart%20effect%20F080.02.pdf

Mahboubi, Hossein, Kasra Ziai, Hamid R. Djalialian, "Customized web-based sound therapy for tinnitus." *International Tinnitus Journal*, Volume 17, No. 1, 2012. http://www.tinnitusjournal.com/detalhe_artigo.asp?id=496

Mahmoudian, Saeid, Mohammad Farhadi, Saeid Gholami, et al., "Pattern of brain blood perfusion in tinnitus patients using technetium-99m SPECT imaging." *Journal of Research in Medical Sciences*, Volume 17, March 2012. https://www.ncbi.nlm.nih.gov/pmc/articles/PMC3527041/

Malamed, Connie, "20 Facts You Must Know About Working Memory." The eLearning Coach. (Accessed 2016.) http://theelearningcoach.com/learning/20-facts-about-working-memory/

Marder, Jenny, "Neuroscience may offer hope to millions robbed of silence by tinnitus." NewsHour Productions, November 6, 2013. http://www.pbs.org/newshour/updates/science-july-dec13-tinnitus_11-06/

Marijuana Doctors, "Medical Marijuana and Tinnitus." (Accessed 2017.)
https://www.marijuanadoctors.com/content/ailments/view/102?ailment=tinnitus

Markou, Konstantinos, Panagiota Lalaki, Nikolaos Barbetakis, et al., "The efficacy of medication on tinnitus due to acute acoustic trauma." *Scandinavian Audiology*, 2001.
https://www.ncbi.nlm.nih.gov/pubmed/11318462

Marquize, Kelly, (edited by Paul Arnold), "The Role of Glutamate in OCD." Health Guide Info, December 18, 2010. http://www.healthguideinfo.com/ocd-treatment/p99790/

Martin, Psy.D., Ben, "In-Depth: Cognitive Behavioral Therapy." *Psych Central*, May 17, 2016.
https://psychcentral.com/lib/in-depth-cognitive-behavioral-therapy/

Massachusetts Eye and Ear, "Sudden Deafness." (Accessed 2016.)
http://www.masseyeandear.org/for-patients/patient-guide/patient-education/diseases-and-conditions/sudden-deafness

Massachusetts Institute of Technology, Research Laboratory of Electronics, "Introduction to Cochlear Micromechanics." (Accessed 2016.)
http://umech.mit.edu/hearing/intro/intro.html

Mattson, Mark P., "Neuroprotective signaling and the aging brain: Take away my food and let me run." *Brain Research*, Volume 886, Issue 1-2, December 15, 2000.
http://www.ncbi.nlm.nih.gov/pubmed/11119686

Maurer, Robert, "There's No Such Thing As Stress: Here's What's Really Bothering You." *Work Smart*, February 8, 2016. http://www.fastcompany.com/3056310/work-smart/theres-no-such-thing-as-stress-heres-whats-really-bothering-you

Max Planck Institute (Source), "Living Near a Forest Keeps Your Amygdala Healthier." Neuroscience News, October 13, 2017.
http://neurosciencenews.com/forest-amygdala-health-7737/

Mayo Clinic, "Epilepsy - Diagnosis & Treatment." (Accessed 2017.) https://www.mayoclinic.org/diseases-conditions/epilepsy/diagnosis-treatment/drc-20350098

Mayo Clinic Staff, "Electroconvulsive therapy (ECT)." Mayo Clinic. (Accessed 2017.)
http://www.mayoclinic.org/tests-procedures/electroconvulsive-therapy/basics/definition/prc-20014161

Mayo Clinic Staff, "Positive thinking: Stop negative self-talk to reduce stress." Mayo Clinic, February 18, 2017. http://www.mayoclinic.org/healthy-lifestyle/stress-management/in-depth/positive-thinking/art-20043950

Mayo Clinic Staff, "Tinnitus - Symptoms and Causes." Mayo Clinic, August 4, 2017.
http://www.mayoclinic.org/diseases-conditions/tinnitus/symptoms-causes/dxc-20180362

Mazurek, Birgit, HeideMarie Haupt, Heidi Olze, et al., "Stress and tinnitus - from bedside to bench and back." *Frontiers in System Neuroscience*, June 11, 2012.
https://www.ncbi.nlm.nih.gov/pmc/articles/PMC3371598/

Mazurek, Birgit, Timo Stöver, HeideMarie Haupt, et al., "The role of cochlear neurotransmitters in tinnitus." *HNO*, December 2007. http://www.ncbi.nlm.nih.gov/pubmed/17943261

McEwen, B.S., S. Chattarji, D.M. Diamond, et al., "The neurobiological properties of tianeptine (Stablon): from monoamine hypothesis to glutamatergic modulation." *Molecular Psychiatry*, Volume 15, 2010.
http://www.nature.com/mp/journal/v15/n3/full/mp200980a.html

McGill University, "Parts of the Brain that Slow Down or Speed Up in Depression." The Brain From Top to Bottom. (Accessed 2016.)
http://thebrain.mcgill.ca/flash/i/i_08/i_08_cr/i_08_cr_dep/i_08_cr_dep.html

Bibliography

McGovern Institute for Brain Research. "Long-distance Brain Waves Focus Attention." ScienceDaily. *ScienceDaily*, June 2, 2009.
https://www.sciencedaily.com/releases/2009/05/090528142829.htm

McGreevey, Sue, "Eight weeks to a better brain." Harvard Gazette, January 21, 2011.
http://www.thealternativedaily.com/study-meditation-actually-increases-frontal-cortex-and-boosts-frontal-lobe-activity/

McIlwain, Lori, "Autism & Sound Sensitivity: More Than Just a Mild Issue." National Autism Association, April 17, 2015. http://nationalautismassociation.org/autism-sound-sensitivity-more-than-just-a-mild-issue/

McNary, Trisha, "Frontal Lobe Enhancing Exercises." LiveStrong, September 11, 2017.
http://www.livestrong.com/article/523499-frontal-lobe-strengthening-exercises/

Mederios, Luisa Nascimento, Tanit Ganz Sanchez, "Tinnitus and cell phones: the role of electromagnetic radiofrequency radiation." *Brazilian Journal of Otorhinolaryngology*, Volume 82, Issue 1, January-February 2016.
http://www.sciencedirect.com/science/article/pii/S1808869415001639

Med-Health, "Olive Oil for Ear Wax." (Accessed 2016.)
http://www.med-health.net/Olive-Oil-Ear-Wax.html

Med-Health, "Serotonin Rich Foods." (Accessed 2017.)
http://www.med-health.net/Serotonin-Rich-Foods.html

MedHelp Communities, waking up with severe tinnitus after operation on head. July 4, 2011.
http://www.medhelp.org/posts/Head--Traumatic-Brain-Injury/Tinnitus/show/1550350

"Medical Hypnotherapy." Elite Hypno, 2011 (Accessed 2016.)
http://www.elitehypno.com/medical-hypnosis.html

Medical News Today, "Insomnia: Studies Suggest Calcium and Magnesium Effective." September 8, 2009. http://www.medicalnewstoday.com/releases/163169.php

Medical News Today, "The Brain Activity Behind Tinnitus Uncovered." (Accessed 2016.)
http://www.medicalnewstoday.com/releases/93609.php

Medical Xpress, "Study identifies the key cellular mechanisms behind the onset of tinnitus." May 10, 2012.
https://medicalxpress.com/news/2012-05-key-cellular-mechanisms-onset-tinnitus.html

Medline Plus, "Audiometry." (Accessed 2016.)
https://www.nlm.nih.gov/medlineplus/ency/article/003341.htm

MedLine Plus, "Hypothalamic dysfunction." U.S. National Library of Medicine. (Accessed 2016.)
https://medlineplus.gov/ency/article/001202.htm

Meeri, Kim, "Blue light from electronics disturbs sleep, especially for teenagers." *The Washington Post*, September 1, 2014. https://www.washingtonpost.com/national/health-science/blue-light-from-electronics-disturbs-sleep-especially-for-teenagers/2014/08/29/3edd2726-27a7-11e4-958c-268a320a60ce_story.html?utm_term=.8741f18d0347

Melina, Remy, "Why Do Medical Researchers Use Mice?" Live Science, November 16, 2010.
http://www.livescience.com/32860-why-do-medical-researchers-use-mice.html

Meng, Zhaoli, Shixi Liu, Yun Zheng, John S. Phillips, "Repetitive transcranial magnetic stimulation for tinnitus." Cochrane ENT Group, October 5, 2011.
https://www.ncbi.nlm.nih.gov/pubmedhealth/PMH0016221/

Mental Health Daily, "Alpha Brain Waves: 8 Hz to 12 Hz." (Accessed 2016.)
http://mentalhealthdaily.com/2014/04/11/alpha-brain-waves-8-hz-to-12-hz/

Mental Health Daily, "Five Types Of Brain Waves Frequencies: Gamma, Beta, Alpha, Theta, Delta." (Accessed 2016.) http://mentalhealthdaily.com/2014/04/15/5-types-of-brain-waves-frequencies-gamma-beta-alpha-theta-delta/

Mercola, DO, Joseph M., "Aspartame: By Far the Most Dangerous Substance Added to Most Foods Today." November 6, 2011. http://articles.mercola.com/sites/articles/archive/2011/11/06/aspartame-most-dangerous-substance-added-to-food.aspx

Mercola, Joseph, "How Sugar Harms Your Brain Health and Drives Alzheimer's Epidemic." The Epoch Times, July 25, 2014. https://www.theepochtimes.com/how-sugar-harms-your-brain-health-and-drives-alzheimers-epidemic_815311.html

Mercola, DO, Joseph M., "How the Cycles of Light and Darkness Affect Your Health and Well-Being." January 19, 2014. http://articles.mercola.com/sites/articles/archive/2014/01/19/sleep-light-exposure.aspx

Merzenich, Dr. Michael, "Acetylcholine Release Amps Up Brain's Plasticity." March 5, 2015. https://www.onthebrain.com/2015/03/acetylcholine-release-amps-brains-plasticity/

Meyer, Martin, Matthias S. Luethi, Patrick Neff, et al., "Disentangling Tinnitus Distress and Tinnitus Presence by Means of EEG Power Analysis." *Neural Plasticity*, Volume 2014. https://www.hindawi.com/journals/np/2014/468546/

Michaels, Sean, "Retuning the brain may cure tinnitus, finds study." The Guardian, January 19, 2011.
http://www.theguardian.com/music/2011/jan/19/retuning-brain-may-cure-tinnitus

Miller, Sara G., "Ringing Ears and Chronic Pain Share Unexpected Link."
Live Science, September 23, 2015.
http://www.livescience.com/52267-tinnitus-chronic-pain-brain-changes.html

Millichap, J. Gordon, Michelle M. Yee, "The Diet Factor in Attention Deficit/Hyperactivity Disorder." *Pediatrics*, Volume 129, Issue 2, February 2012.
http://pediatrics.aappublications.org/content/129/2/330

MindSparke, "Adult Neurogenesis - Hippocampus." (Accessed 2016.)
http://mindsparke.com/adult_neurogenesis_hippocampus.php

Misophonia, "The Symptoms & Triggers of Misophonia." (Accessed 2016.)
http://www.misophonia.com/symptoms-triggers/

Moderation Management, "Alcohol consumption limits." (Accessed 2016.)
http://moderation.org/readings/otherlimits.html

Molendjik, Marc L., Judith P.M. Haffmans, Boudewijn A.A. Bus, et al, "Serum BDNF concentrations show strong seasonal variation and correlations with the amount of ambient sunlight." *Public Library of Science ONE*, Volume 7, Number 11, November 2, 2012. http://www.ncbi.nlm.nih.gov/pubmed/23133609

Molteni, R., R.J. Barnard, Z. Ying, et al., "A High-Fat, Refined Sugar Diet Reduces Hippocampal Brain-Derived Neurotrophic Factor, Neuronal Plasticity, and Learning." *Neuroscience*, Volume 112, Number 4, 2002. https://www.ncbi.nlm.nih.gov/pubmed/12088740/

MomtoGG (Member), "Teen Daughter Gets 'Accidental Relief' from Tinnitus." Tinnitus Talk, September 28, 2016. https://www.tinnitustalk.com/threads/teen-daughter-gets-accidental-relief-from-tinnitus.17757/

Moriya, Junji, Rui Chen, Jun-Ichi Yamakawa, "Resveratrol improves hippocampal atrophy in chronic fatigue mice by enhancing neurogenesis and inhibiting apoptosis of granular cells." *Biological and Pharmaceutical Bulletin*, Volume 34, Number 3, 2011. https://www.ncbi.nlm.nih.gov/pubmed/21372384

Mosley, Michael, Mimi Spencer, "the 5:2 fast diet." The Fast Diet. (Accessed 2017.)
https://thefastdiet.co.uk

Mowatt, Jens, "Which neurotransmitters promote neurogenesis?" Quora, August 1, 2015.
https://www.quora.com/Which-neurotransmitters-promote-neurogenesis?share=1

MSG Truth, "Food For Thought." (Accessed 2016.) http://www.msgtruth.org/foodfor.htm

Mu, Yangling, Fred H. Gage, "Adult hippocampal neurogenesis and its role in Alzheimer's
disease." *Molecular Degeneration*, December 2011. https://molecularneurodegeneration.
biomedcentral.com/articles/10.1186/1750-1326-6-85

Mudd, MD, Pamela, F. Robert Glatz, MD, Kathleen C.M. Campbell, Ph.D., et al., "Ototoxicity."
Medscape, March 14, 2016.
http://emedicine.medscape.com/article/857679-overview

Müller, Nadia, Isabel Lorenz, Berthold Langguth, Nathan Weisz, "rTMS Tinnitus Induced Relief is
Related to an Increase in Auditory Cortical Alpha." *Public Library of Science ONE*, February
4, 2013. http://journals.plos.org/plosone/article?id=10.1371/journal.pone.0055557

Murphy, Patricia, W.M. Burnham, "The ketogenic diet causes a reversible decrease in activity
level in Long-Evans rats." *Experimental Neurology*, Volume 201, Issue 1, September
2006. https://www.ncbi.nlm.nih.gov/pubmed/16750194

Musazzi, Laura, Giorgio Racagni, Maurizio Popoli, "Stress, glucocorticoids and glutamate
release: Effects of antidepressant drugs." *Neurochemistry International*, Volume 59,
Issue 2, August 2011. http://www.sciencedirect.com/science/article/pii/S0197018611001690

Myers, Ph.D., CCC-A, Paula J., James A. Henry, Ph.D., CCC-A, Tara L. Zaugg, AuD, Caroline J.
Kendall, AuD, "Tinnitus Evaluation and Management Considerations for Persons with
Mild Traumatic Brain Injury." American Speech-Language-Hearing Association, April 2009.
http://www.asha.org/Articles/Tinnitus-Evaluation-and-Management-Considerations-for-
Persons-with-Mild-Traumatic-Brain-Injury/

myNoise, "Aural Scan." (Accessed 2017.)
https://mynoise.net/NoiseMachines/auralScannerNoiseGenerator.php

myNoise, "Waterfall Noise." (Accessed 2016.)
https://mynoise.net/NoiseMachines/waterfallNoiseGenerator.php

Nagler, Dr. Stephen, "Thoughts on TRT ..." Tinnitus Talk, January 19, 2015.
https://www.tinnitustalk.com/threads/thoughts-on-trt.7863/#post-90756

Nall, RN, BSN, CCRN, Rachel, (Reviewed by Debra Sullivan, PhD, MSN, RN, CNE, COI),
"Blood Glucose Management: Checking For Ketones." Healthline, May 30, 2017.
https://www.healthline.com/health/type-2-diabetes/facts-ketones?m=2#causes1

Nall, Rachel (Reviewed by University of Illinois-Chicago, College of Medicine), "Repetitive
Transcranial Magnetic Stimulation." Healthline, September 19, 2016. http://www.healthline.
com/health/depression/repetitive-transcranial-magnetic-stimulation#Overview1

NaSCN, "Construction on the new downtown Target," August 15, 2012. https://www.reddit.com/r/
Portland/comments/y9u1r/construction_on_the_new_downtown_target/c5tvp2v

National Institute for Health Research Nottingham, Biomedical Research Centre,
"Auditory examples - sounds of tinnitus." (Accessed 2016.)
http://www.hearing.nihr.ac.uk/public/auditory-examples-sounds-of-tinnitus

National Institute on Deafness and Other Communication Disorders, "Tinnitus: Is this what
happens when the brain's gatekeeper breaks down?" March 16, 2011.
http://www.nidcd.nih.gov/news/releases/11/Pages/031611.aspx

National Institute of Neurological Disorders and Stroke. "Brain Basics: Understanding Sleep." (Accessed 2016.) https://www.ninds.nih.gov/Disorders/Patient-Caregiver-Education/Understanding-Sleep#2

National Sleep Foundation, "A good workout can help you get great shut-eye." (Accessed 2017.) https://sleep.org/articles/exercise-affects-sleep/

Natural Endocrine Solutions, "Intermittent Fasting and Thyroid Health." July 28, 2014. http://www.naturalendocrinesolutions.com/articles/intermittent-fasting-thyroid-health/

Nauert, Ph.D., Rick, "Neurofeedback Trains Brain Waves, Restores Brain Function." (Accessed 2017.) http://psychcentral.com/news/2012/10/26/neurofeedback-trains-brain-waves-restores-brain-function/46720.html

Neal, Meghan, "The Many Colors of Sound." *The Atlantic,* February 16, 2016. https://www.theatlantic.com/science/archive/2016/02/white-noise-sound-colors/462972/

Neurogistics, "What are Neurotransmitters?" (Accessed 2016.) https://www.neurogistics.com/the-science/what-are-neurotransmitters

NeurOptimal, "Neurofeedback Training & Therapy at Home." (Accessed 2017.) https://neuroptimal.com/home-neurofeedback/

Neuroscience News, "Heavy Cannabis Use Associated With Reduced Dopamine Release." April 14, 2016. http://neurosciencenews.com/striatum-dopamine-marijuana-4059/

Neuroscientifically Challenged, "Know your brain: Amygdala." June 24, 2014. http://www.neuroscientificallychallenged.com/blog/know-your-brain-amygdala

Neuroscientifically Challenged, "Know your brain: Striatum." February 15, 2015. https://www.neuroscientificallychallenged.com/blog/know-your-brain-striatum

Newson, Greg, "Low GABA Levels - Increase GABA Naturally." Vitality & Wellness Centre, October 22, 2013. http://www.vitalityandwellness.com.au/health-blog/low-gaba-levels-increase-gaba-naturally

Nicolas-Puel, Cécile, Ruth Lloyd Faulconbridge, Matthieu Guitto, et al., "Characteristics of Tinnitus and Etiology of Associated Hearing Loss: A Study of 123 Patients." *International Tinnitus Journal,* Volume 8, No. 1, 2002. http://www.tinnitusjournal.com/articles/characteristics-of-tinnitus-and-etiologyof-associated-hearing-lossa-study-of-123-patients.pdf

Nield, David, "Scientists Think They've Found The Answer to What Causes Ringing in The Ears." Science Alert, September 25, 2015. http://www.sciencealert.com/scientists-think-they-ve-found-the-answer-to-what-causes-ringing-in-the-ears

Noble, William, "Tinnitus self-assessment scales: Domains of coverage and psychometric properties." Hearing Journal, Volume 54 - Issue 11, November 2001. http://journals.lww.com/thehearingjournal/Fulltext/2001/11000/Tinnitus_self_assessment_scales__Domains_of.6.aspx

Noh, Hae Sook, Hee Po Lee, Dong Wook Kim, et al., "A cDNA microarray analysis of gene expression profiles in rat hippocampus following a ketogenic diet." *Molecular Brain Research,* Volume 129, Issues 1-2, October 2004. http://www.ncbi.nlm.nih.gov/pubmed/15469884

Noise Addicts, "Hearing Test - Can You Hear This?" (Accessed 2016.) http://www.noiseaddicts.com/2009/03/can-you-hear-this-hearing-test/

Noise Addicts, "Poll Results for Frequency Hearing Test." January 23, 2011. http://www.noiseaddicts.com/2011/01/poll-results-for-frequency-hearing-test/

Noise Help, "Noise and Noise Pollution FAQ." (Accessed 2016.) http://www.noisehelp.com/noise-pollution-faq.html

Bibliography

Noise Help, "Noise Dose Chart: Noise Exposure Limits." (Accessed 2016.)
http://www.noisehelp.com/noise-dose.html

Noise Help, "Noise Level Chart." (Accessed 2016.)
http://www.noisehelp.com/noise-level-chart.html

Nootriment Editorial Staff, "GABA Agonist Effects, Side Effects and Natural
Supplements." (Accessed 2016.) https://nootriment.com/gaba-agonist/

Nordqvst, Joseph, "Coffee: Heath Benefits, Nutritional Information." Medical News Today, April 7,
2016. https://www.medicalnewstoday.com/articles/270202.php

Novella, MD, Steven, "Is There a Treatment for Tinnitus." Science-Based Medicine, November
14, 2012. https://sciencebasedmedicine.org/is-there-a-treatment-for-tinnitus/

Nutrition Data, "Foods highest in Total Omega-3 fatty acids." Self. (Accessed 2017.)
http://nutritiondata.self.com/foods-000140000000000000000.html

Nutrition Review, "Silencing Tinnitus - New Research Seeks to Reduce Ringing in Ears."
July 20, 2014. https://nutritionreview.org/2014/07/silencing-tinnitus-new-research-seeks-
to-reduce-ringing-in-ears/

Oberman, Lindsay M., Joseph P. McCleery, Vilanayur S. Ramachandran, Jaime A. Pineda,
"EEG evidence for mirror neuron activity during the observation of human and robot
actions: Toward an analysis of the human qualities of interactive robots."
Neurocomputing, Volume 70, Issues 13-15, August 2007.
http://www.sciencedirect.com/science/article/pii/S092523120600511X

OHSU Ear, Nose and Throat, "Tinnitus Program." (Accessed 2016.)
http://www.ohsu.edu/xd/health/services/ent/services/tinnitus-clinic/index.cfm/

Okomoto, Hidehiko, Henning Stracke, Wolfgang Stoll, Christo Pantev, "Listening to tailor-made
notched music reduces tinnitus loudness and tinnitus-related auditory cortex activity."
Proceedings of the National Academy of Sciences of the United States of America,
December 2009. http://www.pnas.org/content/107/3/1207.abstract

Oregon Health & Science University, "Tinnitus Facts." OHSU Ear, Nose & Throat.
(Accessed 2016.)
http://www.ohsu.edu/xd/health/services/ent/services/tinnitus-clinic/tinnitus_facts.cfm

Organic Facts, "List of Essential Oils." (Accessed 2017.)
https://www.organicfacts.net/health-benefits/essential-oils

"Overactive neurons can cause tinnitus." Auris, Number 4, 2012.
http://www.hear-it.org/Overactive-neurons-can-cause-tinnitus

Oz, MD, Mehmet, "Is there a recommended amount of sun exposure?" (Accessed 2017.)
https://www.sharecare.com/health/healthy-skin/is-recommended-amount-sun-exposure

Packer, Rowena M.A., Tsz Hong Law, Emma Davies, et al., "Effects of a ketogenic diet on
ADHD-like behavior in dogs with idiopathic epilepsy." Epilepsy & Behavior, Volume 55,
February 2016. https://www.ncbi.nlm.nih.gov/pubmed/26773515

Paddock, Ph.D., Catharine, "Tinnitus less common in women who drink more coffee." Medical
News Today, August 8, 2014. https://www.medicalnewstoday.com/articles/280775.php

"Paired VNS™ treatment uses Vagus Nerve Stimulation (VNS) paired with tones."
MicroTransponder, Inc. (Accessed 2017.)
http://www.microtransponder.com/en-gb/tinnitus/physicians/clinical-experiences

Paleo Leap, "The Paleo Guide to Ketosis." (Accessed 2017.)
http://paleoleap.com/paleo-guide-to-ketosis/

Pallavi, Panchu, "Auditory acuity in type 2 diabetes mellitus." *International Journal of Diabetes in Developing Countries*, Volume 28, Number 4, October-December 2008. https://www.ncbi.nlm.nih.gov/pmc/articles/PMC2822154/

Paparella Ear Head & Neck Institute, "Tinnitus and Insulin Resistance." (Accessed 2017.) http://www.pehni.com/patient_ed/dn_tinnitusinsulin.htm

Pappas, Stephanie, "A Good Night's Rest: The Best Sleep Apps." Live Science, January 23, 2015. http://www.livescience.com/49552-best-sleep-apps.html

Pascual-Leone, Professor Alvaro, Belen Rubio, Professor Frederico Pallardó, MD, et al., "Rapid-rate transcranial magnetic stimulation of left dorsolateral prefrontal cortex in drug-resistant depression." The Lancet, Volume 348, Issue 9022, July 27, 1996. https://www.sciencedirect.com/science/article/pii/S0140673696012196

Pedersen, Traci, "New Blood Test May Detect Traumatic Brain Injury." PsychCentral. (Accessed 2017.) https://psychcentral.com/news/2015/08/02/new-blood-test-may-detect-traumatic-brain-injury/88415.html

Perkins, M.Ed., Cynthia, "How to Increase GABA and Balance Glutamate." May 28, 2014. http://www.holistichelp.net/blog/how-to-increase-gaba-and-balance-glutamate/

Perkins, RN, Sharon, "List of Foods for Sulfite Sensitivity." SFGate. (Accessed 2017.) http://healthyeating.sfgate.com/list-foods-sulfite-sensitivity-3306.html

Perry, Mike, "Stop that damned ringing." Salon, May 6, 1999. http://www.salon.com/1999/05/06/tinnitus/

Persson, A., S.C. Sim, S. Virding, et al., "Decreased hippocampal volume and increased anxiety in a transgenic mouse model expressing the human CYP2C19 gene." *Molecular Psychiatry*, Volume 19, 2014. http://www.nature.com/mp/journal/v19/n6/full/mp201389a.html

Peters, MD, Brandon, "Common Side Effects from Light Box Therapy and Ways to Alleviate Them." VeryWell, March 22, 2016. https://www.verywell.com/side-effects-from-light-box-therapy-3015328

Petre, B., S. Torbey, J.W. Griffith, et al., "Smoking increases risk of pain chronification through shared corticostriatal circuitry." *Human Brain Mapping*, February 2015. http://www.ncbi.nlm.nih.gov/pubmed/25307796

"Phantom Limb Pain." Video, University of Texas at Dallas, 2012. https://vimeo.com/52858652

Phonak, "Manage Your Tinnitus Effectively." (Accessed 2017.) https://www.phonak.com/com/en/hearing-aids/tinnitus-treatment.html

Pietrangelo, Ann (Reviewed by Suzanne Falck, MD), "Sudden Sensorineural Hearing Loss (SSHL)." Healthline, June 2, 2017. http://www.healthline.com/health/sensorineural-deafness#Overview1

Pigeon, Dr. Stéphane, "How to Use Sound Machines." myNoise. (Accessed 2017.) https://mynoise.net/howToUseSoundMachines.php

Pigeon, Dr. Stéphane, "myNoise Screencasts." myNoise. (Accessed 2017.) https://mynoise.net/screencasts.php

Pigeon, Dr. Stéphane, "Online Audiogram Hearing Test." (Accessed 2016.) http://www.audiocheck.net/testtones_hearingtestaudiogram.php

Pigeon, Dr. Stéphane, "Online Hearing Test and Audiogram Printout." (Accessed 2017.) https://hearingtest.online/

Pinterest, "Famous People with Hearing Loss and Tinnitus." https://www.pinterest.com/TinnitusHub/famous-people-with-hearing-loss-and-tinnitus/

Pizer, Ann, "Hands and Knees Balance." VeryWell, Yoga Poses, March 17, 2017.
https://www.verywell.com/hands-and-knees-balance-3567081

Pizer, Ann, "How to Do Plank Pose." VeryWell, Yoga Poses, November 7, 2016.
https://www.verywell.com/how-to-do-plank-pose-3567104

Posit Science, "Sleep Loss Infographic." Brain HQ. (Accessed 2017.) http://blog.brainhq.com/
wp-content/uploads/2015/09/89a2209b16e829ceec4a62663d501684.png

Progesterone Therapy, "Seasonal affective disorder treatment." (Accessed 2017.)
http://www.progesteronetherapy.com/seasonal-affective-disorder-treatment.html

Progressive Health, "Find Out What Supplements Help Insomnia." (Accessed 2017.)
http://www.progressivehealth.com/try-these-natural-sleep-aids.htm

Pugh, Rachel, Richard J. Budd, S.D.G. Stephens, "Patients' reports of the effects of
alcohol on tinnitus." British Journal of Audiology, Volume 29, Number 5, 1995.
https://www.ncbi.nlm.nih.gov/pubmed/8838550

Pujol, Rémy, Jing Wang, Sam Irving, "Acoustic Trauma." Journey Into the World of Hearing,
October 30, 2016. http://www.cochlea.eu/en/pathology/surdites-neuro-sensorielles/
traumatisme-acoustique

Ranker, "Famous People with Tinnitus." (Accessed 2016.)
http://www.ranker.com/list/famous-people-with-tinnitus/celebrity-lists

Rankin, Dr. Lissa, "10 Signs You Have WAY Too Much Cortisol." mindbodygreen, May 13, 2013.
http://www.mindbodygreen.com/0-9527/10-signs-you-have-way-too-much-cortisol.html

Rauschecker, Josef, Elisabeth S. May, Audrey Madoux, Markus Ploner, "Frontalstriatal Gating of
Tinnitus and Chronic Pain." Trends in Cognitive Sciences, Volume 19, Issue 10, October
2015. http://www.cell.com/trends/cognitive-sciences/fulltext/S1364-6613(15)00179-5

Rendeiro, Catarina, David Vauzour, Marcus Rattray, et al., "Dietary levels of pure flavonoids
improve spatial memory performance and increase hippocampal brain-derived
neurotrophic factor." Public Library of Science ONE, May 28, 2013.
http://centaur.reading.ac.uk/33643/1/PlosOne.pdf

Renter, Elizabeth, "How To Increase Dopamine Levels: Foods To Eat And What To Do To Feel
Good." Natural Society, September 29, 2012.
http://naturalsociety.com/how-to-increase-dopamine-levels-foods/

reph (Member), "Tinnitus Overview, Sleep Tips, Habituation," Tapatalk Tinnitus Support Message
Board, June 4, 2005. https://www.tapatalk.com/groups/tinnitussupport92262/tinnitus-
overview-sleep-tips-habituation-t438.html

RESPeRATE, "How It Works." (Accessed 2017.) http://www.resperate.com/sleep/

Rivas, Anthony, "What Causes Tinnitus? Brain Scans Show Multiple Areas Are Responsible For
Perpetual Ringing." Medical Daily, April 26, 2015. http://www.medicaldaily.com/what-
causes-tinnitus-brain-scans-show-multiple-areas-are-responsible-perpetual-330794

Roberts, Larry E., Graeme Moffat, Michael Baumann, et al., "Residual Inhibition Functions
Overlap Tinnitus Spectra and the Region of Auditory Threshold Shift." Journal of the
Association for Research in Otolaryngology, Volume 9, Number 4, December 2008.
https://www.ncbi.nlm.nih.gov/pmc/articles/PMC2580805/

Roberts, Larry E., "Residual inhibition." Progress in Brain Research, Volume 166, 2007.
https://www.ncbi.nlm.nih.gov/pubmed/17956813

Robinhood76, "Pack: Dogs everywhere sounds." Free Sounds, November 6, 2008.
http://freesound.org/people/Robinhood76/packs/4026/

Robins, Wendy, "Essential Oil Skin Patch Testing" AromaWeb. (Accessed 2016.)
https://www.aromaweb.com/articles/essential-oil-skin-patch-test.asp

Rodriguez-Gil, M.Ed., Gloria, "The Sense of Smell: A Powerful Sense."
California Deafblind Services, Volume 11, Number 2, Spring 2004.
https://www.tsbvi.edu/seehear/summer05/smell.htm

Rugnetta, Michael (Contributor), "Neuroplasticity." Encyclopædia Britannica, June 15, 2017.
https://www.britannica.com/science/neuroplasticity

Russell, Roger, "Listening and Hearing." (Accessed 2016.)
http://www.roger-russell.com/hearing/hearing.htm

Salvi, Richard, Edward Lobarinas, W. Sun, "Pharmacological Treatments for Tinnitus: New and Old." *Drugs of the Future*, May 1, 2009.
https://www.ncbi.nlm.nih.gov/pmc/articles/PMC3136369/

Salvi, Richard, Suzanne Kraus, Berthold Langguth, Edward Lobarinas, et al., "Tinnitus and Hearing Loss and Changes in Hippocampus." Seminars in Hearing, 32, 2011.
https://www.researchgate.net/publication/273420163_Tinnitus_and_Hearing_Loss_and_Changes_in_Hippocampus

Salviati, Massimo, Francesco Saverio Bersani, Samira Terlizza, et al., "Tinnitus: clinical experience of the psychosomatic condition." *Neuropsychiatric Disease and Treatment*, v. 10, 2014. https://www.ncbi.nlm.nih.gov/pmc/articles/PMC3925227/

"Salicylate Sensitivity." (Accessed 2017.) http://salicylatesensitivity.com/

Salk Institute. "Cannabinoids remove plaque-forming Alzheimer's proteins from brain cells." ScienceDaily. *ScienceDaily*, June 29, 2016.
https://www.sciencedaily.com/releases/2016/06/160629095609.htm

Saunders, James C., "The Role of Central Nervous System Plasticity in Tinnitus."
Journal of Communication Disorders, July-August 2007.
http://www.ncbi.nlm.nih.gov/pmc/articles/PMC2083119/

Savastano, M., G. Brescia, G. Marioni, "Antioxidant therapy in idiopathic tinnitus: preliminary outcomes." Archives of Medical Research, May 2007.
http://www.ncbi.nlm.nih.gov/pubmed/17416295

Schecklmann, Martin, Michael Landgrebe, Berthold Langguth, "Phenotypic Characteristics of Hyperacusis in Tinnitus." January 31, 2014. PLoS ONE9(1): e86944.
https://doi.org/10.1371/journal.pone.0086944

Scheve, Tom, "What are endorphins?" HowStuffWorks, (Accessed 2016.)
http://science.howstuffworks.com/life/endorphins.htm

Schiffer, Thorsten, Stefanie Schulte, Billy Sperlich, et al., "Lactate infusion at rest increases BDNF concentration in humans." Neuroscience Letters, Volume 488, Issue 3, January 25, 2011. http://www.sciencedirect.com/science/article/pii/S0304394010014898

Schlee, Winfried, Nadia Mueller, Thomas Hartmann, et al., "Mapping Cortical Hubs in Tinnitus."
BioMed Central Biology, 2009. https://bmcbiol.biomedcentral.com/articles/10.1186/1741-7007-7-80

Schotz, Wolfgang, Christian Kürschner, "A Reconsideration of Cognitive Load Theory."
Educational Psychology Review, December 2007, Volume 19, Issue 4.
https://doi.org/10.1007/s10648-007-9053-4

Schulz, Jörg B., Jörg Lindenau, Jan Seyfried, Johannes Dichgans, "Glutathione, oxidative stress and neurodegeneration." *The FEB Journal*, Volume 267, Issue 16, August 2000.
http://onlinelibrary.wiley.com/doi/10.1046/j.1432-1327.2000.01595.x/full

Schwertly, Scott, "The Science of Procrastination: Why You Should Start That Presentation Today." LinkedIn SlideShare, October 13, 2014. https://blog.slideshare.net/2014/10/13/the-science-of-procrastination-why-you-should-start-that-presentation-today

Scicurious, "Fighting stress with adenosine antagonists." *Scientific American*, June 10, 2013. http://blogs.scientificamerican.com/scicurious-brain/fighting-stress-with-adenosine-antagonists/

Scott, MS, Elizabeth, "Cortisol and Stress." VeryWell, May 15, 2017. https://www.verywell.com/cortisol-and-stress-how-to-stay-healthy-3145080

Searchfield, Grant D., Jeanie Morrison-Low, Kim Wise, "Object identification and attention training for treating tinnitus." *Progress in Brain Research*, Volume 166, 2007. http://www.sciencedirect.com/science/article/pii/S0079612307660439

Sedley, William, Jehill Parikh, Richard A.E. Edden, et al., "Human Auditory Cortex Neurochemistry Reflects the Presence and Severity of Tinnitus." *Journal of Neuroscience*, November 4, 2015. http://www.jneurosci.org/content/35/44/14822.abstract

Seegert, Liz, "The Keto Diet is Gaining in Popularity, but Is It Safe?" Healthline, June 7, 2016. http://www.healthline.com/health-news/keto-diet-is-gaining-popularity-but-is-it-safe-121914#1

Segal, M.A., Robert, Lawrence Robinson, "Choosing Healthy Fats." HelpGuide, October 2017. http://www.helpguide.org/articles/healthy-eating/choosing-healthy-fats.htm

Seidman, Michael D., "Glutamate Antagonists, Steroids, and Antioxidants as Therapeutic Options for Hearing Loss and Tinnitus and the Use of an Inner Ear Drug Delivery System." *International Tinnitus Journal*, Volume 4, Number 2, 1998. http://www.tinnitusjournal.com/detalhe_artigo.asp?id=294

SharpBrains, "Can brain training work? Yes, if it meets these 5 conditions." May 22, 2013. https://sharpbrains.com/blog/2013/05/22/does-brain-training-work-yes-if-it-meets-these-5-conditions/

SharpBrains, "Study: High television viewing and low physical activity can significantly worsen long-term cognitive function." July 28, 2015. https://sharpbrains.com/blog/2015/07/28/study-high-television-viewing-and-low-physical-activity-can-significantly-worsen-long-term-cognitive-function/

Shin, J.B., F. Streijger, A. Beynon, et al., "Hair bundles are specialized for ATP delivery via creatine kinase." *Neuron*, February 1, 2007. https://www.ncbi.nlm.nih.gov/pubmed/17270734

Shore, Susan E., Larry E. Roberts, Berthold Langguth, "Maladaptive plasticity in tinnitus — triggers, mechanisms and treatment." *Nature Reviews Neurology*, Volume 12, 2016. http://www.nature.com/nrneurol/journal/v12/n3/full/nrneurol.2016.12.html

Shrikant, Nithya, "8 Incredible Yoga Asanas That Will Help You Cure Tinnitus." Stylecraze, September 19, 2017. http://www.stylecraze.com/articles/yoga-asanas-to-cure-tinnitus-hearing-problems/

Shulman, Abraham, Matthew J. Avitable, Barbara Goldstein, "Quantitative Electroencephalography Power Analysis in Subjective Idiopathic Tinnitus Patients: A Clinical Paradigm Shift in the Understanding of Tinnitus, An Electrophysiological Correlate." *International Tinnitus Journal*, Volume 12, No. 2, 2006. http://www.tinnitusjournal.com/detalhe_artigo.asp?id=99

Simoens, Veerle L., Sylvie Hebért, "Cortisol suppression and hearing thresholds in tinnitus after low-dose dexamethasone challenge." BioMed Central Biology, March 26, 2012. https://bmcearnosethroatdisord.biomedcentral.com/articles/10.1186/1472-6815-12-4

Simons, Daniel J., "Inattentional blindness." Scholarpedia, 2007. http://www.scholarpedia.org/article/Inattentional_blindness

Sindhusake, D., P. Mitchell, P. Newall, et al., "Prevalence and characteristics of tinnitus in older adults: the Blue Mountains Hearing Study." *International Journal of Audiology*, July 2003. http://www.ncbi.nlm.nih.gov/pubmed/12916702

Singleton, Bonnie, "Tart Cherry Juice & Sleep." LiveStrong, October 3, 2017. https://www.livestrong.com/article/410380-tart-cherry-juice-gout/

Slajerova, Martina, "Keto Diet Guide." KetoDiet Blog, June 24, 2014. https://ketodietapp.com/Blog/post/2014/06/24/Practical-Guide-to-Keto-Paleo-Diet-for-Health-and-Long-Term-Weight-Loss

Smart Drugs For Thought, "Idebenone: What Is Idebenone?" (Accessed 2016.) https://www.smartdrugsforthought.com/what-is-idebenone/

Smart Drugs For Thought, "Nootropic Research." (Accessed 2016.) https://www.smartdrugsforthought.com/nootropic-research/

Smith, Darren, "$500,000 Default Judgment Issued Against Defendant Over Barking Dog." Jonathan Turley, February 15, 2015. https://jonathanturley.org/2015/02/15/500000-default-judgment-issued-against-defendant-over-barking-dog/comment-page-1/

Smith, Paul F., Yiwen Zheng, "Cannabinoids, cannabinoid receptors and tinnitus." *Hearing Research*, Volume 332, February 2016. http://www.sciencedirect.com/science/article/pii/S0378595515300368

Smith, BPharm, Yolanda, "Ketogenic Diet Side Effects." News-Medical Life Sciences, October 19, 2015. https://www.news-medical.net/health/Ketogenic-Diet-Side-Effects.aspx

Smithdeal, Charles, "Tinnitus, Insulin, and Diabetes." Ezine Articles, June 27, 2011. http://EzineArticles.com/6383076

Smithson, Toby, "What are simple carbohydrates?" Sharecare. (Accessed 2017.) https://www.sharecare.com/health/carbohydrates/what-are-simple-carbohydrates

Society for Neuroscience. "Specific brain areas, mechanisms associated with depression, anxiety." ScienceDaily. *ScienceDaily*, November 11, 2013. https://www.sciencedaily.com/releases/2013/11/131111161428.htm

Soloway, RN, BSN, MSEd, DABAT, Rose Ann Gould, "Essential Oils: Poisonous When Misused." National Capital Poison Center. (Accessed 2016.) https://www.poison.org/articles/2014-jun/essential-oils

SoniModul Clinic, "Our Therapeutic Offer." (Accessed 2017.) https://sonimodul.ch/home/about-us/therapeutic-offer/

Sound Therapy International, "Why classical music can provide relief for tinnitus." PR Wire. (Accessed 2016.) http://prwire.com.au/pr/53634/why-classical-music-can-provide-relief-for-tinnitus

Stanley, Andrea, "8 Natural Sleep Aids That Really Work." Fitness. (Accessed 2017.) http://www.fitnessmagazine.com/health/sleep/natural-sleep-aids/?page=1

Starkey Hearing Technologies, "Test your hearing today." (Accessed 2017.) https://www.starkey.com/online-hearing-test#!/GreetingPrimary

Starkey Hearing Technologies, "The Tinnitus Handicap Inventory (THI): A Quick and Reliable Method for Measuring Tinnitus Outcomes." Starkey Research & Clinical Blog, December 2, 2012. http://blog.starkeypro.com/the-tinnitus-handicap-inventory-thi-a-quick-and-reliable-method-for-measuring-tinnitus-outcomes/

Statistic Brain, "Sleeping Disorder Statistics." (Accessed 2017.) http://www.statisticbrain.com/sleeping-disorder-statistics/

Stephens, D., "Detrimental effects of alcohol on tinnitus." *Clinical Otolaryngology & Allied Sciences*, Volume 24, Issue 2, April 1999. http://www.ncbi.nlm.nih.gov/pubmed/10225155

Bibliography

Stolzberg, Daniel, Richard J. Salvi, Brian L. Allman, "Salicylate toxicity model of tinnitus." *Frontiers in System Neuroscience*, January 19, 2012. http://www.ncbi.nlm.nih.gov/pmc/articles/PMC3341117/

Swain, A.R., S.P. Dutton, A.S. Truswell, "Salicylates in food." *Journal of the American Dietetic Association*, August 1985. https://www.ncbi.nlm.nih.gov/pubmed/4019987

Sweetow, Ph.D., Robert W., "An Integrated Approach to Tinnitus Management." Audiology Online, February 4, 2013. http://www.audiologyonline.com/articles/integrated-approach-to-tinnitus-management-11598

Sun, Wei, Jianzhong Lu, Erin Laundrie, "Neurotransmitter Modulation Relates with Tinnitus Signal Generation and Management." *Journal of Otology*, Volume 2, Issue 2, December 2007. http://www.sciencedirect.com/science/article/pii/S1672293007500164

Tan, Ph.D., Gabriel, John Thornby, Ph.D., D. Corydon Hammond, Ph.D., et al., "Meta-Analysis of EEG Biofeedback in Treating Epilepsy." *Journal of Clinical EEG and Neuroscience*, Volume 4, Issue 3, July 1, 2009. http://www.eeginfo.com/research/epilepsy_main.jsp

Technical University of Munich, "Ringing in the ears and chronic pain enter by the same gate." EurekAlert! September 23, 2015. https://www.eurekalert.org/pub_releases/2015-09/tuom-rit091715.php

Techopedia, "Blue Noise." (Accessed 2016.) https://www.techopedia.com/definition/27896/blue-noise

Techopedia, "Gray Noise." (Accessed 2017.) https://www.techopedia.com/definition/27898/gray-noise

Techopedia, "Violet Noise." (Accessed 2016.) https://www.techopedia.com/definition/27897/violet-noise

Techopedia, "White Noise." (Accessed 2016.) https://www.techopedia.com/definition/10964/white-noise

Tehranipour, Maryam, "The effect of hyperglycemia on hippocampus neuronal density in female rats." Pharmacologyonline. Volume 3, 2010. https://www.researchgate.net/publication/288584003_The_effect_of_hyperglycemia_on_hippocampus_neuronal_density_in_female_rats

The Alternative Daily, "Study: Meditation Actually Increases Frontal Cortex and Boosts Frontal Lobe Activity." April 22, 2013. http://www.thealternativedaily.com/study-meditation-actually-increases-frontal-cortex-and-boosts-frontal-lobe-activity/

The ASMR, "What Is ASMR?" (Accessed 2017.) https://www.theasmr.com/what-is-asmr-meaning/

The Better Sleep Guide, "Five Stages of Sleep." (Accessed 2017.) http://www.better-sleep-better-life.com/five-stages-of-sleep.html

The Brain From Top to Bottom, "Anxiety Neurotransmitters." (Accessed 2016.) http://thebrain.mcgill.ca/flash/d/d_04/d_04_m/d_04_m_peu/d_04_m_peu.html

The Brain Made Simple, "Welcome to Your Kid Friendly Guide to the Brain." (Accessed 2016.) http://brainmadesimple.com/

The Endocrine Society, "High blood sugar causes brain changes that raise depression risk." Medical Xpress, June 23, 2014. https://medicalxpress.com/news/2014-06-high-blood-sugar-brain-depression.html

The Failsafe Diet, "Salicylate Content of Foods." (Accessed 2017.) http://www.failsafediet.com/the-rpah-elimination-diet-failsafe/salicylate-content-of-foods/

The GoodRx Pharmacist, "Seizure Medication Potiga Discontinued." July 27, 2017. https://www.goodrx.com/blog/seizure-medication-potiga-discontinued/

The Guardian, "Retuning the brain may cure tinnitus, finds study." 2011. https://www.theguardian.com/music/2011/jan/19/retuning-brain-may-cure-tinnitus

The Guardian, "Warning over experimental brain boost." (Accessed 2017.) https://www.theguardian.com/science/2014/dec/09/warning-experimental-brain-boost-equipment-research-oxford?CMP=share_btn_tw

The Henry Spink Foundation, "The Tomatis Method." (Accessed 2016.) http://www.henryspink.org/the_tomatis_method.htm

The Listening Centres, "The Listening Therapy successfully treats: Tinnitus." (Accessed 2016.) http://www.listeningcentre.co.uk/tinnitus.php

The National Organization for Hearing Research Foundation, "Inner Ear Cell Regeneration." http://nohrfoundation.org/regeneration

The Nutrition Source, "Carbohydrates and Blood Sugar." (Accessed 2017.) https://www.hsph.harvard.edu/nutritionsource/carbohydrates/carbohydrates-and-blood-sugar/

The Paramus Post, "Supplement may protect against hearing loss." April 18, 2007. http://www.paramuspost.com/article.php/20070413201049969

The Science of Parkinson's Disease, "Food For Thought." September 18, 2017. https://scienceofparkinsons.com/2017/09/18/food/

The Telegraph, "Coroner slams delays over tinnitus sufferer who stabbed himself to death." April 12, 2012. http://www.telegraph.co.uk/news/health/news/9198029/Coroner-slams-delays-over-tinnitus-sufferer-who-stabbed-himself-to-death.html

"Tinnitus." Video, University of Texas at Dallas, 2012. https://vimeo.com/52861200

Tomatis Developpement SA, "Tomatis Method - Its Function." (Accessed 2017.) http://www.tomatis.com/en/tomatis-method/its-function.html (Link redirects to https://www.tomatis.com/en/technology)

Tonkin, Amanda, "A recipe for optimal hearing health." Healthy Hearing, March 4, 2014. https://www.healthyhearing.com/report/51870-A-recipe-for-optimal-hearing-health

Traynor, Robert, "Stem Cell Research in Hearing - Old Age Hearing Loss - Part III." Hearing Health & Technology Matters, October 25, 2012. http://hearinghealthmatters.org/hearinginternational/2012/stem-cell-research-in-hearing-old-age-hearing-loss-part-iii/

Traynor, Robert, "The Effect of Automobile Air Bag Deployment on Hearing." Hearing Health & Technology Matters, October 31, 2012. http://hearinghealthmatters.org/hearinginternational/2012/the-international-threat-of-air-bags/

Trivedi, Yatri, "How to Enable 'Stereo Mix' in Windows and Record Audio from Your PC." How-To Geek, February 10, 2016. https://www.howtogeek.com/howto/39532/how-to-enable-stereo-mix-in-windows-7-to-record-audio/

Tsukinoki, K., J. Saruta, "Role of stress-related brain-derived neurotrophic factor (BDNF) in the rat submandibular gland." Acta Histochemica et Cytochemica, Volume 45, October 31, 2012. https://www.ncbi.nlm.nih.gov/pubmed/23209335

Tuck, "Explanation of Neurotransmitters." February 20, 2017. https://www.tuck.com/neurotransmitters/

Tull, Ph.D., Matthew, "What You Should Know About the Effect of PTSD on the Brain." Verywell, June 25, 2017. https://www.verywell.com/the-effect-of-ptsd-on-the-brain-2797643

UCLA Ahmanson-Lovelace Brain Mapping Center, "Putting Feelings Into Words Produces Therapeutic Effects In The Brain." Medical Xpress, June 22, 2007. https://medicalxpress.com/news/2007-06-words-therapeutic-effects-brain.html

UCLA Mindful Awareness Research Center, "Free Guided Meditations." (Accessed 2017.) http://marc.ucla.edu/body.cfm?id=22

Bibliography

University at Buffalo. "Breakthrough in tinnitus research could lead to testable model." ScienceDaily. *ScienceDaily*, May 12, 2015. https://www.sciencedaily.com/releases/2015/05/150512152646.htm

University of California - Berkeley. "Tinnitus discovery could lead to new ways to stop the ringing: Retraining the brain could reanimate areas that have lost input from the ear." ScienceDaily. *ScienceDaily*, September 13, 2011. https://www.sciencedaily.com/releases/2011/09/110912144247.htm

University of California - Irvine. "Low-pitch Treatment Alleviates Ringing Sound Of Tinnitus." ScienceDaily. *ScienceDaily*, February 15, 2007. https://www.sciencedaily.com/releases/2007/02/070214221229.htm

University of California at San Diego, "Growth factor protects key brain cells in Alzheimer's models." Medical XPress, February 8, 2009. https://medicalxpress.com/news/2009-02-growth-factor-key-brain-cells.html

University of Illinois at Urbana-Champaign, "Emotion processing in the brain changes with tinnitus severity." ScienceDaily. *ScienceDaily*, December 14, 2015. http://www.sciencedaily.com/releases/2015/12/151214145956.htm

University of Utah, Department of Mathematics, "Caffeine Content of Popular Drinks." (Accessed 2017.) http://www.math.utah.edu/~yplee/fun/caffeine.html

University of Washington-Seattle, "Brain Plasticity - An Overview." Edited by Eric H. Chudler, Ph.D. (Accessed 2016.) https://faculty.washington.edu/chudler/plast.html

University of Western Sydney. "Chronic Tinnitus And Its Impact On Demanding Cognitive Tasks." ScienceDaily. *ScienceDaily*, March 10, 2006. http://www.sciencedaily.com/releases/2006/03/060310101636.htm

Unterrainer, Josef, Karoline V. Greimel, Max Leibetseder, "Are Demographic and Socioeconomic Factors Predictive for Perceived Tinnitus Impairment?" *International Tinnitus Journal*, Volume 7, No. 2, 2001. http://www.tinnitusjournal.com/detalhe_artigo.asp?id=203

U.S. Department of Labor, Occupational Health and Safety Administration, "Occupational Noise Exposure." (Accessed 2016.) https://www.osha.gov/SLTC/noisehearingconservation/index.html

U.S. Department of Labor, "OSHA Technical Manual: Noise." Section III, Chapter 5. (Accessed 2017.) https://www.osha.gov/dts/osta/otm/new_noise/

U.S. Department of Transportation, Federal Highway Administration, "Construction Noise Handbook." June 28, 2017. http://www.fhwa.dot.gov/environment/noise/construction_noise/handbook/handbook03.cfm

U.S. Food & Drug Administration, "FDA Drug Safety Communication: FDA determines 2013 labeling adequate to manage risk of retinal abnormalities, potential vision loss, and skin discoloration with anti-seizure drug Potiga (ezogabine); requires additional study." June 15, 2015. http://www.fda.gov/Drugs/DrugSafety/ucm349538.htm

Vann, MPH, Madeline R., (Reviewed by Niya Jones, MD, MPH), "Is Anxiety Hereditary?" Everyday Health, August 24, 2015. http://www.everydayhealth.com/news/is-anxiety-hereditary/

Vanneste, Ph.D., Sven, Dirk De Ridder, M.D., Ph.D., "Deafferentation-based pathophysiological differences in phantom sound: Tinnitus with and without hearing loss." *NeuroImage*, April 1, 2016. https://www.ncbi.nlm.nih.gov/pubmed/26708013

Vanneste, Ma, Msc, Phd, Sven, Dirk De Ridder, MD, PhD, "Noninvasive and Invasive Neuromodulation for the Treatment of Tinnitus: An Overview." *Neuromodulation*, Volume 15, Issue 4, July 1, 2012.
http://onlinelibrary.wiley.com/doi/10.1111/j.1525-1403.2012.00447.x/abstract

Vanneste, Ph.D., Sven, Paul van de Heyning, Dirk De Ridder, M.D., Ph.D., "The neural network of phantom sound changes over time: a comparison between recent-onset and chronic tinnitus patients." *European Journal of Neuroscience*, Volume 34, Number 5, September 2011. https://www.ncbi.nlm.nih.gov/pubmed/21848924

VetInfo, "Do Dogs Dream? What Sleep Research Reveals." (Accessed 2016.)
https://www.vetinfo.com/do-dogs-dream.html

Vimeo, "What is Brain HQ?" Posit Science channel. (Accessed 2016.)
https://vimeo.com/190944852

VitaSouth, "Natural Sources of Glutamate." (Accessed 2016.)
http://www.vitasouth.com/pages/Natural-Sources-of-Glutamate.html

Vizuete, Adriana Fernanda, Daniela Fraga de Souza, Maria Cristina Guerra, et al., "Brain changes in BDNF and S100B induced by ketogenic diets in Wistar rats." *Life Sciences*, Volume 92, Issues 17-19, May 2013.
http://www.sciencedirect.com/science/article/pii/S0024320513001720

Watson, Stephanie, "Hearing Aid Basics." HowStuffWorks. (Accessed 2016.)
http://health.howstuffworks.com/medicine/modern-technology/hearing-aid6.htm

Webb, Jonathan, "Tinnitus mapped inside human brain." April 23, 2015.
http://www.bbc.com/news/science-environment-32414876

WebMD, "12 Basic Yoga Poses," Reviewed by William Blahd, MD, August 17, 2017.
http://www.webmd.com/fitness-exercise/ss/slideshow-yoga-pose-basics

WebMD, "Electroencephalogram (EEG)." (Accessed 2017.)
http://www.webmd.com/epilepsy/electroencephalogram-eeg-21508?page=3

WebMD, "Epilepsy, Children, and the Ketogenic Diet." (Accessed 2017.)
http://www.webmd.com/epilepsy/epilepsy-guide-8/ketogenic-diet

WebMD, "Hearing Tests." (Accessed 2017.)
http://www.webmd.com/a-to-z-guides/hearing-tests#1

WebMD, "Light Therapy." (Accessed 2017.) http://www.webmd.com/a-to-z-guides/light-therapy

WebMD, "Neck Exercises - Topic Overview." (Accessed 2017.)
https://www.webmd.com/pain-management/tc/neck-exercises-topic-overview

WebMD, "Overview of Biofeedback." (Accessed 2017.)
http://www.webmd.com/a-to-z-guides/biofeedback-therapy-uses-benefits#1

WebMD, "Slideshow: Top Concentration Killers." Reviewed by William Blahd, MD, June 16, 2016. http://www.webmd.com/add-adhd/ss/slideshow-top-concentration-killers

WebMD, "Sugar Shockers: Foods Surprisingly High in Sugar." (Accessed 2017.)
http://www.webmd.com/food-recipes/features/sugar-shockers-foods-surprisingly-high-in-sugar#1

WebMD, "What Is a Cortisol Test?" (Accessed 2017.)
https://www.webmd.com/a-to-z-guides/cortisol-test#1

WebMD, "What Is a Salicylate Allergy?" (Accessed 2017.)
http://www.webmd.com/allergies/guide/salicylate-allergy

WebMD, "What is Sulfite Sensitivity?" Reviewed by William Blahd, MD, July 23, 2016.
http://www.webmd.com/allergies/guide/sulfite-sensitivity

Bibliography

Weiler, Elmar W.J., Klaus Brill, Ken H. Tachiki, Dieter Schneider, "Neurofeedback and Quantitative Electroencephalography." *International Tinnitus Journal*, Volume 8, Number 2, 2002. http://www.tinnitusjournal.com/articles/neurofeedback-and-quantitative-electroencephalography.pdf

Widex, "Sensorineural Hearing Loss - What Is It?" (Accessed 2017.) http://www.widex.com/en/hearing-loss/types-of-hearing-loss/sensorineural-hearing-loss

Widex, "The Widex Sound." (Accessed 2017.) http://www.widex.com/en/the-widex-sound

wikiHow, (Review by Alison Buchanan), "How to Do the Warrior Pose in Yoga." (Accessed 2017.) https://www.wikihow.fitness/Do-the-Warrior-Pose-in-Yoga

wikiHow, "How to Reduce Cortisol." (Accessed 2017.) http://www.wikihow.com/Reduce-Cortisol

Wikipedia, "Bark (sound)." (Accessed 2016.) https://en.wikipedia.org/wiki/Bark_(sound)

Wikipedia, "Cortico-striato-cortico loop." (Accessed 2017.) https://en.wikipedia.org/wiki/Cortico-striato-cortical_loop

Wikipedia, "Hyperesthesia." (Accessed 2016.) https://en.wikipedia.org/wiki/Hyperesthesia

Wikipedia, "Legality of cannabis by U.S. jurisdiction." (Accessed 2016.) https://en.wikipedia.org/wiki/Legality_of_cannabis_by_U.S._jurisdiction#By_state

Wikipedia, "Limbic system." (Accessed 2016.) https://en.wikipedia.org/wiki/Limbic_system

Wikipedia, "Neurobiological effects of physical exercise." (Accessed 2016.) https://en.wikipedia.org/wiki/Neurobiological_effects_of_physical_exercise

Wikipedia, "Nociception." (Accessed 2017.) https://en.wikipedia.org/wiki/Nociception

Wikipedia, "Oxidative stress." (Accessed 2016.) https://en.wikipedia.org/wiki/Oxidative_stress

Wikipedia, "Striatum." (Accessed 2016.) https://en.wikipedia.org/wiki/Striatum

Wikipedia, "Suprachiasmatic nucleus." (Accessed 2017.) https://en.wikipedia.org/wiki/Suprachiasmatic_nucleus

Williams, Mark, Christian Hauptmann, Nitesh Patel, "Acoustic CR neuromodulation therapy for subjective tonal tinnitus: a review of clinical outcomes in an independent audiological practice setting." *Frontiers in Neurology*, March 17, 2015. http://journal.frontiersin.org/article/10.3389/fneur.2015.00054/abstract

wiseGEEK, "What Is a Mu Wave?" (Accessed 2016.) http://www.wisegeek.com/what-is-a-mu-wave.htm

wiseGEEK, "What is EEG Neurofeedback?" (Accessed 2017.) http://www.wisegeek.com/what-is-eeg-neurofeedback.htm

wiseGEEK, "What is Excitotoxicity?" (Accessed 2016.) http://www.wisegeek.com/what-is-excitotoxicity.htm

wiseGEEK, "What is Grey Noise?" (Accessed 2016.) http://www.wisegeek.com/what-is-grey-noise.htm

wiseGEEK, "What is Magnolol?" (Accessed 2016.) http://www.wisegeek.com/what-is-magnolol.htm

wiseGEEK, "What is Neural Plasticity?" (Accessed 2016.) http://www.wisegeek.org/what-is-neural-plasticity.htm

wiseGEEK, "What is Taurine Deficiency?" (Accessed 2016.) http://www.wisegeek.com/what-is-taurine-deficiency.htm

wiseGEEK, "What is the Auditory Cortex?" (Accessed 2016.) http://www.wisegeek.org/what-is-the-auditory-cortex.htm

wiseGEEK, "What is the Role of Neurotransmitters in the Brain?" (Accessed 2016.) http://www.wisegeek.com/what-is-the-role-of-neurotransmitters-in-the-brain.htm

Wishnia, Steven, "Smoke vs. Snack: Why Edible Marijuana is Stronger Than Smoking." Leafly, June 13, 2014. http://www.thedailybeast.com/articles/2014/06/13/smoke-vs-snack-why-edible-marijuana-is-stronger-than-smoking.html

Wolters Kluwer Health, "Magnolia bark extract." Drugs, 2009. https://www.drugs.com/npp/magnolia-bark-extract.html

Wong, ND, Cathy (Reviewed by Richard N. Fogoros, MD), "Health Benefits of Eleuthero." VeryWell, August 19, 2017. https://www.verywell.com/health-benefits-of-eleuthero-89449

Wong, ND, Cathy, "The Benefits of Chamomile." VeryWell, September 11, 2017. https://www.verywell.com/chamomile-for-a-sounder-slumber-89328

Wong, ND, Cathy (Reviewed by Richard N. Fogoros, MD), "The Benefits of Medium Chain Triglycerides." VeryWell, September 5, 2017. https://www.verywell.com/the-benefits-of-medium-chain-triglycerides-90054

Wong, ND, Cathy, (Reviewed by Richard N. Fogoros, MD) "The Many Uses for Lemon Balm." VeryWell, August 31, 2017. https://www.verywell.com/the-health-benefits-of-lemon-balm-89388

Wu, Jin-Ji, Yanji Cui, Yoon-Sil Yang, et al., "Modulatory effects of aromatherapy massage intervention on electroencephalogram, psychological assessments, salivary cortisol and plasma brain-derived neurotrophic factor." *Complementary Therapies in Medicine*, Volume 22, Issue 3, June 2014. http://www.sciencedirect.com/science/article/pii/S0965229914000582

Xu, Ying, Baoshan Ku, Lu Tie, et al. "Curcumin reverses the effects of chronic stress on behavior, the HPA axis, BDNF expression and phosphorylation of CREB." *Brain Research*, Volume 22, Issue 1, November 29, 2006. https://www.sciencedirect.com/science/article/pii/S0006899306027144

Yeoman, Matthew, "Brain Health, Neuroplasticity and How it May Relate to Puzzles." February 14, 2014. https://www.passionforpuzzles.com/2014/02/brain-health-neuroplasticity-and-how-it-may-relate-to-puzzles.php

Yoga Journal, "List of Yoga Poses: A-Z Asana Guide." (Accessed 2017.) https://www.yogajournal.com/pose-finder

Yogis Anonymous, "Experience real yoga classes. Anywhere." (Accessed 2017.) https://yogisanonymous.com

YouTube, "After watching this, your brain will not be the same I Lara Boyd I TEDx Vancouver." TEDx Talks channel, December 15, 2015. https://www.youtube.com/watch?v=LNHBMFCzznE

YouTube, Audacity installation tutorials search results. (Accessed 2016.) https://www.youtube.com/results?search_query=install+audacity

YouTube, Audacity not recording tutorials search results. (Accessed 2016.) https://www.youtube.com/results?search_query=audacity+not+recording

YouTube, "Back to Silence." Tinnitus Talk Support Forum channel, March 3, 2016. https://www.youtube.com/watch?v=wNjDBOJfMfY

YouTube, "Beethoven - Für Elise (60 Minute Version)." Ludwig van Beethoven channel, September 20, 2013. https://www.youtube.com/watch?v=Lkcvrxj0eLY

YouTube, "British Tinnitus Association - Sounds of Tinnitus." jackpirat8 channel, July 17, 2011. https://www.youtube.com/watch?v=2mV-Z54fiBo

YouTube, "Brown Noise 8 Hours, for Relaxation, Sleep, Studying and Tinnitus." Mind Amend channel, March 9, 2015. https://www.youtube.com/watch?v=GSaJXDsb3N8

Bibliography

YouTube, "Can You Be Hypnotized? The Lemon Test." Morpheus Hypnosis channel, November 22, 2011. https://www.youtube.com/watch?v=x7wr_y-ThPs

YouTube, "Cool Hearing test." ScienceForum channel, October 2, 2011. https://www.youtube.com/watch?v=h5l4Rt4Ol7M

YouTube, "David Letterman with William Shatner - March, 1996!" videoholic ULTIMATE channel, July 28, 2013. https://www.youtube.com/watch?v=yCdx8aueK9I

YouTube, "Decibel Meter of Roaring Crowd Noise - Century Link Field: Seahawks Packers NFC Championship." Bosch Voyage channel, January 19, 2015. https://www.youtube.com/watch?v=AZrr7wjb8ZE

YouTube, "Dr. Russell Blaylock: Excitotoxins - The Taste That Kills." chroniclewatch channel, July 10, 2011. https://www.youtube.com/watch?v=tTSvlGniHok

YouTube, "Ear Organ of Corti." animacionesplus channel, August 4, 2010. https://youtu.be/1JE8WduJKV4

YouTube, "Eat, Fast, and Live Longer BBC Documentary." Daily Content channel, July 10, 2015. https://www.youtube.com/watch?v=Ihhj_VSKiTs

YouTube, "Experimental Tinnitus Sound Treatment." medexamtoolscom channel, May 12, 2013. https://www.youtube.com/watch?v=ibWYcDSbcwg

YouTube, "Fix Audacity not recording!" GotGuides channel, December 24, 2013. https://www.youtube.com/watch?v=SI7xyuKbAKk

YouTube, "Guided Meditation to ease Anxiety, Worry, Overthinking & Urgency." Positive Meditation Positive Energy Magazine channel, May 8, 2013. https://www.youtube.com/watch?v=xoYnqvadurg

YouTube, "How Old Are Your Ears? (Hearing Test)." AsapSCIENCE channel, August 13, 2013. https://www.youtube.com/watch?v=VxcbppCX6Rk

YouTube, "HYPNOSIS in Dentistry." rothsteven77 channel, May 5, 2010. https://www.youtube.com/watch?v=ErKU1rPQqmY

YouTube, "Hypnosis Test - Find Out If You Can Be Hypnotized." newlifeclinicsct channel, March 8, 2012. https://www.youtube.com/watch?v=H_J0D0c5LIM

YouTube, "I have tinnitus and I want to die." De Monitor channel, March 5, 2015. https://www.youtube.com/watch?v=HGcUJ2Dg3uo

YouTube, "Mozart Classical Piano Study Music & Alpha Waves: ULTIMATE Concentration, Mozart K.448 Study Music." H4 Happiness - Study Music, Relaxing Music channel, November 24, 2015. https://www.youtube.com/watch?v=CiaV_4KQJcQ

YouTube, "Mozart - Sonata for Two Pianos in D, K. 448 [complete]," Am4d3usM0z4rt channel, October 26, 2011. https://www.youtube.com/watch?v=tT9gT5bqi6Y

YouTube, "Music star Will.i.am speaks about his Tinnitus." sixesfullofnines channel, January 13, 2014. https://www.youtube.com/watch?v=JojiB_zSKW4

YouTube, "Neck Massage: Do It While You View It." Rich Poley channel, February 12, 2009. https://www.youtube.com/watch?v=duSNnBnqFts

YouTube, "Om Gurvay Namaha-Vyanah." Vyanah Music for Relaxation channel. May 15, 2008. https://www.youtube.com/watch?v=UukINnU0F_I

YouTube, "Rafaele Joudry interview - Tinnitus Relief - Sound Therapy International." SoundTherapyWorld channel, February 19, 2012. https://www.youtube.com/watch?v=NePxKfJu2V8

YouTube, "Remodeling Sensory and Motor Circuits in the Brain: New Insights from Hearing Loss and Tinnitus." UWTV channel, July 18, 2014. https://www.youtube.com/watch?v=tFqr0rk9FC4

YouTube, "selective attention test." Daniel Simons channel, March 10, 2010.
https://www.youtube.com/watch?v=vJG698U2Mvo

YouTube, "Stop telling people there is no cure for tinnitus!" Julian Cowan Hill channel,
August 22, 2013. https://www.youtube.com/watch?v=TFgu0q2otEc

YouTube, "Stress, Portrait of a Killer - Full Documentary (2008)." interface channel,
October 16, 2011. https://www.youtube.com/watch?v=eYG0ZuTv5rs

YouTube, "Ten Hours of Ambient Sound - Blue Noise." Dale Snale channel, February 12, 2013.
https://www.youtube.com/watch?v=WSCU_t3o7Kl

YouTube, "The Exact Moment I Got Tinnitus." Jacob Everett channel, April 27, 2014.
https://www.youtube.com/watch?v=kjMLtbzoE6A

YouTube, "Three-Minute Mindfulness Meditation." David O'Grady channel, April 8, 2012.
https://www.youtube.com/watch?v=cDflnqo0TQs

YouTube, "Tinnitus Short Film - 24.7.52.10." kieo32 channel, May 22, 2008.
https://www.youtube.com/watch?v=BN1xIXye6s4

YouTube, "Vyanah, Music For Meditation & Inner Balance."
Vyanah Music for Relaxation channel. (Accessed 2017.)
https://www.youtube.com/channel/UCu_14PpxWo-m1PWGhpxZoVQ

YouTube, "Why fasting bolsters brain power: Mark Mattson at TEDx Johns Hopkins University."
TEDx Talks channel, March 18, 2014. https://www.youtube.com/watch?v=4UkZAwKoCP8

YungLean (Member), "Fake It Until You Make It." Tinnitus Talk, January 4, 2015.
https://www.tinnitustalk.com/threads/fake-it-until-you-make-it.7590/

Zhang, Si Yi, Donald Robertson, "A study of tea tree oil ototoxicity." *Audiology & Neuro-Otology*,
March 2000. https://www.ncbi.nlm.nih.gov/pubmed/10720822

Zhang, Yun, William M. Pardridge, "Conjugation of brain-derived neurotrophic factor to a
blood-brain barrier drug targeting system enables neuroprotection in regional brain
ischemia following intravenous injection of the neurotrophin."
Brain Research, Volume 889, Issues 1-2, January 2001.
http://www.sciencedirect.com/science/article/pii/S0006899300031085

Zheng, Yiwen, Peter Reid, Paul F. Smith, "Cannabinoid CB1 Receptor Agonists Do Not
Decrease, but may Increase Acoustic Trauma-Induced Tinnitus in Rats." *Frontiers in
Neurology*, March 18, 2015. https://www.ncbi.nlm.nih.gov/pubmed/25852639

Zimmer, Carl, "The Brain: 'Ringing in the Ears' Actually Goes Much Deeper Than That."
Discover, October 27, 2010.
http://discovermagazine.com/2010/oct/26-ringing-in-the-ears-goes-much-deeper

INDEX

33780222R00268

Made in the USA
San Bernardino, CA
26 April 2019